CLINICS IN DEVELOPMENTAL MEDICINE NO. 109

FITS AND FAINTS

Clinics in Developmental Medicine No. 109

FITS AND FAINTS

JOHN B. P. STEPHENSON

Royal Hospital for Sick Children
Glasgow

1990
Mac Keith Press
OXFORD: Blackwell Scientific Publications Ltd.
PHILADELPHIA: J. B. Lippincott Co.

©1990 Mac Keith Press
5a Netherhall Gardens, London NW3 5RN

First published 1990

British Library Cataloguing in Publication Data

Stephenson, John B.P.
  Fits and faints
  1. Man. Nervous system. Diseases
  I. Title
  616.8

ISBN 0 521 411963

Printed in Great Britain at The Lavenham Press Ltd., Lavenham, Suffolk
Mac Keith Press is supported by **The Spastics Society, London, England**

To

Henri Gastaut

**epileptologist
and nonepileptologist
extraordinary**

AUTHOR'S APPOINTMENTS

JOHN B. P. STEPHENSON,
M.A., B.M., D.C.H., F.R.C.P.,
F.R.C.P.G.

Consultant in Paediatric Neurology;
Physician-in-charge, EEG Department,
Fraser of Allander Unit, Royal Hospital for
Sick Children, Yorkhill, Glasgow G3 8SJ.
Honorary Clinical Lecturer in Child Health
(Paediatric Neurology), University of
Glasgow.

CONTENTS

ACKNOWLEDGEMENTS

The late Robert Shanks and John Stobo Prichard first fired me with enthusiasm for understanding those convulsions which are distinct from epilepsy. Space does not permit adequate acknowledgement of all those other individuals at home and abroad who have helped through conversation, discussion, correspondence (often protracted) and the sharing of case reports. I include here also the many parents who gave graphic and accurate accounts of their children's attacks.

Several people have let me see original material, and I am particularly grateful to Stephen Ashwal, Agatino Battaglia, Jackson Braham, Neil Gordon, Donald Hadley, Cesare Lombroso, Jim Manson, Yvonne Navelet, Fred Plum and David Southall.

The influence of France is strong in the dedication and in the foreword. Henri Gastaut pioneered many of the concepts developed in this book and never failed to provide wise replies to my attempts at penetrating questions. It is a great honour to have Jean Aicardi agree to write some words of introduction, though knowing his critical mind I have a certain trepidation in not knowing in advance what he is going to say!

Many authors have been kind enough to send me reprints of their work, and I acknowledge the additional help of the libraries of the University of Glasgow and the Royal Society of Medicine, and of the British Library Document Supply Centre.

All my present and erstwhile colleagues in Glasgow have been supportive in relation to this modest venture. Much of the work would not have been possible without the technical expertise and willing cooperation of Geraldine Block and Hilary Reidpath of the EEG Department of the Royal Hospital for Sick Children. Dr Robert McWilliam assisted in the study of reflex anoxic seizures, in addition to his major contribution to the measurement of intracranial pressure.

For statistical help I acknowledge with thanks Kenneth Clarke and my son Philip Stephenson of the University of Glasgow.

I am more than grateful to Jean Hyslop, Medical Artist, University of Glasgow, and to the staff of the Department of Medical Illustration, Royal Hospital for Sick Children, for help with the figures.

Diane Henderson typed the manuscript with speed, precision and cheerfulness, and I thank her deeply. Cynthia Young, my secretary, gave additional welcome help.

Dr Christopher Rittey kindly reviewed the manuscript.

Pat Chappelle of Mac Keith Press processed the text with patient tolerance and meticulous attention. I should also thank Martin Bax, Senior Editor, for trusting me with the book.

Finally I give the largest thankyou to Philippa and my family. I hereby resolve to remove the papers from some of the floors!

FOREWORD

There is currently a large overdiagnosis of epilepsy in children who present with loss of consciousness, falls or other paroxysmal motor or psychic phenomena. As pointed out by Jeavons (1983), as many as 20 to 30 per cent of patients diagnosed as having epilepsy have in fact non-epileptic attacks. Yet, it is extremely important to avoid making a wrong diagnosis of epilepsy, not only because of the stigma attached to the label of 'epileptic' but also because the side-effects of anti-epileptic drugs are frequent and should not be inflicted on patients who cannot draw benefit from their use.

John Stephenson's book is concerned precisely with this problem. Stephenson analyses the common and less common causes for the misdiagnosis of epilepsy and especially emphasizes the problems posed by anoxic seizures, a field in which he has prominently contributed over the years. This monograph is undoubtedly the most comprehensive source of information available about the various types of anoxic attacks, their clinical and EEG features, mechanisms and prognosis.

Over 140 case histories illustrate the whole gamut of fits and faints—from the common breath-holding spells and swoons to the active form of the Munchausen syndrome by proxy (suffocation or strangulation of an infant by an adult), through the bizarre forms of syncope such as those which are self-induced by a Valsalva manoeuvre—and bring the flavour of real life into an exhaustive, yet highly readable account. Special attention is paid to the occurrence of true epileptic seizures induced by anoxia, a phenomenon that is probably less rare than the slim literature available would suggest and one that easily leads to diagnostic errors.

This monograph strikingly confirms that everything that shakes or faints need not be epilepsy. Incidentally, I was pleased to read that what is often referred to as 'hot water epilepsy' or 'bathing epilepsy' in many instances may well be reflex anoxic seizure.

What makes this book especially appealing is even more the medical philosophy it conveys than the wealth of data it contains, however lavish this may be. This is indeed a beautiful illustration of what constitutes the essence of clinical medicine: making sense of the apparently meaningless and giving shape to the amorphous, through a methodic gathering of facts and a rigorous processing of the information collected, selecting the essential and pruning out irrelevant details. Such an intellectual process should take into account all sources of information including that obtained through more or less sophisticated technical tools. In the field of paroxysmal disorders, however, information comes above all from the clinical history, because the events that constitute the essential part of the disease are not usually observed, and because what is seen clinically or by neurophysiological techniques outside the paroxysm itself generally gives no clue to the nature of the paroxysmal event and may indeed be misleading (thus, the finding of spikes on interictal record is no guarantee of the epileptic nature of an attack). It is true, therefore, that the diagnosis is as good as the history.

The importance of history-taking is marvellously demonstrated in the detailed history revealed in Stephenson's Case 4.8. It is fascinating to read the succession of precise, well-oriented yet not leading questions and their answers, and to realize that this leads ineluctably to the correct diagnosis as surely as fingerprints and cigarette butts lead the detective to the culprit in a crime story. Yet such invaluable material all too often remains buried in the parents' minds just because doctors do not bother to try to understand and find it easier to camouflage intellectual laziness behind a rampart of electroencephalograms and CT scans.

Stephenson's monograph shows the right track and furthermore provides some astute practical clues to help establish a full communication between patients and doctors. Among these are a glossary of lay terms corresponding to our medical jargon, and some sound advice that miming seizures for the parents is a useful practice, an experience shared by other physicians who deal with seizure patients.

This is a delightful book that anyone involved in clinical medicine in general and child neurology in particular will enjoy reading. It is also a useful book that will really help the reader to deal practically with his or her patients with faints or turns. Not the least benefit will be to alleviate the unnecessary burden that a wrong diagnosis of epilepsy imposes on the patient. There are few greater satisfactions for the physician than to rid a patient of both a stigmatizing label and the prospect of a prolonged and perhaps poorly tolerated treatment, and to achieve this as a result of a fascinating intellectual process that requires nothing more nor less than the best of his or her clinical acumen.

JEAN AICARDI
DÉPARTEMENT DE PÉDIATRIE
HÔPITAL ENFANTS MALADES
PARIS

REFERENCE

Jeavons, P.M. (1983) 'Non-epileptic attacks in childhood.' *In* Rose, F.C. (Ed.) *Research Progress in Epilepsy*. London: Pitman.

1
INTRODUCTION

This book is about fits, faints and 'funny turns' (Bower 1974*a,b*). It deals mainly with the young, but not exclusively so. It is not a textbook of epilepsy but rather emphasizes those conditions which tend to be relegated to 'differential diagnosis' (Strandjord 1987) or dismissed in a few lines. Certain of these conditions are common and will be encountered by anyone involved in the practice of clinical medicine in its widest sense. Others are admittedly rare, but important nonetheless to those who suffer them.

Around 25 years ago I met a young boy in what was then known as the Casualty department ('Accident and Emergency'). On his card was written 'known epileptic'. He had a history of frequent seizures, unresponsive to 'anticonvulsants'. He certainly twitched and his consciousness was impaired, but all his attacks were in the morning, an hour or so after he ought to have been up and about. Not only that, but they usually occurred at weekends or after a public holiday. Further probing revealed that on these occasions he had missed his evening meal, and that when his parents, rising late, entered his room, they noticed a strange, sweetish smell. He had, of course, ketotic hypoglycaemia, and not epilepsy at all: dietary manipulations easily eliminated his seizures (Stephenson and Hainsworth 1966).

As Jeavons (1983) and others have emphasized, 'known epileptic' means nothing of the kind. Either it is not epilepsy, or the epilepsy is insufficiently understood—otherwise, why the consultation? The term 'anticonvulsant' incorporates a similar elision of thought. What the doctor means is *anti-epileptic*, hindering or preventing epileptic seizures. To use the term anticonvulsant for a drug such as ethosuximide, which stops non-convulsant epileptic absences, is semantically incorrect. Far more dangerous is to prescribe an anticonvulsant, *thinking inwardly that this means anti-epileptic*, to a patient with a convulsive seizure, *when it has not been established that the seizure was an epileptic one in the first place*.

The conception that seizures are not necessarily epileptic may be new or strange to some. This view will be elaborated in Chapter 2 and throughout the book. The most common and in my opinion the most important non-epileptic seizure is the fainting fit or anoxic seizure. By that, one must not imagine the stereotype of a swooning adolescent girl but rather a proper, obvious convulsive seizure. Yet this anoxic seizure is no longer to be regarded as lurking in the 'borderland of epilepsy' (Gowers 1907): it resides in a totally distinct and different territory. Interconnections do exist between anoxic and epileptic seizures, as will be demonstrated in Chapters 11 and 12, but the differences should not be blurred.

With the specialization of medicine, neurologists tend to see patients with 'fits' and cardiologists those with 'faints'. Paediatricians and general practitioners have the advantage of seeing both. The seizures which most other specialists see are fainting fits, albeit not always recognized. An ophthalmologist, for example, is astonished to find his patient slump, lose consciousness, urinate and jerk during the application of a laser to the eye (McNamara 1984). Immediately, the blood pressure is taken and found to be 120/80 and the pulse 82, so the doctor thinks 'how can it be a faint?' When the heart stops, the brain stops, and it is this sort of fit which this book is primarily about. Epilepsy takes second place, not because of its lesser importance but because others have dealt with it well, and few have dealt with the other side of the looking-glass. Your author hopes that the view will not be too distorted.

2
EPILEPTIC AND NON-EPILEPTIC SEIZURES: WORDS AND MEANINGS

'When I use a word,' Humpty Dumpty said in a scornful tone, 'it means just what I choose it to mean – neither more nor less.' (Lewis Carroll: *Through the Looking Glass.*)

To discuss fits and faints it is first necessary to agree on the meanings of the words as we use them now (Table 2.I). We should no more be the prisoners of the origins of our language than we ought to be prisoners of our genes (Dawkins 1976). The word 'seizure' has the same semantic derivation as 'epilepsy', from επιλαμβανειν (epilambanein), to seize (Temkin 1971), and, unfortunately, many medical writers still use it in this way. To them, 'epileptic seizure' is a tautology: all seizures are by definition epileptic. However, language evolves. To quote Aicardi (1986), 'It has been slowly realized that all seizures marked by loss of consciousness, involuntary movements, or disturbances of sensorium are not of the same origin, that they may be the result of different mechanisms, and that they have widely different outcomes and implications.' As Gumnit (1987) puts it, 'Another major area of terminology that has become confusing is the problem of "epileptic seizures" and "nonepileptic seizures". The term epileptic seizure refers to sudden change in the electrical activity of the brain, usually accompanied by subjective or objective changes in behaviour. Nonepileptic seizures are sudden changes in objective or subjective behaviour which do not have at their root an independent sudden change in the electrical activity of the brain. Nonepileptic seizures can be divided into physiological non-CNS events, such as syncope, cardiac standstill, etc., and

TABLE 2.I
Meanings of words

Label	Origin	Medical slang	Current definition
Seizure	Invasion by demons, attack	Epileptic fit	Episode of (transient) alteration of cerebral function: needs further specification as epileptic, anoxic, toxic, psychic, etc.
Fit	Conflict, fight	Epileptic seizure	Motor seizure (tonic etc.), epileptic or non-epileptic
Convulsion	Pulled together	Infantile seizure (implying not epileptic)	Tonic, clonic, or tonic-clonic seizure, epileptic or non-epileptic
Faint	Feint, feign	Vasovagal or vasodepressor syncope	Syncopal episode
Syncope	Cut off	Transient loss of consciousness	Consequence of acute cerebral hypoxia

psychogenic seizures.' In fact there is nothing very new about this: Gastaut has for many years differentiated seizures into those which are epileptic, anoxic, toxic, metabolic, psychic, and hypnic (Gastaut 1968, 1973, 1974; Gastaut and Broughton 1972).

Epileptic seizures

Epileptic seizures ideally should be defined electroclinically. On the one hand there must be clinical manifestations, and on the other there must be an excessive discharge of a population of cerebral neurons (Gastaut 1973, Aicardi 1986), even though in clinical practice this electrical discharge must be inferred from the details of the history. If, as is usually the case (except in certain simple partial epileptic seizures—Devinsky *et al.* 1989), these abnormal neuronal discharges spread to some or all of the cerebral cortex directly under the vault of the skull, and if, as is seldom possible, recording electrodes are attached during the seizure, then particular changes in the EEG will specify that the seizure is an epileptic one.

Epilepsy

Epilepsy (see Chapter 6) implies recurrent unprovoked epileptic seizures, or at any rate epileptic seizures provoked only by everyday stimuli. No-one would regard as epilepsy a series of epileptic seizures provoked by electroconvulsive therapy. Most would not regard as epilepsy a series of epileptic seizures each associated only with high fever in a young child. However, recurrent epileptic seizures induced by television or the visual display unit of a computer would fall within the rubric of epilepsy. As Aicardi (1986) has pointed out, it is common sense that for all epileptic seizures there will be factors that tend to provoke and factors that tend to inhibit the genesis of the seizure. Epilepsy has recently been redefined (Rodin 1987) as 'a disturbance of brain function characterized by excessive fluctuations in its electrochemical balance that express themselves at their height in spontaneously recurring seizures. The clinical manifestations of the seizure depend upon the point of origin, extent, and speed and spread of electrical discharges. The etiology is unknown, but its appearance is facilitated by brain damage and/or hereditary factors.'

In practice it is useful to make exceptions and to exclude from the definition of epilepsy recurrent epileptic seizures confined to the first weeks of life, and 'cluster seizures' in which several epileptic seizures occur within a short period of time (less than six weeks) and do not recur. Childhood epilepsies, even with these exceptions, are not necessarily permanent: if the description 'an epileptic' is to be used at all, it should be reserved for the child with an epilepsy which is not likely to remit. Epilepsy and epileptic syndromes in childhood have been well described in recent publications (O'Donohue 1985; Roger *et al.* 1985; Fejerman and Medina 1986; Aicardi 1986, 1988).

Non-epileptic seizures

Non-epileptic seizures are seizures which, while they may be epileptiform, that is to say look very like epileptic seizures (Temkin 1971), have an entirely different mechanism. By far the most important mechanism is the anoxic one, which will be discussed in detail in later chapters.

Anoxic seizures

Anoxic seizures (Chapter 7) may be generalized or focal. In brief, *generalized anoxic seizures* result when there is a sudden loss of oxygen supply to the cerebral hemispheres and upper brainstem, this generally implying an abrupt failure of cerebral perfusion by oxygenated blood (Gastaut 1974). Short-lasting hypoxia or ischaemia leads to loss of consciousness and postural tone, and an appearance commonly described as fainting or simple syncope, but for which the terms 'anoxic absence' or 'atonic seizure' could equally well be applied. Longer anoxia (and for the moment anoxia is equated with oligaemia or ischaemia) leads to a motor seizure or convulsion, the so-called 'convulsive syncope' (Gastaut 1973). Two things make for additional confusion here. One is that, where the mechanism of the anoxic motor seizure has been brainstem herniation due to a paroxysm of increased intracranial pressure (see Chapter 10), then the terms 'decerebrate seizure' or 'cerebellar seizure' have been used instead (Gastaut 1973). The other is that, as we shall see in Chapter 11, there is a 'new' seizure type, the *anoxic-epileptic* seizure (Stephenson 1983a, Gastaut *et al.* 1987, Aicardi *et al.* 1988, Battaglia *et al.* 1989), which is even more convulsive than the purely anoxic convulsive syncope, and which combines anoxic and epileptic mechanisms. For these and other reasons the term anoxic seizure is preferred for an episode of anoxic origin, with a qualification regarding the form of the seizure much as one qualifies an epileptic seizure as absence, tonic-clonic and so forth. *Focal anoxic seizures* are better known as transient ischaemic attacks.

Psychic seizures

Psychic seizures (Chapter 13) are second only to anoxic seizures in importance. Such non-epileptic seizures of psychological origin have also attracted confused and confusing terminology. The term 'pseudoseizure' has been used for these events in the past (Holmes *et al.* 1980, Gulick *et al.* 1982), but as we shall see the anoxic seizure is at least as important if not more important as a form of pseudo-epileptic seizure. Many prefer the term *psychogenic seizure* (Ramani 1987), but Gastaut's term *psychic seizure* (Gastaut 1973) is more specific and less likely to be confused with psychogenic or self-induced epileptic seizures (Aicardi and Gastaut 1985). 'Active' psychic seizures are those in which the patient has symptoms or objective evidence of altered behaviour, while 'passive' psychic seizures exist only in the mind of the mother (Meadow 1984).

Toxic seizures

Toxic seizures are those predominantly motor reactions, often dystonic, recognized as sequelae to an increasing number of drugs (Shafrir *et al.* 1986). Admittedly most doctors do not use the term 'toxic seizure', but its use may aid the memory in difficult diagnostic situations.

I do not favour a separate category of *metabolic seizure*, because frequently seizures of metabolic origin have an obvious epileptic mechanism, but obviously metabolic disorders are inevitably considered in *aetiology*.

Hypnic seizures

'Hypnic seizure' is the term used by Gastaut (Gastaut and Broughton 1972) to describe those non-epileptic seizures which are *primarily* disorders of sleep. It could be that these are in total very frequent, but only occasionally do they raise important diagnostic and management issues (see Chapter 15). Such primary sleep disorders have to be distinguished from sleep-associated seizures which have other mechanisms (epileptic, anoxic, etc.).

Finally there are a number of paroxysmal events, jerks, stiffenings and so forth, some of which may be called 'convulsions', which defy classification into any of the types of seizure so far described. They will be found as *'miscellaneous'* in Chapters 5 and 14.

Conclusions

How then should the terms or labels in Table 2.I be used?

Seizure is now a term of limited specificity and has to be further qualified, as epileptic, anoxic or psychic. 'Seizure disorder' adds no further diagnostic precision.

Fit is more of a slang word, but may be helpful in talking to patients or parents especially to contrast a fainting fit (anoxic seizure) from an epileptic fit.

Convulsion is even more in the vocabulary of slang. It is used in a non-specific manner to describe any motor seizure of whatever mechanism, and is sometimes employed by parents or professionals when the only 'motor' phenomenon witnessed is passive upward conjugate deviation of the eyes. In parts of North America in particular, the term 'convulsive disorder' seems to have become popular as a synonym for epilepsy. It is hard to see how this habit can generate anything but confusion.

Whereas *syncope* has a precise meaning, the consequence of acute cerebral hypoxia or metabolic arrest however caused, the term *faint* is often endowed with a more specific connotation than is justified. One has heard it said, for example, that asystole never occurs in fainting. Actually this means that asystole never occurs in pure vasodepressor syncope (Engel 1962). As we shall see, asystole is a regular feature of reflex fainting fits of vagal type (reflex anoxic seizures).

If Humpty Dumpty is consistent, and the meaning of terms is agreed, this is a first step toward discussing what actually happens to our patients.

3
SIZE OF THE PROBLEM

We have surprisingly few data on the incidence or prevalence of the disorders discussed in this book (Keränen 1987). Patently, not everything that is referred to as 'epilepsy' is so, as indicated by Tables 3.I to 3.IV, which give a crude breakdown of patients referred to my outpatient clinic at the Royal Hospital for Sick Children, Glasgow, during the years 1973–1986.

Although those with a final diagnosis of epilepsy of one sort or another are in the majority, those with afebrile anoxic events form a substantial proportion, which I do not think is based on biased referral. Evidence from general practice has suggested a lifetime prevalence of about 20 per 1000 for single and more frequently repeated seizures, and 17 per 1000 for recurrent seizures (Goodridge and Shorvon 1983). Those authors noted that 7.8 per 1000 patients were receiving anticonvulsant treatment at the time of their survey and that 5.3 per 1000 had active epilepsy, defined as having had a seizure within the past two years. Goodridge and Shorvon recognized that the diagnosis of epilepsy was a clinical one and that syncopal and psychogenic episodes had to be distinguished, but they accepted as epileptic seizures those regarded as definitely so by neurologists or paediatricians, or by themselves. The prevalence of non-epileptic seizures was not given in that study.

Two longitudinal studies have thrown some light on the question of relative prevalence. In the National Child Development Study (Ross *et al.* 1980, Ross and Peckham 1983), 6.7 per cent of the 1958 cohort had experienced at least one episode of altered consciousness. This was diagnosed as 'established' epilepsy in 4.1 per 1000. The other categories in declining order of frequency were as follows: febrile convulsions without later afebrile seizures, 22.3 per 1000; transitory afebrile convulsive episodes not occurring after age 5 years, 20.6 per 1000; breath-holding attacks, faints without convulsions, or temper tantrums, 18.1 per 1000; epilepsy reported by doctor but unsubstantiated, 2.5 per 1000; febrile convulsions with later spontaneous afebrile seizures, 1.3 per 1000; convulsions with meningitis or encephalitis, 0.8 per 1000; convulsions reported by parent but not to general practitioner or hospital, 0.8 per 1000; and non-epileptic blank spells confirmed by general practitioner or hospital, 0.5 per 1000. The significant omission from this list is that there was no category for faints *with* convulsions.

In their analysis of the Child Health and Education Study, Golding and Butler (1983) reported that of the 1970 cohort three per 1000 had 'idiopathic epilepsy', seven per 1000 had 'symptomatic convulsions' and nine per 1000 had faints and breath-holding. Unfortunately, although one of their illustrations showed a different age distribution for the onset of faints and for breath-holding, the number of those with faints and the number of those with breath-holding was not given and the terms were not defined.

Rossiter *et al.* (1970) reported preliminary findings in a defined population, but

TABLE 3.I

Paroxysmal disorders referred as ?epilepsy

Disorder	N	%
Epileptic	821	53.5
Anoxic	370	24.1
Febrile, uncertain**	109	7.1
Miscellaneous neurological	81	5.3
Psychic	65	4.2
'Funny'*	57	3.7
Hypnic**	33	2.1
Total	1536	100.0

*See Chapter 14; **see Chapter 15.

TABLE 3.II

Anoxic events* referred as ?epilepsy

Event	N
Vasovagal or 'reflex' non-convulsive syncope	137
Convulsive syncope after early childhood	73
Reflex anoxic seizures	97
Blue breath-holding (prolonged expiratory apnoea)	24
Mixed (blue and white) or white breath-holding	18
Valsalva-type breath-holding	2
Convulsive breath-holding (mechanism uncertain)	9
Cardiogenic	5
Anoxic-epileptic seizures**	5
Total	370

*See Chapters 8 and 9 for further details; **see Chapter 11.

so far the fine details of the different anoxic and epileptic seizures in their Australian population have not yet been published. However, these authors found an incidence of convulsions 'due to breath-holding' of 8.1 per 1000.

The frequency with which a convulsive syncope is observed in blood donors should give an idea of the minimal prevalence of anoxic seizures of reflex vagal type. In their *prospective* study Lin *et al*. (1982) noted convulsive syncope in 42 per cent of those with reactions, that is to say in 0.5 per 1000 donors. It was notable that in their *retrospective* study only 12 per cent of syncopal reactions were noted to be convulsive.

The population incidence or prevalence of psychic seizures and of most of the other disorders to be discussed is not known. Some of these conditions, although uncommon—such as the febrile tonic seizures which signify herniation ('coning') in pyogenic meningitis (Horowitz *et al*. 1980)—are sufficiently important to warrant epidemiological studies.

TABLE 3.III

Psychic episodes* referred as ?epilepsy

Type of episode	N
Day-dreams	19
Gratification/eidetic imagery	13
Anxiety attacks	12
Miscellaneous	10
Motor seizures ('pseudo', simulated)	8
Meadow syndrome	3
Total	65

*See Chapter 13 for further details.

TABLE 3.IV

Miscellaneous neurological disorders referred as ?epilepsy

Disorder	N
Paroxysmal vertigo	34
Tics	16
Non-progressive neurological*	22
Unexplained	9
Total	81

*Progressive disorders have not been analysed—see Chapter 14.

Fainting fits and epileptic fits

Extensive and continuing clinical experience in the outpatient clinic, in the wards, in the intensive care unit and in the EEG department indicate that the most common difficult clinical problem is the distinction between anoxic and epileptic seizures, between fainting fits and epileptic fits. Many reports in the literature attest to this difficulty (*e.g.* Symonds 1950; Williams 1950; Lloyd-Smith and Tatlow 1958*a,b*; Gastaut 1958; Lennox and Lennox-Buchtal 1960; Keipert 1969; Duvernoy *et al.* 1980; Gordon 1982; Ballardie and Murphy 1983; and discussions in Aicardi 1986 and Gilliatt and Roberts 1986). In his Hower Award address on the future of clinical child neurology, Aicardi (1987) said: '. . epidemiological studies require a correct diagnosis as the basis of patient selection. This type of study will probably assume increasing importance as limited resources must be allocated to the correct measures, and selecting the wrong target can represent the waste of considerable money and effort.' In the field of seizures, he went on, 'Simplicity is a good thing but should not be used at the expense of accuracy or even of truth. The real world is infinitely complex and only the abilities of our minds are limited.' It will always be easier to make a correct diagnosis by a personal consultation but it is hoped that this book will make it easier for epidemiological studies to clarify the contribution of the tendency to epileptic and non-epileptic seizures to morbidity and mortality. In the absence of such data, the author makes no apology for giving maximum emphasis to what seems to be the most common major problem, the reflex anoxic seizure or vagal cardio-inhibitory fainting fit (Stephenson 1978*a*).

4
HISTORY ACQUISITION

John Stobo Prichard* impressed upon me the adage:

> *'What . . ?'—history; 'Where . . ?'—examination.*

In the diagnosis of paroxysmal disorders, fits, faints and whatever, 'What . . ?' is paramount and the history is all-important. Complete acquisition may be impossible, but no effort is too great in attempting to approach this goal.

Prolonged interrogation

The diagnosis is as good as the history. The objective is to elicit a sequence which, replayed in the mind's eye, is as good as or better than a split-screen video recording with full polygraphy. With experience, a few minutes may be enough for a watertight history, but your author still finds that an hour may be necessary, first to disentangle, and then to weave the threads of a true likeness of the hitherto undiagnosed seizure. The historical approach (and its difficulties) are illustrated in the 140 case histories in this book. Aspects of some of the essentials follow.

Individual assessment

It is self-evident that the age, sex, health and syndrome diagnosis of the individual are important in determining the most likely diagnoses of paroxysmal events. Details of some of these are given in Chapter 15.

Family history

Virtually all the points which will be made about the acquisition of the history apply with equal force to the history of seizures in relatives. As Jeavons (1983) has emphasized, one of the main reasons for a misdiagnosis of epilepsy (in the sense of making this diagnosis when the patient has something completely different) is a 'family history of epilepsy'. It is just as imperative not to accept that the mother or father has 'known epilepsy' or the brother or sister 'febrile convulsions' as it is not to accept that the patient before one is 'a known epileptic'. Case histories at the end of this chapter (4.2, 4.3, 4.4) and elsewhere illustrate this point.

Setting

It is absolutely necessary to discover the setting in which the episode, or episodes, have occurred. Were they in the awake state, or in drowsiness, or in sleep—and if so in what stage of sleep? What was the patient doing; what were other people doing; what was happening just before the episode occurred? Was it at rest, during

---

*The late John Stobo Prichard was for many years Chief of Neurology at the Hospital for Sick Children, Toronto, and was the first President of the International Child Neurology Association.

exercise, while eating, at the lavatory, in bed, at school, at the hairdresser's, or in the course of any other of the myriad of human activities? With only a small amount of additional information, the setting may give the diagnosis. For example, if a tonic seizure occurs in a child in the setting of a normal school, the diagnosis is almost certainly that of (vaso)vagal syncope (Chapter 15).

Stimulus
It is equally important to discover if there appears to have been an immediate stimulus to initiate the apparent seizure. Although the numerous triggers to reflex epilepsy (Gastaut and Tassinari 1966) are—apart from television (and computer-associated visual display units) and startle—rare, in the case of syncope and certain other paroxysmal events a recognizable stimulus is the rule rather than the exception. Like other aspects of the history this item may need to be elicited, in the sense of squeezed out from the memory of the informants. Sometimes the existence of triggers may be denied but if one allows undirected talk then a significant pointer may emerge (*e.g.* see Case 15.24).

Prodrome
Feelings of unease are described by older patients before certain types of epileptic seizure and likewise parents of young children may notice difficult behaviour beforehand. A type of irritability is well known before the onset of migraine. Apprehension or a 'distant' feeling may precede certain syncopes.

Aura
In general, the term aura is more applicable to non-epileptic than to epileptic seizures. The 'aura' preceding certain epileptic seizures with focal origin is actually the beginning of the first of a series of epileptic seizures, being a 'partial epileptic seizure' in the modern terminology. The auras preceding certain syncopes are equally complex but sometimes it is difficult to decide whether the symptoms represent an aura or a stimulus. For example, in syncopes of a vagal mechanism discussed in later chapters, abdominal pain may be a trigger but may also be the first symptom of a vagal discharge.

Onset
What happens at the onset of an ictus is often of great diagnostic importance. In the descriptions of witnesses, this detail may be omitted or suppressed in favour of the more dramatic events which follow. Mental force is needed to concentrate on this 'moment of time'.

Ictal course
Even in rather short seizures a good deal may happen. It is commonly necessary to decelerate the witness's descriptive tale and to suggest a simile such as the slow-motion replay of the scoring of a goal. The duration of the seizure may be markedly exaggerated but estimates may be improved by using a stop-watch and having the witness replay the events in his or her mind, indicating the start and finish (see, for

TABLE 4.I

Everyday words for seizure phenomena

Absence	Atonic	Clonic
day-dream	faint	twitch
stare	swoon	jerk
blank	sag	flick
trance	flop	(fast, slowing down)
daze	fall	
	drop	
	crash	
	collapse	

Complex motor	Myoclonic	Spasm
thrash	jerk	spasm
toss about	twitch	stretch
jactitate (ballismus)	jack-knife	shrug
	jump	shoot out
	hiccup	
	'face in the cornflakes'	
	shock	

Tonic	Vibratory	Unspecified
stiff	vibrate	spell
rigid	shake	turn
like a board	tremble	fit
twisted	tremor	attack
clawed	rigor	episode
'like Frankenstein'	quiver	convulsion
banana-shaped		seizure
contorted		
cramped		

example, Case 4.7). However, stories of unexpectedly long seizures may not be due to observer panic, they may be true (Cases 4.8, 11.1).

Cessation of seizure
How exactly the seizure ended may give diagnostic clues, for example the gasp at the conclusion of the awake apnoea syndrome (Case 15.6) or the beetroot flush after cardiac standstill (Case 7.3).

Immediate postictal state
It is well known that transient neurological deficits may follow unilateral or partial (focal) epileptic seizures. It seems less well known that a fully developed generalized tonic-clonic epileptic seizure (grand mal) is followed by stupor. Although superficially similar, this is quite different from the intense desire to sleep which may follow convulsive syncope when there has been a pure anoxic seizure. It may be surprisingly hard to elicit a distinctive story (Case 15.38). In the context of acute illness, it is of immense importance to recognize that postictal inability to localize pain may mean not that the seizure was epileptic (such as a febrile

convulsion with an epileptic mechanism) but rather that it was a manifestation of impaired cerebral perfusion requiring urgent attention (Case 15.46).

After-effects
The discovery that urination has occurred, or the emergence of headache, are not of diagnostic value, as these occur after various epileptic and anoxic seizures. A prolonged confusional state commonly, but by no means always, signifies a preceding epileptic seizure (*e.g.* Case 4.9).

History from both witness and patient
Ideally, all these historical details should be extracted both from the patient and from the witness or witnesses. In adult medicine, the latter is often difficult unless extraordinary efforts are made to contact those who may have seen what happened. In paediatrics, the opposite may happen in that parents are questioned but the child's perceptions are ignored. Even at the age of 2 years a child may come out with helpful comments, and a school-age child may, with patience, be persuaded to produce genuinely useful information. However, in the case of psychic seizures following sexual abuse the critical part of the story is normally omitted (Case 13.1).

History from a second witness
As Meadow (1984) has emphasized, mothers may sometimes invent (Case 13.2) or induce (Case 8.6) seizures in their children. When this clinical situation is *possible* it is important to interview other witnesses who have seen the actual *onset* of a seizure, since it is common for a mother who is suffocating her child to allow her husband, and nursing and medical staff, to see the middle and end of the seizure (Case 8.7).

Delayed history
In any branch of medicine, if one has not obtained a diagnosis through the sequence history, necessary examination and necessary investigations, then one goes back to the history and starts again. With seizures and suchlike there may be an additional difficulty in that a full history is not available from the onset because of the nature of the seizure. For example, an older child was brought in, stuporous, having been found confused, and twitching on the right, in a woodwork class at school. Not until some days later could he remember the onset as being with the classroom rotating and growing larger, giving a clue as to the origin of the epileptic seizures.

Miming
The use of mime is an essential extension of the verbal history in motor seizures. Some of the words commonly used in describing seizure phenomena (Table 4.I) may lead to a misinterpretation of the precise posture and the rate, force and regularity of movements. Natural inhibitions make for difficulties in having a witness mime a seizure in all its detail. Sometimes this inhibition is indeed justifiable (I asked a father in front of medical students to mime his young

13

daughter's seizures, mistakenly believing that she had simple myoclonic jerks. In due course he threw himself to the ground, stiffened, and jerked violently for three quarters of a minute. 'You asked for it!' he said. Embarrassment was mutual); but mostly the effort is worthwhile (Case 15.38). It will be recognized that parents do not necessarily wish to perform such mimes in front of their children.

When inhibitions prove too much (as they frequently do), and particularly in a child suspected of having an epilepsy with multiple seizure types, then providing a choice of mimes—'Which does he have?'—may be productive. Various types of absence, jerk, spasm and stiffening can be demonstrated seriatim.

Replication

The reproduction of a seizure in front of the witness and determining whether it is identical to natural attacks may be of great diagnostic value. Laboratory involvement is not necessary in many instances at the outset, although certain commonsense precautions are necessary if falling is anticipated. The easiest epileptic seizure to reproduce is the simple absence, having the child blow a tissue or imitate one's strong hyperventilation (beware tetany in the examiner!). The brief stiffening of the uncommon but therapeutically most important startle epilepsy is not too difficult to stage-manage (Case 15.24). An ability to generate humour may allow the reproduction of cataplexy (Case 14.4). Patience in allowing the young infant to drift off to sleep reveals benign myoclonus (Case 15.2). Blue breath-holding attacks (prolonged expiratory apnoea) may be provoked by a sudden, unexpected and noxious but harmless stimulus (such as a pinch to the toe) (Gauk *et al.* 1963), and in fact this may be easier if the child is not connected to elaborate recording apparatus (Case 8.1). It is likewise probably easier to induce cardiac asystole and convulsive syncope with the child unattached, but when this is necessary it is more useful for these reflex anoxic seizures to be reproduced under EEG and ECG control, preferably with video-recording in addition (for further details see Chapter 9).

Video-recording

The increasing availability of portable video cameras which can be used in the home may allow the capture on film of seizures which it has been impossible to describe with sufficient accuracy or to reproduce in circumstances in which some method of intensive monitoring (Gumnit 1987) is practicable.

'Bugging'

Covert video surveillance has been undertaken to confirm that suffocation is the explanation of the seizures in Meadow syndrome (Rosen *et al.* 1983, Southall *et al.* 1987*c*, Williams and Bevan 1988). In practice this may pose considerable administrative problems, and other diagnostic methods may be as effective (Case 8.7).

The EEG

I do not believe that there should be a 'routine' EEG in paediatrics (or indeed at any other age) any more than there ought to be a routine physical examination.

How much the EEG technician does and in what way depends on the *problem*.

If the problem is, 'Is there evidence of accidental benzodiazepine overdose?' then all that is needed is a brief run with a limited number of channels to look for generalized fast (beta) activity. If there is a question of a focal lesion, special and detailed montages may have to be used. Under varying circumstances provocations such as strong hyperventilation, stroboscopic activation (with monocular occlusion, and at fast and slow rates), pattern stimulation, the use of sleep recording, sensory stimuli or ocular compression, or the use of additional medications may all help to elucidate the EEG itself. The technician may also use polygraphy, monitoring ECG, respiration, eye movements, surface EMG and limb displacement.

The conclusion depends both on the problem and on a knowledge of the overall neurological state. This includes: (i) information about the age and sex, and (in the case of newborns) the gestational age; (ii) a detailed history of the paroxysmal events of the seizures and suchlike, and up-to-date information on medication; (iii) a note of abnormal neurological findings; and (iv) the mention of fever, biochemical upsets or systemic illness at the time of the recording.

The way the conclusion is written also depends on whom it is addressed to. It is, or ought to be, a personal communication between two clinicians, and not simply a summary of amplitudes and frequencies. It may be conventional to preface the conclusion by a statement as to whether it is a normal or abnormal recording, but it is imperative to remember that 'abnormal record' does not have any more specific meaning than 'abnormal neurological examination', and may mean less.

There are many types of EEG abnormality with varying degrees of specificity. A recording may be abnormal in one way or another if the child is too hot or too cold; is metabolically deranged; is drugged; is unconscious; recently had a seizure; is in a seizure at the time; has a brain illness, brain injury or brain malformation; has a gene for febrile convulsions or a gene for epilepsy which s/he does not manifest; has or has had a type of epilepsy; is at an age when paroxysmal discharges are more likely to be seen on the EEG; or if s/he has a statistically unusual EEG profile without pathological significance. The best-known EEG abnormality correlated with epilepsy is the short-duration, high-amplitude electrical discharge known as the spike. However, it must be remembered that more people have spikes in their EEG who do not have epilepsy than those who do.

It has been argued (Goodin and Aminoff 1984) that, providing one pays attention to the prior probability of the diagnosis of epilepsy (in the jargon, the prevalence), then the EEG may in fact be a powerful tool for epilepsy diagnosis. Goodin and Aminoff pointed out that if the possibility of epilepsy is no greater in one's patient than in the general population, then an EEG showing spikes will not make a diagnosis of epilepsy likely. However, if the clinician regards the chances of epilepsy as evens (*i.e.* a 50 per cent probability) before the EEG, then EEG spikes will increase the probability to 90 per cent, making the diagnosis highly likely.

Using the standard method of determining sensitivity, specificity, positive predictive value and negative predictive value (see Stephenson and King 1989), it can be further shown that with intermediate levels of probability the absence of EEG spikes or a normal EEG in no way excludes the diagnosis of epilepsy, but if the prior probability is very low and on a par with the prevalence in the general population, then a normal EEG will further reduce the probability and to a degree 'exclude' epilepsy.

There are several difficulties about these arguments: one is the soundness of the clinician's judgement on the prior probability of epilepsy. Another is that in certain conditions in which one may want to know whether epilepsy is present, spikes may be a common feature even in the absence of epileptic seizures, as for example in various types of cerebral palsy. An important group in which EEGs are often requested is the population of children who have had one or more febrile seizures (Chapter 15). In such children the likelihood of finding EEG spikes is much higher than the likelihood of later epilepsy (Aicardi 1986, Wallace 1988). No great good comes in discovering these spikes, and difficulties in explaining them to parents certainly follow. A recent study compared interictal sharp EEG transients in those suffering neonatal seizures and in a comparison group who experienced apnoea but who were neurologically well (Clancy 1989). Unfortunately, the study did not include a group of neurologically abnormal neonates who did not have epileptic seizures, so that statistical inferences which could help in diagnosis are not available.

The EEG may be of great help in defining the type of epilepsy once the diagnosis of epilepsy has been made on clinical grounds, and it is of increasing value in helping with the diagnosis of many acute and chronic disorders of childhood such as haemorrhagic shock encephalopathy syndrome, subacute sclerosing panencephalitis, lissencephaly or pachygyria, or the syndromes of Angelman or Rett. However, it can be a hazardous investigation when it is done for the wrong reasons and reported by someone not closely in touch with clinical realities. As Aicardi (1987) put it, 'Clinical medicine is basically an intellectual process whereby data from all sources, whether strictly clinical (in the restricted sense) or from the laboratory and other technical tools, is integrated and shaped into a meaningful profile.' The EEG is one such laboratory or technical tool and must be requested and interpreted with the utmost caution and wisdom.

Ictal EEG capture
The diagnosis of epileptic and non-epileptic seizures may certainly be advanced if an EEG can be recorded during the episode (Blumhardt 1986, Aminoff *et al.* 1988*a*), bearing in mind that in the majority of *simple* partial epileptic seizures, surface EEG manifestations may not be seen (Devinsky *et al.* 1989). Greater diagnostic certainty may be possible if the EEG and other parameters are monitored with simultaneous video-recording (Holmes *et al.* 1980, Rosen *et al.* 1983, Kellaway 1987, Ramani 1987, Duchowny *et al.* 1988). The investment that is involved in the more elaborate of these recording methods emphasizes the prime importance of history acquisition as the initial diagnostic step.

Case histories
CASE 4.1
A 10-year-old was referred with the following story. 'This girl had an attack which has been

16

well described as a grand mal seizure by witnesses while at the hairdresser's. She has had several fainting attacks in the past, but these have been of a quite different nature. She is said to have had a cyanotic episode with twitching after a pertussis vaccine as a child.'

According to her mother she was standing in front of a mirror getting her hair cut. The hairdresser felt her swaying but the child had no warning. She went down onto the floor on her side, pulled her hands up (flexed) into a shaking position as if trying to grasp at her face, her knees bent, and her feet started 'going' (jerking) and her hands and legs shaking, with her eyes staring into mid-air. After some minutes her eyes opened and she looked very pale. In the past she had had a number of limp faints and she had had a cyanotic episode with a fit of coughing when she had whooping cough disease at the age of 2 years.

Comment. 'Grand mal' was excluded once the history had been obtained in detail. Note how whooping cough disease had become 'pertussis vaccine encephalopathy' in the mind of the referring doctor, setting the scene for a later diagnosis of epilepsy. The presenting seizure was typical of vagocardiac syncope provoked by hair-cutting (see Chapter 15, p. 159).

CASE 4.2
There was much concern that this 10-year-old boy had epilepsy 'like his father'. He had two episodes in which he felt faint, dropped, became stiff and wet himself, then was able to answer questions within 15 seconds. On both occasions he was pale. His father's 'epilepsy' had begun 12 years before when he was about 20 and had attended eight family funerals in six weeks. His fits were blackouts preceded by a feeling of butterflies in his stomach and lightheadedness. He felt he should continue his phenytoin tablets in case he lost his driving licence, despite having had no episodes for 10 years.

Comment. A family history of epilepsy is a potent inhibitor to the diagnosis of vagal syncope (Jeavons 1983). In this case it is likely that the father's attacks were also syncopal, but he is now irretrievably 'epileptic'.

CASE 4.3
The father of a 3-year-old girl with typical reflex anoxic seizures was regarded as an 'epileptic'. His first fit occurred when he was aged 14 years after he had fallen off his bicycle onto his head. All the episodes are similar. He sees lights and then gets a sensation over him that he must lie down. His eyes go right up into his eyelids, his mouth 'goes funny' and he shakes all over for around 30 seconds to a minute—during this, and for a minute or so after, his breathing becomes very snorty; then he comes to and goes into a deep sleep for an hour or so. When he reawakens he feels very well, as if it were the best sleep he ever had in his life, though he is also very thirsty and very white. He thought they occurred if he forgot to take his phenobarbitone. One episode happened while he was involved in a heated argument with somebody. Another was when he was watching a horror film on TV—a door opened in a house as a monster was about to eat somebody and he got such a fright that he fell off his chair and had a fit. A more recent episode occurred as he was sitting in church at a christening. When he felt it coming on he saw the flashing lights and reached for the phenobarbitone which he kept in his pocket. He rushed out of the church and walked about in the fresh air until it went off.

Comment. The history details suggest that this man had vagal-mediated convulsive syncopes like his daughter but, as with the father in Case 4.2, he is now an established 'epileptic'.

CASE 4.4
An 18-month-old girl was referred because of shivering attacks. These had no pathological significance, and the child was only referred because her mother was supposed to have

epilepsy. In fact the mother's story was as follows. She had had a small number of attacks in which everything would seem far away visually, and at the same time voices and noises would have a hollow sound as if she was in a hollow chamber, and she would have to lean against a wall. These episodes were brought on by being hot in the kitchen when cooking or ironing. After an EEG she had been told that she had temporal lobe epilepsy, was put on carbamazepine and had lost her driving licence.

Comment. It was the family history of 'epilepsy' which prompted this consultation. Her story seems typical of vasovagal syncope, but her misdiagnosis is a natural consequence of 'Please investigate' and 'EEG please to exclude epilepsy'. The family doctor is in the best position to correlate the diagnoses in different generations in the same family (pending advances in the genetic field!) and to preserve a critical outlook over lifetimes.

CASE 4.5
A 10-year-old boy was sitting in a car. His father was driving so did not see everything that happened. First the boy mumbled some words which did not make sense and then he arched his back, went completely stiff and became unconscious for about 90 seconds; he then recovered, feeling tired. He remembered seeing black spots in front of his eyes immediately before passing out and was sweaty afterwards.

Comment. This is a particular example of a general difficulty in which the event, the seizure or whatever, is not seen or is incompletely witnessed. In this case the boy's aura and his immediate postictal recall indicated an anoxic seizure, presumably vagally mediated.

CASE 4.6
A 4-year-old boy had reflex anoxic seizures for two years induced by falls or frights. He would go pale, roll his eyes, and become stiff, with saliva coming out of his mouth. Some of them occurred for no apparent reason, when he was sitting on his chair having dinner, but according to his father a consistent stimulus was the smell of something burning.
    Ocular compression (see pp. 83–89) induced an asystole of 15 seconds with EEG flattening for nine seconds, and an anoxic seizure characterized by flexion, downward eye jerks, snorting, deviation of the eyes to the right, upward eye deviation, and further snorting before recovery. His father said that this seizure was very mild, and like the start of one of the natural ones.

Comment. It was not clear at first whether the smell which the boy spoke of was an aura or a stimulus. Although the other triggers were typical of reflex anoxic seizures (see Chapters 8 and 9), it was helpful to the family to expand the history by reproducing the attack.

CASE 4.7
An intelligent 21-month-old boy had episodes of crying without sound and becoming blue, from the neonatal period. The most dramatic episode occurred after his MMR (measles/mumps/rubella) immunization when he bumped his head. His parents found him lying face down, cyanosed and flaccid, with his eyes rolled up and apnoeic. They thought the duration of the episode must have been about two minutes, but when they mimed it and were timed by a stopwatch the duration came out as 12 seconds. The parents were concerned as to whether they could ever let the child out of their sight.

Comment. In this case of blue breath-holding attacks ('prolonged expiratory apnoea'—see Chapter 8) the parents' perception of time was evidently exaggerated, albeit their stopwatch-timed recollection may have been over-short. However, parents' estimation of the duration of attacks can be remarkably accurate (*e.g.* see Cases 11.1 and 11.2).

18

CASE 4.8

All the seizures in this 20-month-old girl had been precipitated by a bang to the head, but her story of jerking for a minute-and-a-half in each attack, constant urination, and the fact that she went 'lifeless' for about 45 minutes before coming round again had suggested the possibility—or indeed probability—of epilepsy. Indeed in one of the episodes twitching was said to have gone on for 15 minutes.

Ocular compression was carried out with the mother present and the procedure was videotaped. The resting EEG and ECG were normal. Ocular compression after a latency of less than one second induced an asystole with 28.5 seconds of EEG flattening, during which there was tonic extension. Following the return of high-voltage slow delta activity, two abrupt extensions of the upper limbs occurred (see Fig. 7.1, p. 44), with latencies of six seconds and 13 seconds. Mouth movements ('automatism') occurred 60 seconds after the return of the EEG, and 10 seconds later she was crying and the EEG promptly returned to the normal frequency of about eight per second. The child then seemed miserable but went to sleep again for an hour or so.

During this seizure the mother was in a considerable state of panic and behaved as if she thought the child was dead. Later she said that she was very pleased that the seizures had been reproduced and witnessed. Her conversation with the author was also recorded on videotape and is reproduced, in edited form, below.

Doctor: She's not your only child?
Mother: No, I've got three children.
Doctor: And does anybody have faints or fits or 'turns'?
Mother: I do, I faint.
Doctor: And what's the provocation?
Mother: Tiredness, heat, exhaustion, illness, pregnancy.
Doctor: And what happens in your faints?
Mother: I black out completely.
Doctor: Just go limp?
Mother: Completely limp.
Doctor: With a warning?
Mother: Yes, I normally get spots in front of my eyes which get bigger and bigger and just blank me out.
Doctor: Is it always standing up, or can you faint sitting or lying down?
Mother: I think it's always been standing up.
Doctor: What age did it start?
Mother: From puberty I would say.
Doctor: And nobody else in the family?
Mother: Nobody else in the family has fainting. My husband has allergies.
Doctor: Yes. When did your child start having episodes?
Mother: She was 12 months exactly.
Doctor: And how many in total?
Mother: Approximately 12. A dozen.
Doctor: Are they all the same?
Mother: They've all been the same, apart from the last one where the convulsions actually lasted 15 minutes, and the other ones they lasted for only two minutes.
Doctor: And she's never had a turn without what you call a convulsion with twitching; there's always been twitching in every single one?
Mother: Yes, but to some degree, a greater or lesser degree; some fits have been worse than others and we can't decide . . It's nothing to do with the bang on the head, sometimes she can get a big bang from falling off a chair and she'll have a mild fit maybe or she could fall off a chair and have a big fit.

Doctor: Can you describe very exactly what occurs in one of the typical episodes?

Mother: She will get a bang on the head, could be a heavy bang, like she walked into a swing once and had a big bang, or another time she just slipped and banged her head very slightly on the tiled bathroom floor. She lets out a scream and she doesn't take her breath in again. It seems as if she can't, as if her throat is paralysed, and her eyes go back in her head, she goes very straight, often her spine arches, she goes very stiff and she tries to breathe in, she sometimes makes a strange gurgling noise in her throat, but not always, but she is trying to take her breath in, but it seems that she can't. After, I'm not sure, maybe 40, 50, 60 seconds she does manage to take a little gasp and then maybe another 10 seconds later she'll manage to take another little gasp. So the breathing is shallow, and when she manages to take these short breaths then she starts to convulse and her arms and legs twitch and her eyes are back in her head and the movements of her body are quite uncontrollable and involuntary.

Doctor: And what's happening in this convulsion?

Mother: Her arms and legs are twitching.

Doctor: Yes, right.

Mother: Jerking, jerking and she throws her arms and legs out and jerks like that.

Doctor: So there is a large number of jerks, I mean there's more than 10 jerks and there's lots of . . .

Mother: Gosh, I've never counted how many. To tell the truth it's very difficult for me, I become very upset. I try to be observant and my husband's been with me and we do discuss it afterwards, but it's hard to be objective.

Doctor: Are they rapid jerks, I mean are they jerks like three-per-second jerks just now, is it that sort of speed or sort of occasional big things?

Mother: I'd say it was more the latter.

Doctor: And her eyes, they're sticking up all the time for the whole two minutes?

Mother: Her eyes back in her head completely for the whole two minutes.

Doctor: And that follows the original business of being stiff?

Mother: Yes.

Doctor: What are the colour changes from the very beginning, if there are colour changes?

Mother: She goes . . . as she gets less and less breath, she goes bluer and bluer as the oxygen . . .

Doctor: How blue? Not black?

Mother: No, no. She's gone blue enough for us to worry about her breathing and her oxygen and we have resuscitated her.

Doctor: Is it just blue or is it blue and pale at the same time?

Mother: Well I suppose she's pale with a bluish tinge, she normally has very good colour and she does go very pale. Yes, but I would say she was more blue than pale.

Doctor: When does the paleness become dominant?

Mother: When she is coming out of the fit, it leaves her very, very pale, drained of colour completely. I would say that you wouldn't notice the paleness while she is having the fit, you would notice the bluish, mauvish tinge about her face, especially around her mouth and her lips as she becomes short of oxygen. I haven't noticed her being particularly pale, I only notice how pale she is afterwards.

Doctor: And then she's asleep?

Mother: She comes to after two minutes and she's very pale, she's very bad-tempered, she's very listless. Oh, I'm sorry, I've got it confused. She has this convulsion for about two minutes and then when she starts to breathe again normally—deep breaths—she lapses into unconsciousness completely, she's totally limp and lifeless and floppy. And she will come round from that after about 10 minutes

20

—she wakes up and lets out a cry and she's miserable, and she's fed up and she's still very, very pale. She normally has something to drink and then she will go to sleep, and she will sleep sometimes for two hours, a very tired, exhausted sleep even though she may have just woken up from her morning nap, and when she wakes up she's perfectly okay. That's the general picture. Today she didn't lapse into that unconscious state after the fit. The thing that happened today, I would say perhaps has happened once before. We weren't sure she'd banged her head or not, we think she may have walked into the door. We were in the room with her but didn't see exactly what happened, and she, I think, maybe jerked her arms and legs once, but generally it was just the stiffness and the arching of the spine and then the lapsing into unconsciousness after. She struggled to breathe and when she could breathe she lapsed into unconsciousness and her eyes went back in her head again, in this fit, but that was the only time when she hasn't really convulsed properly. All the other occasions she's convulsed.

Doctor: The convulsing really is this long time? I mean, sometimes you panic, you think that time stands still and this could take a long time, but you really think it is as long as two minutes?

Mother: Yes, my husband times it. Yes, two minutes always.

Doctor: But it's more than half-a-dozen jerks—I mean, one, two, three, four, five, six—there's more than that, there's lots of jerks?

Mother: No, maybe there's only about half-a-dozen. It's not a rapid twitch, her whole body doesn't shake, it's jerks out of her arms and legs.

Doctor: The one that lasted 15 minutes you didn't see, this was the one precipitated by . . .

Mother: A blow to the mouth, of the roof. My mother saw it, a GP saw it and, yes, my mother said it lasted for 15 minutes. She was convulsing, jerking her arms and legs.

Doctor: You don't know how fast that was?

Mother: Quite violently for 15 minutes. That was the last one she had.

Doctor: And the only treatment she's had, she had Tegretol, carbamazepine?

Mother: Yes, she took Tegretol for five days. After four days she came out in a livid rash.

Doctor: And she hasn't had any other type of treatment?

Mother: No she hasn't. Only Valium to bring her out of a fit, once.

Doctor: And have you recovered from today's episode?

Mother: Just about. I'm vague about the movement, I really can't be sure what sort of movement it is. As far as I know, it's very long extended movements of the arms and legs, they're just stretched out like that.

Doctor: They're not little twitches, but big, the whole limb, the limb stretching out in a sort of big jerk?

Mother: I would say yes.

Doctor: I was going to ask you if what you saw today was like the beginning of the ones in which she had the jerks, because she didn't do an awful lot of jerking. She did about two jerks, with her arms sticking out a bit. Were these jerks anything similar to the ones she has?

Mother: Yes they were, very similar, yes.

Doctor: They were the same kind?

Mother: That was the same thing. I would say she probably did more than that though, normally, and she wouldn't come out of it as quickly.

Doctor: Tell me the main difference between this one and the normal one.

Mother: I would say the one she had today was a mild one compared to the ones that she normally has.

Doctor: Because you were getting in a great panic, absolutely horror struck, and I was thinking that you were thinking that it's even worse than the normal one, but it was . . .

Mother: I always do.

Doctor: So this is mild compared with the normal one?

Mother: It's mild, it lasted for less time.

Doctor: Because I thought you were acting as if this had never happened to you before.

Mother: Even though she's had 12 fits it doesn't mean to say I can get used to it.

Doctor: Okay, that's for the benefit of anyone else who watches this film. Just an extra question. The sort of not-breathing she was doing in the turn we induced by pressing her eyes—was it a similar sort of thing to what you call holding her breath?

Mother: Yes, only I think on previous occasions in some of the fits she's held her breath for much longer than that. My husband has actually counted 60 seconds.

Doctor: Yes, okay.

Mother: I asked the GP when I saw him after she'd gone off to hospital, I asked him what he thought it was and he said as far as he was concerned he had seen many cases of epilepsy and she was having a typical grand mal.

Doctor: And what did the paediatric neurologist say?

Mother: There wasn't a paediatric neurologist at the hospital. I saw a young unqualified paediatrician, he couldn't tell me anything.

Doctor: You've seen a paediatric neurologist?

Mother: Yes.

Doctor: What did he think?

Mother: Initially he thought it was 70 per cent likely to be epilepsy, an odd chance that the remaining 30 per cent could be reflex anoxic seizures, but he said not all the symptoms I described fitted the pattern of the reflex anoxic seizures, therefore he inclined towards epilepsy, and also looking at my case history which shows that the paternal great grandmother had epilepsy and I had problems—complications in pregnancy—and he said the whole picture sort of balanced out to look as if it was epilepsy.

Doctor: No, it's not.

Mother: It's not? Definitely, you can really conclusively say it's not epilepsy?

Doctor: Yes.

Mother: I don't really know what reflex epileptic seizures are. I'm delighted, yes.

Later, the doctor who had witnessed the episode of jerking for 15 minutes wrote with a description:

'The grandmother contacted me yesterday with your request for information regarding the incident. I am not the family's general practitioner but was called to the house where the child was by a friend of mine.

'I was confronted with an unconscious child whom I thought to be in the clonic phase of a grand mal convulsion; unconscious, stiff, slightly twitching, not cyanosed.

'Mother was at the hairdresser's and granny was climbing the wall [panicking].

'When I realised that this present episode had lasted at least 15 minutes till then I decided IV diazepam was indicated—four mg caused her to stop twitching and relaxed her limbs.

'At this point two burly ambulance men appeared and in view of the situation and my lack of past history here I decided it would be safer to allow the local paediatricians to observe her. Just after the girl had been whisked off mother arrived back in even more of a state than granny, eventually explaining that the girl was seeing distinguished neurologists up and down the country and what was I doing giving her Valium of all things!

'Grandmother has since explained that you consider these episodes to be hypoxic do's of some sort. I can only say that when I saw the girl that day she was convulsing in exactly the same way small children do when they have febrile convulsions.'

At around Christmas time some 18 months later the mother wrote: 'You may remember that I brought my daughter to see you as she was having very severe debilitating fits. I thought you may be interested to know that after seeing you she had one more fit the following week and then no more until she had a very mild fit at Easter this year brought on by a loud sudden noise. This was her last fit and we feel that she has grown out of them . . . I don't know what you did to her on our visit but I am extremely grateful.'

Comment.   This case is described at some length because it illustrates a number of aspects of history acquisition. Despite the recognition that episodes had been precipitated by blows to the head, the referring paediatric neurologist favoured a diagnosis of epilepsy sufficiently strongly to order an EEG and a CT brain scan, and to recommend the initiation of carbamazepine therapy (to which the child quickly became allergic). It is striking how distressed the mother became on witnessing what was the mildest attack the child had ever had, and it is no surprise how she found it difficult to be precise about the details of the convulsive movements. However, from the conversation with her it seems likely that in most attacks the child was having repeated anoxic extensor spasms similar to those recorded and illustrated in Figure 7.1 (p. 44). The history of urinary incontinence and immediate postictal sleep was properly given and taken, and in this instance it was the absence of quantitative data on what happens in anoxic seizures (see Table 7.I, p. 43) which allowed the mis-interpretation. The most difficult part of the story, however, arose from the existence of a novel event. One might attribute the tale of 15 minutes twitching to the mother's state of panic, but the corroborative description of the doctor who visited the house indicates that by that stage it had become a clonic epileptic seizure. This was thus a real epileptic seizure precipitated by a severe syncope, or what I call an anoxic-epileptic seizure (see Chapter 11: also Stephenson 1983, Battaglia *et al.* 1989). Nonetheless, the most important lesson of this case is the prime importance of the setting and stimulus for establishing the basic diagnosis.

CASE 4.9

This 2½-year-old girl was known to have reflex anoxic seizures, as were her sister and cousin. All three had had anoxic seizures reproduced by ocular compression in the EEG department. She was referred again because of what appeared to be a different type of attack over the past several months which was thought to be undoubtedly epileptic. Most episodes did not have an obvious stimulus, but others seemed to have been induced by rather minor noxious stimuli such as her father raising his voice. The most recent episode, precipitated by being told to hurry up, was typical. She first looked dazed and then slumped onto the fire. Her eyes 'went funny' and she stiffened up, made a slavering noise, opened her eyes wide and stared, and kept putting her hand to her mouth and making mouth and lip movements for what appeared to be several minutes until she came out of the attack, crying and looking white.

A repeat ocular compression induced an asystole of 26 seconds with a suppression of EEG activity for 17 seconds, followed by prolonged one- to two-per-second slow-wave activity on the EEG. The anoxic seizure was characterized by upward deviation of the eyes, flexion, a moan, extension, full extension, staring, a snort, another noise, a jerk, another extension and a dazed appearance. Then there were lip movements and further staring and an 'ooh ooh' noise; and then putting her hand to her mouth, looking up and putting her tongue in and out; looking about slightly and looking at her mother but not clearly knowing her; touching the electrodes, crying a little and scratching her ear; looking at her mother, crying and indistinctly speaking; rubbing her eyes; holding out her arms and making gurgly vocalizations and more tongue movements; protruding and licking her lips; and poking her mouth and teeth. Then she started to come back to normal about two minutes afterwards and was normal after about six minutes. Her mother said that this was identical in every detail to the episodes which she had observed at home.

Comment. Not surprisingly, the referring physician mistook this girl's episodes for long complex partial epileptic seizures. The diagnosis of non-epileptic reflex anoxic seizures was not believed until the history was extended by reproducing an identical attack. In this situation it is important (as was done here) to have the details of the history written down before replication is undertaken, to avoid biased interpretation.

CASE 4.10

A 9-year-old boy was said to have had absences during violin lessons for the preceding six months. After one-and-a-half minutes of hyperventilation he demonstrated what looked like an absence and did not respond. However, under video–EEG control, no EEG alteration occurred during unresponsiveness, and at one year follow-up he had been well without therapy.

Comment. The clinical suspicion here was of 'petit mal', that is to say, primary generalized typical absences. It was necessary to extend the history into replication under EEG control to demonstrate that that diagnosis was not possible. (If the symptoms had indicated simple partial epilepsy, exclusion by this method would not have been possible—Devinsky *et al.* 1989.)

CASE 4.11

A 5-year-old boy with known moyamoya disease complained of complete loss of vision for up to an hour after stress, for example after pain to his knee or other unexpected hurts. In fact, this was an improvement, as previously, before vascular surgery, he had loss of head control and bilateral hemiparesis after such stresses.

Comment. Although it is often helpful to extend the history by attempting to replicate a seizure under EEG control, this case is included to emphasize the hazard of hyperventilation during EEG in childhood cerebrovascular disease (Stephenson and King 1989).

5
INTRODUCTION TO DIFFERENTIAL DIAGNOSIS

This chapter mainly consists of tables which expand the propositions introduced in Chapter 2 and serve as a skeleton for discussion of the various seizures and suchlike throughout the book. Table 5.I outlines a number of predominantly motor components and points to their occurrence in various seizure mechanisms. Since this book is concerned particularly with fainting fits, special attention has been paid to tonic seizures, while much less emphasis has been placed on epileptic seizure types for which there is little differential diagnosis.

Absences (Table 5.II)
Absences are commonly epileptic, anoxic or psychic.

Epileptic absences are generalized non-convulsive seizures most typically accompanied by three-per-second regular spike and wave on the EEG. That type of complex febrile convulsion characterized by more than one febrile seizure in the same febrile illness may be an early indication of the presence of the gene for this type of epilepsy (Rocca *et al*. 1987*a*). Epileptic absences with generalized spike and wave occur in both normal individuals and those with mental impairment and other chronic encephalopathies, and have to be distinguished both from atypical absences with other types of EEG accompaniment and from undifferentiated complex partial seizures in which lapse of consciousness is the only obvious feature. The range of epileptic syndromes is well discussed elsewhere (Aicardi 1988), and the epileptic syndromes with typical absences (including juvenile myoclonic epilepsy with absences) are discussed in detail by Panayiotopoulos *et al.* 1989.

Anoxic or syncopal absences have been less well defined but are thought to be milder manifestations of short-lasting cerebral oligaemia. It is difficult to know how common this is compared with loss of vision or loss of tone in similar circumstances. A recently described anoxic absence is that associated with compulsive Valsalva manoeuvres (Gastaut 1980: Gastaut *et al*. 1982, 1987: Aicardi *et al*. 1988; Battaglia *et al*. 1989).

Psychic absences, or at any rate blanks of psychological origin, are clearly common, in the form of day-dreams and, in younger children, of gratification or of what one suspects as eidetic imagery, the viewing of a 'television in the sky' (see p. 143).

Other apparent states of absence may be secondary to excessive sedative medication or be a consequence of disturbed sleep, as in obstructive sleep apnoea.

Atonic seizures (Table 5.III)
Atonic epileptic seizures are one of the forms of epileptic fall or drop seizures. The

TABLE 5.I
Clinical manifestations related to origin of seizures

The three major seizure mechanisms

	Epileptic	Anoxic	Psychic
Absence	} Various epilepsies	} Vasovagal	Gratification
Atonic			'Swoon'
Myoclonic			Tic (some)
Spasm	} Cerebral pathology	} Abrupt cerebral hypoxia	} Meadow syndrome (active)
Tonic			
Vibratory	} T-C; C-T-C*		Anxiety
Clonic		Anoxic-epileptic	Simulated
Complex motor	Frontal, etc.	Abrupt cerebral hypoxia	Gratification

Other paroxysmal events

	Toxic	Hypnic	Miscellaneous
Absence	} Sedatives		Diurnal effect of sleep disorders
Atonic			Cataplexy; cranio-cervical lesions
Myoclonic		Benign sleep myoclonus	Benign myclonus; tic; hyperekplexia
Spasm	} Anticonvulsants; dopamine antagonists		Subacute sclerosing panencephalitis
Tonic		Sleep dystonia	Alternating hemiplegia, tetany
Vibratory	Alcohol		Shuddering (pre-essential tremor)
Clonic			Clonus
Complex motor		Jactatio; *pavor nocturnus* ('night terrors')	Paroxysmal choreoathetosis

*T-C = tonic-clonic; C-T-C = clonic-tonic-clonic

mechanism of epileptic falls includes, singly or in combination, atonic, myoclonic, spasm and tonic components. (Egli *et al.* 1985, Ikeno *et al.* 1985). In the pure atonic epileptic seizure the child falls *in toto*, like a puppet with all the strings simultaneously cut, and the detailed relationship with the EEG spike can best be demonstrated by a split-screen video recording.

Atonic episodes of anoxic origin are common, the best known being found in the vasovagal faint. Loss of tone is indeed the usual early manifestation of any type of acute cerebral ischaemia of any cause, including compulsive Valsalva manoeuvres (Aicardi *et al.* 1988).

TABLE 5.II
Absence types

Epileptic	True, epileptic absences—primary (chilhood and adolescent absence epilepsy; juvenile myoclonic epilepsy with absences), secondary, atypical Complex partial seizures—frontal, temporal
Anoxic	Pre-syncope; arrhythmias
Psychic	Anxiety
Toxic/metabolic	Sedatives (anti-epileptic drugs); toluene inhalation; hypoglycaemia
Hypnic	Sleep deprivation; obstructive sleep apnoea
Miscellaneous	Day-dream (subacute sclerosing panencephalitis—SSPE)

TABLE 5.III
Atonic seizure types

Epileptic	Atonic (myoclonic, spasm and tonic, especially startle-tonic, may simulate) ?Temporal lobe syncope
Anoxic	'Fainting'—vasodepressor, vasovagal (including some reflex syncopes)
Psychic	Simulated; hysteria
Toxic/metabolic	Hypoglycaemia
Hypnic	Narcoleptic cataplexy
Miscellaneous	Arnold–Chiari; other cranio-cervical; cataplexy

Of the other mechanisms of atonic fall, cataplexy is usually obvious because of the emotional precipitation. In the very young, narcolepsy may be less important as an explanation of cataplexy than type C Niemann–Pick disease with vertical supranuclear ophthalmoplegia (Kandt *et al.* 1982). Compressive lesions at the foramen magnum may also allow for this type of atonic fall (Dobkin 1978). Falls in the more elderly have been reviewed elsewhere (Botez and Hausser 1982).

For convenience, Table 5.IV summarizes the features of three common varieties of faint or fall.

Myoclonic seizures (Table 5.V)
Myoclonic phenomena are commonly, but by no means always, epileptic. Myoclonic epilepsies are numerous and complex, and are well described elsewhere (Aicardi 1986).

Myoclonic phenomena have been described as a constituent of anoxic seizures but the veracity of this is uncertain. Lin *et al.* (1982) reported that eight blood donors who had convulsive syncope showed 'violent and brief myoclonic jerks', but detailed recordings are not available. One suspects that many of the so-called myoclonic jerks in these circumstances are spasms, the difference being that a

TABLE 5.IV
Three types of faint or fall

	Epileptic fall	*Syncope*	*Psychic 'faint'*
Provocation	None (or startle)	Yes (may not be recognized)	'Stress'
Pallor	Often	Usually	No
Predominantly tonic	If neurodevelopmentally abnormal	50% of cases	Eyes to the ground
Witnessed	Not necessarily	Not necessarily	Yes

TABLE 5.V
Myoclonic seizure types

Epileptic	Various myoclonic seizures
Anoxic	Reported in convulsive syncopes, but not fully verified
Psychic	Some tics
Toxic/metabolic	Hepatic, renal and pulmonary insufficiency
Hypnic	Benign sleep myoclonus, including neonatal
Miscellaneous	Gilles de la Tourette and 'neurological' tics; benign myoclonus of infancy; hyperekplexia; non-epileptic myoclonus in various neurological diseases

TABLE 5.VI
Spasm types

Epileptic	Infantile spasms; axial spasms in older children (common epileptic fall); periodic spasms; startle epilepsy
Anoxic	Post-opisthotonic phase of anoxic seizure on return of EEG
Psychic	Some tics
Toxic/metabolic	See Table 5.VII
Hypnic	Grimaces and other normal sleep phenomena
Miscellaneous	Subacute sclerosing panencephalitis (post-measles); benign non-epileptic spasms; intussusception

myoclonic jerk has a duration measured in milliseconds and a spasm one measured in hundreds of milliseconds.

The most common non-epileptic myoclonus occurs in sleep: the neonatal form is particularly important (see p. 140). So-called benign 'myoclonus' of infancy (Lombroso and Fejerman 1977) must be distinguished from infantile spasms of epileptic type (see p. 38). Tics present no diagnostic problems. Hyperekplexia, or startle disease (see Chapter 14, p. 141) is recognized by its evolution from a stiff irritable neonate, and has to be distinguished from startle epilepsy (see below). True myoclonus occurs in many other neurological disorders both with and without accompanying epilepsy.

Spasms (Table 5.VI)
Spasms are very brief tonic seizures with a duration of the order of one second.

Spasms of presumed epileptic nature are common. One says 'presumed' because infantile spasms and the similar type of spasms afflicting those beyond infancy are assumed to be epileptic, and are normally classified with the epilepsies, but are likely to have a different mechanism albeit still not well defined. Infantile spasms are well known to all paediatricians but similar spasms, whether axial or involving the limbs as well as the trunk, are a common mechanism of epileptic falls in later childhood (Egli *et al.* 1985). The title 'periodic spasms' has been suggested for a particular, localization-related type of recurrent event (see Gobbi *et al.* 1987).

In so-called startle epilepsy, falls result from spasms induced by sudden unexpected noises (Saenz-Lope *et al.* 1984).

Spasms are a prominent component of anoxic seizures particularly in the period immediately after the restoration of cerebral oxygenation, that is to say commonly after the return of adequate cerebral perfusion. Hence, in the active form of Meadow syndrome (Meadow 1984), spasms may be the visible component of the anoxic seizure once the mother has released the baby from her suffocation.

Of the other non-epileptic spasms, those precipitated by drug sensitivity will be discussed in the section on tonic seizures. The repetitive phenomena of subacute sclerosing panencephalitis are commonly spasms, although there may also be an atonic component.

The most benign variety of spasms is that originally described as 'benign myoclonus of early infancy' (Lombroso and Fejerman 1977) but more recently renamed 'benign non-epileptic infantile spasms' (Dravet *et al.* 1986). Runs of spasms occur in normal children with normal ictal and interictal EEG.

Tonic seizures (Table 5.VII)
Tonic seizures in epilepsy
Tonic fits are one of the characteristic seizures of the abnormal brain and, as has been and will be repeatedly emphasized, tonic seizures in normal individuals are usually anoxic seizures.

Tonic epileptic seizures are commonly but not exclusively generalized, having EEG accompaniments of 'desynchronization' (with a low amplitude and loss of spikes if spikes were previously prominent), or a low- or medium-voltage fast activity, or a higher-voltage fast spike appearance. Such seizures may be the sole epileptic seizure in an individual, and children who have such seizures in the daytime tend to be in the borderline or mildly mentally impaired range of ability. Some cases seem to be familial. Bradyarrhythmia at the onset of a tonic-clonic seizure in which the tonic component overshadows the clonic may lead to initial diagnostic confusion (Cases 12.1, 12.2; and see Mutani *et al.* 1970, Navelet *et al.* 1989). Nocturnal tonic episodes have been described in which there is no EEG change and which may not actually be epileptic seizures but rather some form of dystonia (Lugaresi and Cirignotta 1981, Rajna *et al*. 1983, Maccario and Lustman 1990).

More commonly tonic epileptic seizures occur as part of some sort of polymorphous epilepsy. Either this is the sort of mixed epilepsy of infancy and later childhood which begins with febrile and sub-febrile hemiclonic convulsions, and proceeds via myoclonic jerks and photosensitivity to various other types of partial and secondary generalized epileptic seizures, or it is in the context of the so-called Lennox–Gastaut syndrome in which atypical absences, spasms and possibly myoclonic seizures may occur in the daytime with a preponderance of tonic seizures in the night. Often these tonic epileptic seizures have a strong vibratory component, and the quiver or shaking may be interpreted as indicating that the seizure was a tonic-clonic or 'grand mal'.

On occasion tonic seizures are partial rather than generalized and may be described as a type of partial seizure with complex motor symptomatology. A seizure of that kind may not be uncommon in tuberous sclerosis. Hemitonic seizures may be mistaken for generalized tonic epileptic seizures because if, as is often the case, the child is lying on his or her side then the lack of involvement of the limbs on one side may not be apparent.

A further type of epileptic seizure which may in some individuals be described as tonic, but is more often in the nature of a spasm or even briefer, is that found in 'startle' epilepsy. Such individuals, with a structurally abnormal brain but often normal intelligence and only minimal asymmetrical motor disability, abruptly fall over when startled by sudden sounds or other surprising stimuli. It may not even be recognized that the patient is having epileptic seizures at all but instead s/he is regarded as clumsy and just tending to fall easily. The diagnosis is important because these seizures commonly respond completely to an appropriate dose of carbamazepine (Saenz-Lope *et al*. 1984) (see Case 15.24).

Tonic anoxic seizures
Tonic components, often with opisthotonus, are common in all types of anoxic seizures (see Chapter 7).

Blue breath-holding (prolonged expiratory apnoea) is well known in normal children and as a complication of respiratory disorders, in particular pertussis infection, (Southall *et al*. 1988*b*), but also occurs in association with central nervous malformation and brainstem tumour (Southall *et al*. 1987*a*). Apnoeas also occur in mixed breath-holding attacks with a partial vagal component, in obstructive apnoeas and in association with reflux.

A Valsalva–Weber manoeuvre (see Duvoisin 1961, 1962) may be a frequent occurrence in some mentally impaired children with autistic features. Profound asphyxia results from suffocation in 'active' Meadow syndrome.

Vagal attacks (reflex anoxic seizures) with a reversible cardiac asystole are described in detail elsewhere (see Chapters 8, 9). A tonic seizure in a child at a normal school is likely to be (vaso)vagal convulsive syncope.

Unusual cardiac and circulatory obstructive causes include paroxysmal

TABLE 5.VII

TABLE 5.VII
Tonic seizure types

Epileptic	Common epileptic seizure of the abnormal brain; startle epilepsy
Anoxic	Breath-holding; suffocation; cardiac asystole; ventricular fibrillation; circulatory obstruction; acute intracranial hypertension
Psychic	Simulated/hysteria; invented ('passive Meadow syndrome')
Toxic/metabolic	Dopamine agonists, bethanechol, carbamazepine, etc.; tetany; fatty acid oxidation disorder
Hypnic	Sleep dystonias
Miscellaneous	Brainstem disease; demyelination (multiple sclerosis)
Mechanism unknown	Many febrile seizures; many neonatal seizures; alternating hemiplegia

ventricular fibrillation with or without deafness, valve stenosis, Fallot's tetralogy, cardiomyopathy, and paroxysmal pulmonary hypertension.

An acute increase in intracranial pressure can trigger what might be described as an anoxic seizure of tonic type whether the explanation be acute brain swelling or the acute obstruction of cerebrospinal fluid outflow from tumour or blocked shunt in hydrocephalus.

Other types of tonic attack

Toxic causes are often easier to diagnose but may be difficult when drug adminstration complicates organic illness. Dopamine antagonists or the acetyl-choline agonist bethanechol induce brief tonic episodes, as does carbamazepine overdose. In the case of the former drugs, consciousness is likely to be unimpaired, but with carbamazepine the disturbance of consciousness makes the tonic episodes (Case 5.1) more easily misdiagnosed as epileptic. Strychnine poisoning and tetanus should be recognized in context. The metabolic basis of tetany will not usually present problems, but the sudden onset of a metabolic encephalopathy with a tonic seizure may indicate a fatty acid oxidation disorder requiring a panoply of investigations.

Although there is a psychological or psychogenic element in a number of tonic attacks, primarily psychic tonic seizures are unusual. A type of tonic seizure of hysterical nature in which there is tonic deviation of the eyes toward the ground on whichever side the patient is lying has been described (Henry and Woodruff 1978).

Tonic or dystonic attacks in sleep have been described in otherwise normal individuals. Such episodes are probably non-epileptic (Rajna *et al.* 1983) (Case 5.2). Miscellaneous additional mechanisms are several. Brainstem disease is probably responsible for tonic attacks seen in encephalitis or in the haemolytic uraemic syndrome. Tonic episodes in demyelinating disease do not usually present until adulthood and tend to be very focal (Twomey and Espir 1980). The mechanism of the tonic or hemitonic attacks that may be part of the syndrome of alternating hemiplegia have a mechanism which is as yet unknown. When febrile seizures are tonic it cannot always be determined easily whether the mechanism is epileptic or anoxic, but when a tonic febrile seizure is accompanied by a decline in consciousness, high intracranial pressure has to be suspected (see Chapter 15). In the neonatal period the mechanisms are on the whole still uncertain (Mizrahi and Kellaway 1987).

Tonic seizures in acute illness

It may be helpful to present a small series of children, seen by the present author, in whom tonic seizures of one sort or another were prominent in the presentation of an acute illness. The range of diagnoses is shown in Table 5.VIII.

Of the 32 children in this series, all but 10 were admitted directly to the intensive care unit and several of the others were transferred shortly afterwards. Those whose tonic seizures were epileptic all had various degrees of mental impairment at follow-up. Some had defined cerebral malformations, in others a specific diagnosis was not possible. Six of the children had anoxic seizures. One of these was a 3-year-old girl who had a vagal attack complicating migraine, followed by transient hyperglycaemia. Another was a 4-year-old boy with prolonged expiratory apnoea (blue breath-holding), precipitated by a row with his father during an attack of gastroenteritis, with sufficiently long stupor to warrant admission to the intensive care unit. Two children had manifestations of Meadow syndrome. One of these suffered neurological damage which was improving when he was terminally suffocated by his mother in the ward three weeks after admission (Case 16.3); post-mortem showed pure hypoxic and hypoxic-ischaemic changes in the brain. The other was suffocated by his mother in the ward several times daily and his history and detailed findings are given elsewhere (Case 8.6). A further child was known to have an unusual heart disorder but her typical and severe anoxic seizures were not due to asystole, arrhythmia or obstructive cardiomyopathy. Ictal recording showed that the explanation was paroxysmal pulmonary hypertension and the case history and details are given elsewhere (Case 8.8). The remaining child had a complex cyanotic congenital heart disease and the exact mechanism of the anoxic seizures was not proved.

Toxic seizures were induced by drugs in five children but the clinical features were such that diagnostic confusion was common at the onset. In two cases the tonic episodes were a manifestation of carbamazepine poisoning, and mimicked epilepsy when there was a family history of it. In the child with marked hepatic dysfunction, prochlorperazine was the explanation of the tonic episodes; explanation of the chronic hepatitis was obscure. In a child with acute lymphatic leukaemia, hypertension and meningism, droperidol had been given as a pre-medication for one of the diagnostic procedures. In a further child with severe burns, arterial hypertension and increased intracranial pressure, trimeprazine was the defined culprit.

There were only two children in whom tonic episodes were the initial features of a metabolic disorder. One of these, who had Reye syndrome, did well. The other was a 2-year-old girl who was fasted at another hospital before an anaesthetic for the setting of a fracture of the radius and ulna; postoperatively she had a tonic seizure when looking at a book with her mother. Correction of her hypoglycaemia

TABLE 5.VIII

Tonic seizures presenting as acute illness—diagnosis and outcome

Diagnosis	Outcome scores*					Total
	1	2	3	4	5	
Epileptic	—	5	—	—	—	5
Anoxic	3	1	—	1	1	6
Toxic	5	—	—	—	—	5
Metabolic	1	—	1	—	—	2
Vascular	2	—	1	1	—	4
Infective	7	—	—	1	2	10
Total	18	6	2	3	3	32

*Outcome scores: 1 = normal; 2 = remained delayed; 3 = mild deterioration; 4 = severe deterioration; 5 = died.

did not lead to improvement. The explanation of her severe encephalopathy was later proved to be medium-chain acyl coenzyme A dehydrogenase (MCAD) deficiency.

In the category of vascular disorders I have put those children who had hypertensive encephalopathy, haemolytic-uraemic syndrome and so-called haemorrhagic shock encephalopathy syndrome (HSES).

The remaining 10 children had definite or probable infective disorders. In six there was pyogenic meningitis *(Streptococcus pneumoniae, Haemophilus influenzae* or indeterminate) or meningococcal septicaemia. A viral origin was definite in two children, but disputed in the other two.

All those whose tonic seizures were toxic in origin had a good outcome, although there was commonly diagnostic confusion at the outset. The outcome of those who had tonic epileptic seizures did not seem to depend upon their therapy, and all were delayed later as they had been beforehand (although this may not have been apparent to the parents). The group with severe anoxic seizures included some of those with the most difficult problems, in particular those for whom suffocation by the mother was the cause. Excessively prolonged cardiac arrest in the child with cyanotic congenital heart disease probably explained his neurological deterioration. Nine of the children (five with bacterial infection, one with viral infection, two with metabolic disorders and one with HSES) had intracranial pressure monitoring by the method of McWilliam and Stephenson (1984b; 1985a,b). Monitoring seemed to help management (Balakrishnan *et al.* 1989), but its effect on outcome is not known.

Vibratory clonic and tonic-clonic seizures

A summary of the commoner possibilities is given in Tables 5.IX, 5.X and 5.XI. The major differential diagnosis is 'grand mal', the generalized tonic-clonic epileptic seizure, as discussed in Chapter 6. The even more dramatic 'epileptic-anoxic' seizure is discussed later in Chapter 12. The common major motor anoxic

TABLE 5.IX

Vibratory seizure types

Epileptic	Not certain that can be sole manifestation; seen between the tonic and clonic phases of grand mal seizures and superimposed on generalized tonic seizures
Anoxic	Superimposed on tonic phase in acutely raised intracranial pressure
Psychic	Anxiety
Toxic/metabolic	Intoxications
Hypnic	*Pavor nocturnus* (night terrors)
Miscellaneous	Shuddering (pre-essential tremor)

TABLE 5.X

Clonic seizure types

Epileptic	Pure clonic seizures (*Gelegenheitskrampf*) and hemi-clonic seizures; a component of generalized tonic-clonic seizures and clonic-tonic-clonic seizures
Anoxic	Only as 'anoxic-epileptic' seizures
Psychic	Simulated/hysteria
Toxic/metabolic	(Mechanism commonly is epileptic)
Hypnic	Restless legs
Miscellaneous	Clonus

TABLE 5.XI

Three types of tonic-clonic seizure

	Epileptic tonic-clonic	*Anoxic tonic(-clonic)*	*Psychic tonic-clonic*
Anticonvulsant effect	Yes	No	No
Combativeness	No	No	Often
Incontinence	Sometimes	Sometimes	No
Postictal	Yes	Brief	Occasionally

TABLE 5.XII

Complex motor seizure types

Epileptic	Frontal, prefrontal and certain complex partial seizures
Anoxic	Asymmetrical component of tonic phase
Psychic	Simulated/hysteria
Toxic/metabolic	Variations of asymmetrical tonic reactions
Hypnic	*Jactatio capitis* and suchlike
Miscellaneous	Paroxysmal choreoathetosis

34

TABLE 5.XIII

Confusion/'minor status'

Epileptic	Generalized non-convulsive status (absence status, etc.); partial non-convulsive status (frontal, temporal, etc.); post-epileptic fugue
Anoxic	Status syncopus; post-anoxic seizure chewing phase; confusional migraine
Psychic	Hysterical fugue; schizophrenia; gratification
Toxic/metabolic	Toxic confusional state; hallucinatory drugs; hypoglycaemia, etc.
Hypnic	Hypersomnolence (nocturnal arousal disorders)
Miscellaneous	Organic brain syndromes

seizure is illustrated by many case histories throughout the book and discussed from Chapter 7 onwards. Psychic seizures are discussed in Chapter 13.

Complex motor seizures (Table 5.XII)
Elaborate motor components may be displayed in epileptic seizures of frontal lobe origin, and in certain psychic seizures, particularly those of hysterical manifestation. Other complex motor disorders of different mechanism such as paroxysmal choreoathetosis are discussed in Chapter 14.

Confusion or altered consciousness
Many epileptic and non-epileptic conditions may present with acute or recurrent alterations of consciousness (Table 5.XIII). It is not proposed to discuss any of these in further detail.

Partial or focal seizures
Partial epileptic seizures used to be called 'focal epileptic seizures' and some epileptologists would like them to be so again (Wolf 1985). Complex partial epileptic seizures used to imply complex symptomatology involving 'higher' function without *necessarily* impairment of consciousness. Now complex partial seizures are defined as including impairment of consciousness as a necessary feature, although they may be preceded by simple partial epileptic seizures, that is without impairment of consciousness, whether or not the symptomatology of the simple partial seizure is elementary or elaborate. The range of symptomatology of partial epileptic seizures encompasses the whole gamut of the functions of the cerebrum, with myriad possible manifestations. Unlike certain generalized epileptic seizures, partial epileptic seizures usually imply epilepsy, whether of a benign or at any rate remitting type (at certain stages in childhood) or lesional with a presumptive or definite focal pathology. EEG monitoring can confirm a diagnosis of partial epileptic seizures (Aminoff *et al.* 1988*a*), but cannot exclude the diagnosis of simple partial epileptic seizures because commonly these may not have surface EEG manifestations (Devinsky *et al.* 1989). This large and important area is well discussed in other publications and will not feature in this book except in relation to specific aspects, such as ictal apnoea.

Nor does this book deal with the range of what might be called partial or focal anoxic seizures, particularly transient ischaemic attacks, and it touches only briefly on migraine which has been well discussed elsewhere (Hockaday 1988).

Case histories

CASE 5.1

A 2-year-old boy with no previous history of seizures was admitted after suddenly choking and becoming stiff. He had repeated tonic seizures and extension without regaining consciousness in between, but he localized pain inconstantly. His four older siblings all had some sort of seizures, three of them febrile convulsions, the other hemifacial seizures consistent with benign focal epilepsy of childhood for which she was receiving carbamazepine. It was this that he had managed to steal from the refrigerator in the short time that his mother had gone to another part of the house.

Comment. A family history of epilepsy may lead to a misinterpretation of the significance of syncopes or other paroxysmal events (cf. Cases 4.2, 4.3, 4.4). Confusion is more direct when toxic seizures (repeated tonic extensions) are induced by carbamazepine, prescribed for another member of the family. When this is regarded as 'impossible' it is one of the genuine indications for testing the blood-carbamazepine level.

CASE 5.2

An 18-month-old boy had begun having nocturnal episodes at the age of 6 months, originally every week and now every four weeks. They had always occurred during sleep and were characterized by squealing or crying followed by a general stiffness 'like a banana' (opisthotonus), with the hands going together and the head rolling from side to side, followed by going back to sleep.

Comment. It is a fair guess that several paroxysmal disorders of waking and sleeping have yet to be described. In this child the tonic episodes were presumed to be non-epileptic.

6
EPILEPTIC SEIZURES AND EPILEPTIC SYNDROMES

It is not within the scope of this book to enter in detail into the huge subject of epilepsy and the epilepsies. Sources have been referred to in the introduction, and a comparison of epileptic and non-epileptic seizures of various types has been outlined in the previous chapter. The purpose of this chapter is to put together a very brief but critical outline of epileptic seizures, epilepsy and those clusters of observable phenomena that we call epileptic syndromes (Aicardi 1988).

Definition
Medical students like the pragmatic definition of an epileptic seizure as something that occurs in people with epilepsy. However, if the intelligent medical student is given the definition of epileptic seizures as 'transient clinical events that result from abnormal and excessive activity of a more or less extensive collection of cerebral neurons' (Aicardi 1986), then further probing soon leads to difficulties. As Aicardi pointed out, 'Even from a theoretical point of view, the differentiation of an epileptic discharge from other paroxysmal activities may be difficult. For example, tonic seizures occurring with acute anoxia usually are interpreted as a release phenomenon resulting from the interruption of inhibitory influences from the cortex, which is more sensitive to the lack of oxygen than the brainstem reticular formation. In that situation, what is the nature of the excessive activity of the brainstem neurons responsible for tonic contraction? Could not this activity be considered as an excessive discharge in the grey matter?' While it is the thesis of this book that it is pragmatically useful and theoretically sound to distinguish anoxic (and psychic and so forth) seizures from epileptic seizures, nonetheless it may be that it is artificial to encompass everything that is currently called epileptic within the same definition. For example, episodes which are currently regarded as epileptic seizures occur in the absence of cerebral hemispheres (Danner *et al.* 1985), and the brainstem origin of infantile spasms was suggested by their occurrence in an infant with hydranencephaly (Neville 1972). Elucidating and admitting such distinctions might allow new therapeutic approaches.

Meanwhile, we may perhaps amend the definition to: *Epileptic seizures are clinical events resulting from* or including *abnormal and excessive activity of a more or less extensive collection of cerebral neurons, provided these are extant.*

Occasional epileptic seizures
Occasional epileptic seizures occur in illness or unusual circumstances and do not imply epilepsy. Almost all occasional epileptic seizures are convulsions, either bilateral (symmetrical or asymmetrical) or unilateral. Many occasional convulsions

are not epileptic seizures, as discussed elsewhere in this book, or have a mechanism which is not established.

The best-known situation is febrile illness, which is discussed in Chapter 15. Stress convulsions in adults (Friis and Lund 1974) seem to have a genetic relation to febrile seizures. Many types of disturbance of homeostasis or metabolism are associated with occasional epileptic convulsions. Of particular importance is acute glomerulonephritis where the seizure may be the first manifestation and be accompanied by urination which dissipates the evidence. The diagnosis of hypertensive encephalopathy has to be made by taking the blood pressure *after* a convulsion has finished.

Although non-epileptic seizures are frequent after various chemicals or drug overdose, prominent epileptic seizures may be the presenting feature of lead encephalopathy or piperazine sensitivity in young children (Yohai and Barnett 1989).

Epilepsy and epileptic syndromes

The recognition of clusters of features both in the epileptic seizure or seizures suffered and in the biography of the individual allow the recognition of an epileptic syndrome. This may have heuristic value and assist in therapy and prognostication. Some epileptic syndromes are better established than others and this section will be selective, focusing on epileptic syndromes which are important in differential diagnosis (Bodensteiner *et al.* 1988).

The idealized conception of *West syndrome* is infantile spasms with EEG hypsarrhythmia and developmental regression. The actual runs or salvos of spasms designated 'periodic spasms' or 'periodic events' by Gobbi *et al.* (1987) have a certain ictal similarity, both clinically and on EEG (although there was a tendency to asymmetry and focal features), but the patients they described did not have generalized EEG disruption nor developmental regression. 'Benign infantile spasms' occur in runs in normal individuals with no ictal or interictal EEG change (Lombroso and Fejerman 1977, Dravet *et al.* 1986). Benign myoclonic epilepsy is another epileptic syndrome of infancy (Roger *et al.* 1985) in which runs of jerks may occur. These are distinguished by the fact that they are truly myoclonic, that is to say of millisecond duration, and although the interictal EEG may be normal, if a run is captured on EEG, generalized spike and wave or polyspike and wave will coincide with the jerks.

A less well-defined but important epileptic syndrome of infantile onset has been called 'severe myoclonic epilepsy of infancy' (Roger *et al.* 1985) or polymorphous epilepsy. The hemiclonic febrile-associated convulsions may at first be mistaken for occasional convulsions, before other seizure types emerge and development stagnates. The low threshold to multiple types of stimuli aside from increased temperature may be striking (Morimoto *et al.* 1985). Whether an epileptic syndrome will crystallize from prospective studies of infants who present with tonic(-clonic) epileptic seizures with vagal bradycardia and apnoea remains to be determined. These 'epileptic-anoxic' seizures are discussed in Chapter 12.

Benign Rolandic epilepsy is the best-established epileptic syndrome of partial or focal type and will not be dealt with further. Attempts to increase the range of benign partial epileptic syndromes continue, the latest being 'Benign nocturnal childhood occipital epilepsy' (Panayiotopoulos 1989), a proposal criticized by Aicardi at the conclusion of that article. The constellation of features described was, in the context of normal children without important family history, nocturnal seizures with tonic deviation of the eyes and vomiting, together with occipital spike and slow complexes on eye closure. Attention is drawn to this seizure type because of the vomiting component, which may be seen in epileptic seizures with right-hemisphere pathology (Jacome and FitzGerald 1982, Jacome and Suarez 1987, Kramer *et al.* 1988).

I do not propose to deal with any of the other epileptic syndromes, which have been well discussed elsewhere (*e.g.* Roger *et al.* 1985; Aicardi 1986, 1988; Panayiotopoulos *et al.* 1989), with one exception—'*childhood grand mal*'. The generalized tonic-clonic seizure is the archetypal epileptic fit. In attempts at epidemiological analysis, generalized tonic-clonic seizures may amount to as many as 23 per cent of classified epileptic seizures (Keränen *et al.* 1988), but the methodological difficulties in such studies in children have been emphasized (Leviton and Cowan 1981). I would agree with Aicardi (1986) that in the case of pure generalized tonic-clonic epileptic seizures, as the sole type of seizure, 'the exact frequency of such an occurrence is poorly known and probably varies with the origin of patients and the investigations performed'. Oller-Daurella (1985) found that in his data bank of 3000 patients with epilepsy, there were only 169 cases (5.6 per cent) of pure primary grand mal epilepsy not associated with absences or myoclonus. Of this small number, only 23 per cent began between the ages of 3 and 11 years and only 11 per cent before the age of 3 years. The rarity of this epileptic syndrome is important from the point of view of differential diagnosis. Even though the prognosis for seizure remission in pure grand mal (generalized tonic-clonic) epilepsy is excellent (Brorson and Wranne 1987), life and opportunities are never exactly the same after such a diagnosis has been made. Provided there are not pieces of evidence suggesting other diagnoses—genuine evidence of a focal onset, absences, early morning myoclonus, a tendency for the seizures to occur shortly after waking irrespective of the time of day—and particularly the presence of any kind of stimulus or trigger, then one has to consider the following position. Pure epileptic 'grand mal' is rare; vagal-mediated convulsive syncope is common. This will be elaborated in later chapters with case history examples.

Case histories
CASE 6.1
A 9-month-old boy had frequent daily episodes of a motionless stare with alteration in colour (a slight grey cyanosis), together with possible mouth movements. Ambulatory EEG/ECG during these episodes revealed rhythmic right-sided slow activity approximately in the right temporal area. CT scan was normal. The episodes disappeared with carbamazepine, and when it was withdrawn one year later they did not recur.

Comment. In this case the history suggested the possibility of some sort of syncope but cassette recordings at home favoured true epileptic seizures, which disappeared promptly with carbamazepine. Similar cases have been described by Watanabe *et al.* (1987), and it behoves those who deal with epilepsies in the young both to be aware of the present consensus on epileptic syndromes (Aicardi 1988) and to keep abreast of new developments. Such are beyond the scope of this book.

CASE 6.2
A 12-year-old girl was reported to have had five 'grand mal' seizures in three years. As her mother affirmed, 'I know as I am a nurse.' (She said she had worked for four years on a psychiatric ward and had seen many patients whose episodes had been called grand mal and which were identical to those suffered by her daughter.) The details were that she had a dizzy feeling and felt warm and couldn't see in the two seconds before passing out. Sounds seemed to be in the distance and she turned somewhat pale. Then she would become unconscious and fall; her eyes would be 'in the back of her head' (rolled upwards) and she would be stiff. She would be out for two or three minutes during which she would twitch maybe 10 times and might be doubly incontinent of urine and faeces, but then would wake at once, dazed, and then would sleep very deeply. One of these episodes occurred in the dentist's chair.

Ocular compression induced an asystole of 14 seconds, with an anoxic seizure and an appearance which the mother insisted was identical to the natural attacks.

Comment. 'Everyone with epilepsy ought to have this test.' This comment by the mother after the ocular compression was excusable, if exaggerated. Her daughter had, of course, anoxic (vagocardiac) and not epileptic seizures.

7
ANOXIC SEIZURES OR SYNCOPES

Syncopes are the mechanisms of what I, like Gastaut (1974), call anoxic seizures. Syncope (σὖνχοπή) means 'a cutting off', and what is now implied is an abrupt cutting off of energy substrates to the cerebral cortex. In practice, this usually comes about through a sudden reduction in cerebral perfusion by oxygenated blood, either from a reduction of cerebral blood flow itself or from a drop in the oxygen content (or a combination of the two). The term 'anoxic seizure' (anoxic cerebral seizure) is shorthand for the clinical or electroclinical event that occurs as a result of the cutting off of nutrition to the most metabolically active neurons. It does not imply a total lack of oxygen any more than the term anaemia denotes a complete absence of blood, but it does mean an acute deprivation of supply.

In this and succeeding chapters emphasis will be placed on the common and often diagnostically misleading vasovagal and vagal cardio-inhibitory syncopes. Attention will also be paid to the other cardiac and respiratory mechanisms which are commonly, or rarely, involved. The predominantly tonic non-epileptic seizures which are a danger sign of increased intracranial pressure can be considered, in the same light, as syncopes or anoxic seizures. However, since there is another mechanism which may be involved, that is, impairment of consciousness from direct compression of the brainstem, this subject is considered in a separate chapter (Chapter 10).

Effect of anoxia on the brain
Before turning to the various clinical situations and syndromes, it may be helpful to review the general features of acute cerebral anoxia particularly from the clinical and EEG point of view.

Observations and experiments on mammals in the last century showed that convulsions could be induced by tying the carotid and vertebral arteries (Cooper 1836) or by exsanguination (Kussmaul and Tenner 1859). These were regarded as epileptiform (Temkin 1971) if not epileptic. At around the same time it was shown that reversible cardiac arrest could lead to seizures (Adams 1827, Stokes 1846). The first systematic study of the effect of abrupt interruption of the cerebral blood flow in man was by Rossen *et al.* (1943). In that study, a cervical cuff was abruptly inflated to 600mmHg, with the subject sitting, in a series of volunteers. None of them managed to press the release button, their eyes became fixed and unconsciousness was apparent within about nine seconds.

Clinical features of anoxic seizures
Clinical descriptions of anoxic seizures have been given by many authors (*e.g.* Gastaut and Fischer-Williams 1957, Duvoisin 1962, Gastaut 1974, Stephenson

1978*a*, Lin *et al.* 1982, Aicardi 1986, Kempster and Balla 1986, Aminoff *et al.* 1988*b*).

Premonitory symptoms such as greying out were commonly reported, but amnesia before the onset has also been reported in many patients (Duvoisin 1962), and in one clinical study premonitory symptoms were absent in 15 per cent of cases (Kempster and Balla 1986).

In Table 7.I I have listed 18 features recorded in a consecutive series of 100 children in whom asystole (induced by ocular compression—see Chapter 9) was sufficient to cause flattening of the EEG, that is to say loss of cerebral activity. These features will be considered in order of the frequency in which they were observed, preceded by some comments about loss of posture or atonia (which could not be studied because all the children were supine when the anoxic seizure was induced).

Atonia
This is a consistent finding in syncopes brought about by cardiac asystole (Gastaut 1974) and is the dominant feature of what is commonly regarded as a faint. Duvoisin (1962) found the atonia intermittent so that there was bobbing of the head, and it is evident, therefore, that this feature may be of only momentary duration.

Stiffening
Tonic EMG activity is probably universal if the EEG becomes isoelectric in an anoxic seizure but is not always clinically obvious. This feature may be apparent when the EEG only slows without flattening, and even when there is no appreciable EEG change at all as in some cases of ventricular tachyarrhythmia (Aminoff *et al.* 1988*b*) and sobbing syncope (Gastaut 1968, 1974).

Snort
An unvoiced snoring type inspiration or snort, occurring close to the restoration of cardiac rhythm, was frequent in our patients. Phonation described as 'growling' was noted by Lin *et al.* (1982) in adult blood donors.

Flexed upper limbs
Brief tonic flexion of the upper limbs at the onset of the seizure was a fairly consistent feature in motor seizures whether or not EEG flattening occurred. This was illustrated in a previous publication by the present author (Stephenson 1978*a*, Figs. 3 and 4). A similar flexion was noted by Duvoisin (1962) after Valsalva manoeuvres.

'Jerks'
In the series detailed in Table 7.I 'jerks' were recorded in 60 per cent, and some sort of jerking at the onset and at the conclusion of an anoxic seizure has been reported by most authors. It is probable that the jerks, of which there are rarely more than six, are more in the nature of spasms than myoclonic phenomena. It

TABLE 7.I

Clinical features of anoxic seizures with EEG flattening induced by ocular compression in 100 children

Stiffening	70	Dazed	24	Limb quiver	5
Snort	69	Eyes up	19	Immediate postictal sleep	5
Flexed upper limbs	67	Double extension	14	Agitation/fear	4
Jerks	60	Disorientation	14	Leg twitching	2
Extension	35	Urine incontinence	11	Vomit	2
Eye jerks	33	Adversive head movement	6	True tongue-biting	1

seems that in adults these can be quite violent—they are described by Duvoisin (1962) as 'violent thrashing movements', with 'the initial jerks . . . the most violent, the amplitude [decreasing] progressively . . . normal muscle tone [returning] with the last jerk'. Similarly, Lin *et al.* (1982) described eight patients having 'violent' myoclonic jerks, some convulsive movements 'requiring the patient to be held down'.

Extension
The opisthotonus which is well known in breath-holding attacks (see figure in Gauk *et al.* 1963) was not a usual feature in our series. Likewise a tonic phase of only moderate intensity was noted by Duvoisin (1962).

Eye jerks
Nystagmus, commonly downbeat in type, was probably more frequent than the figure of 33 per cent suggests. This nystagmus was noted by Gastaut (1958): its EEG correlates are described in the next section.

Dazed
The low figure of 24 per cent for this item (but see 'disorientation' below) merely indicates that recovery of consciousness was often apparently instantaneous at the end of the motor phenomena.

Eyes up
Ocular revulsion or upward eye deviation (observed in 19 per cent of episodes) is a passive phenomenon (Gastaut 1974) and may well be more frequent than this figure suggests.

Double extension
These violent extensions, commonly with abduction and upward circumduction of extended upper limbs, may be a dramatic feature of the 'recovery' phase after the cerebral energy supply has been restored. An example has been described in Case 4.8 and is illustrated in Figure 7.1. Aminoff *et al.* (1988*b*) described tonic flexion of the trunk or drawing up of the limbs on restoration of the circulation.

Disorientation
Significant disorientation was experienced in 14 per cent of seizures. In adults with

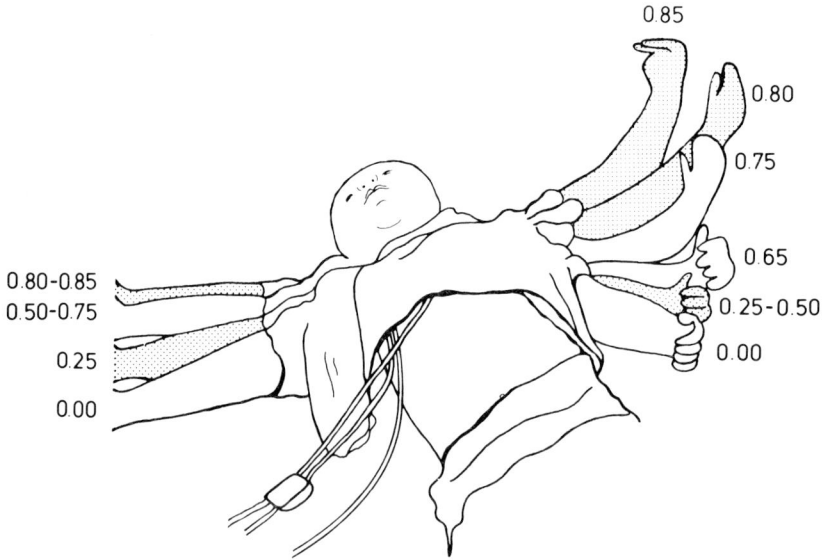

0.85

0.80

0.75

0.65

0.80-0.85

0.50-0.75

0.25-0.50

0.25

0.00

0.00

Fig. 7.1. Film tracings of one of the 'spasms' which supervened after the return of the heartbeat in an anoxic seizure induced by ocular compression in a 20-month-old girl (Case 4.8—see pp. 19–23). Drawings were made from videotape frames over a timespan of 0.85 seconds. Each spasm involved abduction and circumduction of the upper limbs, more obvious on the child's left in this figure. Note hyperextension at the neck, which is the remnant of the tonic phase of the seizure. Over this fixed posture of the neck and trunk are sketched the serial positions of the upper limbs. The numbers refer to the time in seconds after the first frame, which is referenced as 0.00. The excursion of the left upper limb is better appreciated. During the first 0.5 sec. the range of movement is small, but thereafter there is an acceleration so that only 0.05 sec. separates the later postures. The rapidity of abduction is such that it is easy to see how these spasms may have been misnamed 'myoclonic jerks'.

induced ventricular tachyarrhythmias (Aminoff *et al.* 1988*b*) confusion did not last more than 30 seconds even when the duration of loss of consciousness had been 130 seconds. Exceptionally, however, much longer periods of confusion may be observed, as noted clinically and experimentally in Case 4.9.

Incontinence

Urine incontinence is not rare, nor is it confined to females. In our study the incidence was 11 per cent and in the clinical study of adults by Kempster and Balla (1986) it was 23 per cent.

Faecal incontinence is less common, but does occur (Lin *et al.* 1982).

Adversive head movement

It was long ago emphasized (Gastaut and Fischer-Williams 1957) that if tonic activity is asymmetrical then there will be turning of the head to one side and possibly an appearance resembling an asymmetric tonic neck reflex. More subtly, there may be a tonic lateral conjugate deviation of the eyes.

Limb quiver
A vibratory movement may be prominent and may superficially resemble clonic twitching.

Immediate postictal sleep
How much this is a feature of young children is not clear. Many patients may be markedly drowsy after convulsive syncope but in our series 5 per cent passed directly to sleeping without an intermediate phase of apparent awareness.

Agitation/fear
Such emotions may be related to the disorientation or confusion (or possibly to the ocular compression!).

Leg twitching
The lower limb movements were described by Duvoisin (1962) as extensor thrusts. In any given patient they are no more frequent in number than upper limb 'jerks'.

Vomit
Vomiting occasionally occurs at the conclusion and in natural episodes in the pre-syncopal phase (Gastaut 1974). Vomiting has not been described in the *middle* of the anoxic seizure (but see Paulson 1963).

True tongue-biting
Aicardi (1986) has suggested that this does not exist but we have one example which was photographed in confirmation. It was insufficient to lead to a serious laceration.

Other motor phenomena
Irregular facial movements or eyelid flutter without any tonic activity were noted in two of the older patients with ventricular tachyarrhythmia as reported by Aminoff *et al.* (1988*b*).

Autonomic phenomena
Salivation seems to be prominent at the onset, particularly in older patients (Duvoisin 1962, Gastaut 1974).

   Colour changes depend on the mechanism of the syncope and include cyanosis in hypoxic episodes, pallor in various types of systemic hypotension, and postictal flush after cardiac standstill from whatever cause. However, particularly in convulsive syncope brought about by cardiac asystole of vagal origin, pallor may not be observed, as in 15 per cent of the clinical series of Kempster and Balla (1986).

   Sweating ('cold sweat') is common after syncopes of any type, but quantitative data are not available.

Coherent sequence
As stressed in Chapter 4, historical diagnosis depends on the sequential details

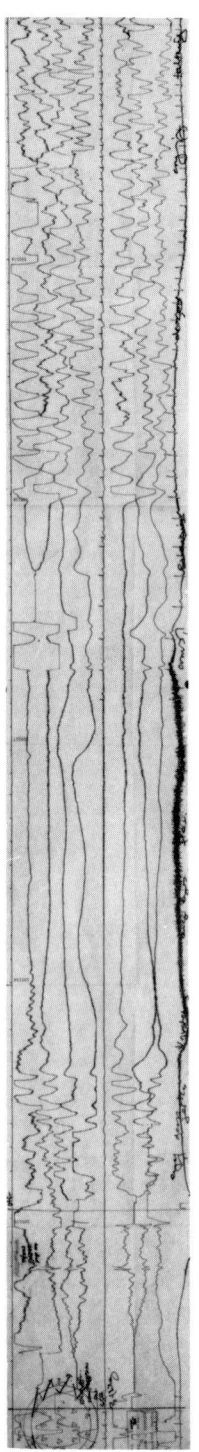

Fig. 7.2. Example of typical 'gestalt' appearance of anoxic seizure induced when ocular compression results in prolonged asystole (30 secs.). Note also the rapid notching of the upper trace at the onset of EEG flattening, this being associated with downbeat nystagmus.

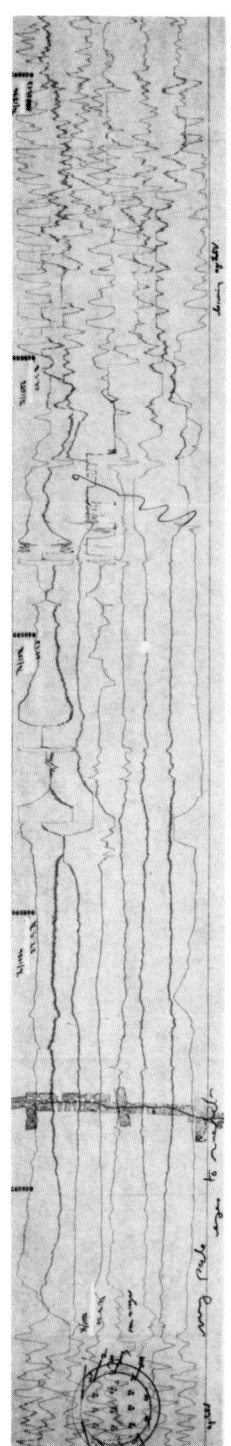

Fig. 7.3. Poor quality EEG with no ECG channel recorded in a 12-year-old girl when having a spontaneous tonic seizure lying supine (Case 9.25). The vertically written numbers are at 10-second intervals. There is approximately 30 seconds of EEG flattening in between bursts of slow waves, with superimposed muscle potentials reflecting the tonic seizure and movement artefacts associated with the convulsion. It can be inferred that this girl had an asystole of about 30 seconds even though no ECG was attached.

from the setting, stimulus and warning (albeit with amnesia) through the ictus with its own sequence, to the termination and the after state. None of the components of the anoxic seizure are unique, but they have a coherent sequence which it is the historian's duty to elicit. Examples are given in the many case histories in this book, and further use of simultaneous video recording will doubtless improve the definition of these serial features.

Time course
The duration of unconsciousness depends to a certain extent on the mechanism of the syncope, and on the age of the patient. With intermittent suffocation, as in Meadow syndrome, it may take up to five minutes before a full anoxic seizure is induced (see Case 8.6). Asystole of less than 10 seconds may lead to convulsive syncope in a young child, whereas asystole may last for 19 seconds without any syncope whatever in an older adult (Stern and Tzivoni 1976). From the data given in Table 7.II (see p. 55), the duration of unconsciousness in an anoxic seizure from vagal cardio-inhibition is likely to be around 10 seconds to one minute. In ventricular tachyarrhythmias it may of course be longer (Aminoff *et al.* 1988*b*). EEG studies have allowed a certain quantitation of these data, and are discussed in the next section.

Electroencephalography in anoxic seizures
Gibbs *et al.* (1935) first showed that hypoxia (breathing pure nitrogen) leads to slowing and increased amplitude of the EEG. Similar findings were obtained on acute mechanical obstruction of the cerebral circulation by Rossen *et al.* (1943). The 'classical' view of the EEG effect of short-lasting anoxia was summarized by Gastaut *et al.* (1961*e*). An orderly series of changes was observed: first desynchronization (which might not be obvious), followed by progressive slowing with increase of amplitude, then abrupt disappearance of the EEG signal, then abrupt return of high-voltage slow activity which increased in frequency and declined in amplitude before returning to the preceding normal appearance.

An example of this appearance is shown in Figure 7.2. Once the gestalt of this sequence is recognized, it is easy to see that the appearance in Figure 7.3 is the same.

Recently, however, Aminoff *et al.* (1988*b*) have questioned the specificity and sensitivity of the EEG appearance. They suggested that the differences might in part be related to the mechanism of the syncope and the age of the patient, so it is worth reviewing the data with these questions in mind.

Ocular compression induced asystole
Most observations on the EEG in anoxic seizures have related to the effect of asystole after ocular compression (Gastaut and Fischer-Williams 1957; Gastaut and Gastaut 1957, 1958; Fildisevski 1961; Gastaut *et al.* 1961*b*; Maulsby and Kellaway 1964; Lombroso and Lerman 1967; Gastaut 1968, 1974; Gastaut and Broughton 1972; Stephenson 1978*a*; Lehovsky *et al.* 1979). Those studies included adults and children, both supine and sitting, and in all cases the 'classical' anoxic appearance

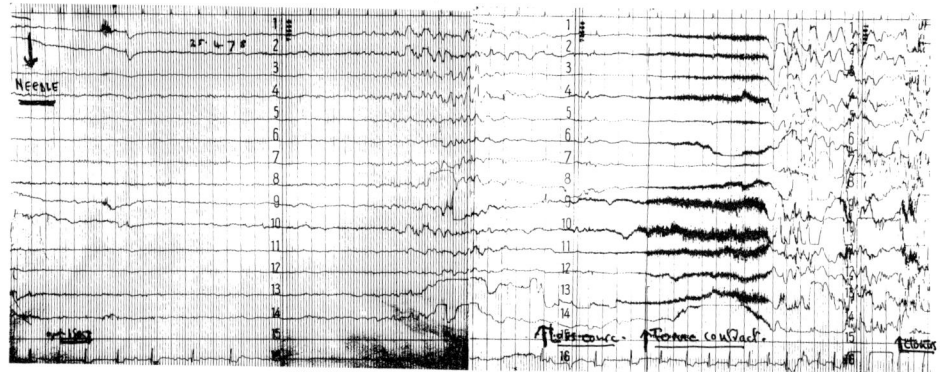

Fig. 7.4. Asystole induced within six seconds of needle insertion in a 23-year-old man (see Braham *et al.* 1981). On this occasion the asystole is only 11 seconds but a tonic seizure results. (Braham, *personal communication*.)

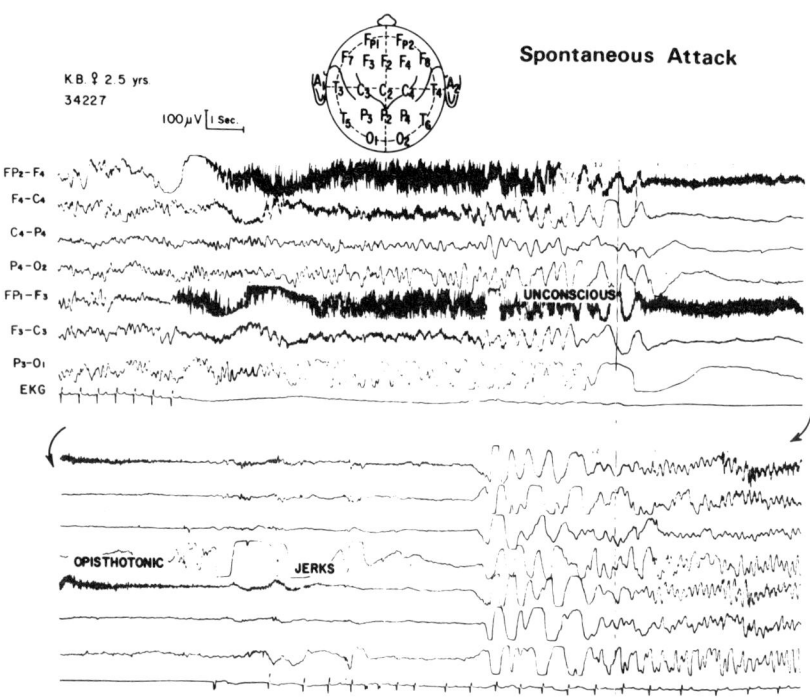

Fig. 7.5. Spontaneous asystole occurring in patient of Lombroso and Lerman (1967) while supine on EEG table. (Reproduced by permission.)

of the EEG was observed. Age-related differences in 'threshold' will be discussed below. (Ocular compression is discussed further in Chapter 9.)

Venepuncture fits
The mechanism of these seizures is reflex vagal cardio-inhibition (see Chapters 9 and 15), and published EEGs in children have again showed 'classical' appearances (Lombroso and Lerman 1967, Roddy *et al.* 1983). Review of the figures of Lloyd-Smith and Tatlow (1958*a*) with respect to a young adult also indicates a 'classical' EEG appearance, a point made strongly by Gastaut (1958) (a riposte by Lloyd-Smith and Tatlow, 1958*b*, was not convincing). Figure 7.4 illustrates the effect of needle insertion on a patient described by Braham *et al.* (1981). The initial EEG slowing which precedes the loss of EEG activity is of lower amplitude than the examples previously discussed but this young adult does follow the 'classical' pattern.

Spontaneous vagal anoxic seizures
EEGs in cases reported by Lombroso and Lerman (1967) and Gastaut (1974), and those illustrated overleaf in Figures 7.5 and 7.6, once again show the same 'classical' pattern.

Postural syncopes
In the report by Stevens and Fazekas (1955) of studies using tilt-testing after administration of hexamethonium in older patients, the illustrations suggest some EEG variability, but as the ECG trace is not shown it is difficult to make firm conclusions. In the patients of Karp *et al.* (1961) in whom tilt-testing was carried out after oral sodium nitrite (normal volunteers aged 17 to 24 years), the full classic appearance was only seen in the patient who had eight seconds of asystole on head-up tilt, with a tonic seizure. Patients with shorter syncopes had only EEG slowing. Similar EEG slowing was found by Forster *et al.* (1942) after sodium nitrite and head-up tilt in young normal adults.

Carotid sinus compression
Carotid sinus compression in older patients may lead to asystole or to vaso-depressor hypotension or both. Furthermore, arterial disease may lead to lateralized cerebral events. Thus, the data are difficult to analyse. In the early report by Forster *et al.* (1942) one supposes that the patients were elderly but their ages were not given. In one anoxic seizure they described, in which the asystolic mechanism was prominent, the tonic seizure occurred with fairly mild slowing of the EEG without flattening. They also reported flattening of the EEG without slowing. In the report of Gastaut *et al.* (1961*d*), vasodepression with the patient erect induced 'classical' appearances but not unexpectedly the results were complex and variable. Nonetheless, Gastaut and his colleagues finally buried the idea of a 'cerebral' type of carotid sinus syncope, showing that all were anoxic in mechanism.

Miscellaneous vagal asystoles
The case of Ossentjuk *et al.* (1966) is unique in that in one instance of sinus arrest

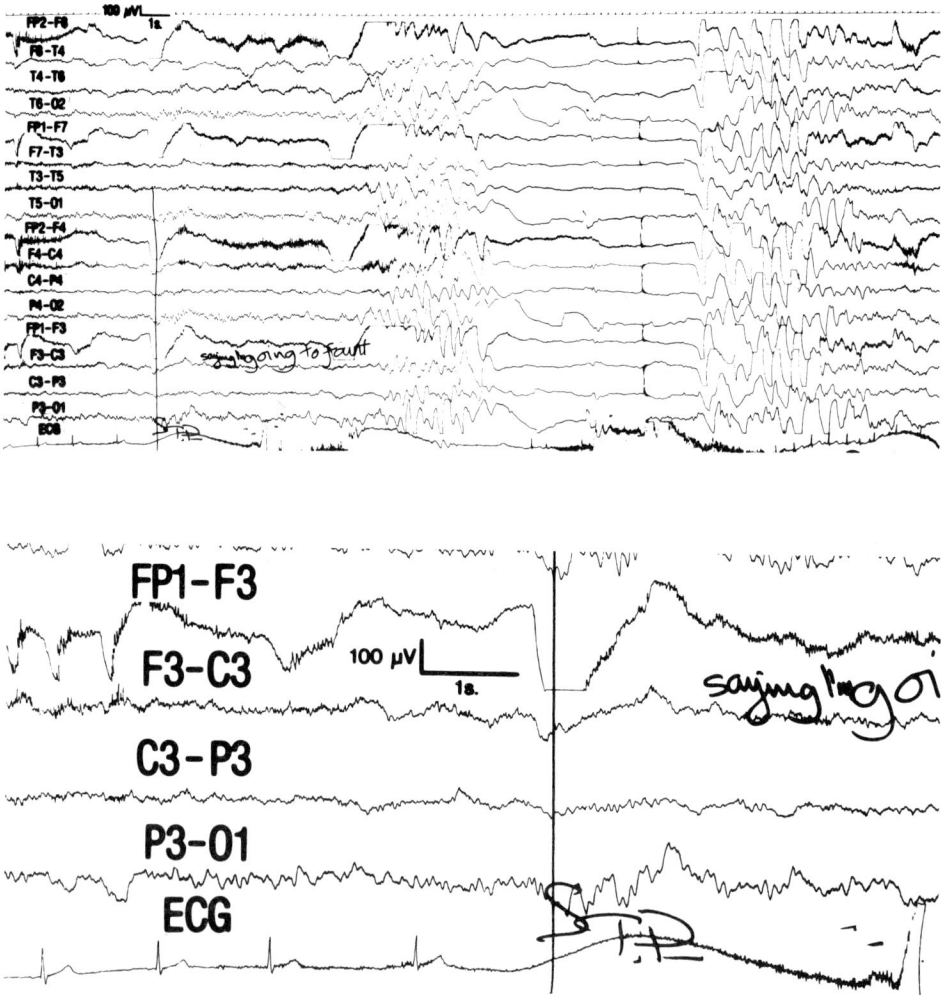

Fig. 7.6. Tonic seizure mediated by vagal asystole occurring without provocation in 9-year-old girl while supine on EEG table (Case 8.10).

(a) Bradycardia has preceded the asystole, but note that she is saying that she is going to faint several seconds after the asystole has begun. The EEG pattern is characteristic of a pure non-epileptic anoxic seizure.

(b) Onset of asystole magnified. The S written at the vertical line indicates that she closed her eyes. Note baseline sway and then development of EMG potentials on the ECG channel after the onset of asystole.

quite high-voltage 'waves' of about two per second developed during prolonged asystole. This will be discussed further in the chapters on anoxic-epileptic seizures (Chapter 11) and epileptic-anoxic seizures (Chapter 12).

Heart disease with asystole (Stokes–Adams)

Reports of EEG findings in true Stokes–Adams attacks with seizures are surprisingly rare. Amyes *et al.* (1953) reported the case of a 30-year-old woman with heart block. In an anoxic seizure during which she was supposedly asystolic (ECG was not recorded with the EEG), diminution of EEG activity (although not necessarily of isoelectric appearance) occurred without slowing before or after. The case of Regis *et al.* (1961) concerned a 30-year-old man with progressive ophthalmoplegia (?mitochondrial disorder) with heart block. During an asystolic seizure a flat EEG appearance developed without dramatic slowing before or after, but there was the usual abrupt high-amplitude slow wave a few seconds after the restarting of the ECG complexes. Lai and Ziegler (1981) recorded slowing during asystole in an adult with atrial fibrillation. Moss and Rockoff (1981) recorded appropriate flattening (arrest 27 seconds, flat EEG 15.5 seconds) in a 62-year-old woman with complete heart block.

Ventricular tachyarrhythmia

Until recently, very limited information was available regarding the EEG in anoxic seizures associated with ventricular tachyarrhythmias. In the case of Tucker and Yoe (1956) a woman of 58 demonstrated slow activity after 13 seconds of paroxysmal ventricular tachycardia and a flat EEG recording after three minutes. Aminoff *et al.* (1988*b*) were able to study this aspect in a quantitative manner because they employed an indwelling automatic cardioverter defibrillator which has to be tested in advance of its natural usage. They studied 14 patients aged 25 to 73 and found that with respect to ventricular fibrillation or ventricular tachycardia the 'classical' anoxic EEG changes were not totally consistent. In particular they found that some patients became unconscious without apparent EEG change. In others attenuation or flattening occurred without associated slow activity. In others, an attenuated EEG had reverted to normal without an intervening period of conspicuous slow (delta) activity.

Valsalva manoeuvre

In contrast to the variability with some types of cardiac arrhythmia, EEG changes with a strong Valsalva manoeuvre leading to an anoxic seizure have tended to be 'classical' in type (*e.g.* Gastaut *et al.* 1961*e*, 1982, 1987; Duvoisin 1962; Aicardi 1986; Aicardi *et al.* 1988). During induced syncope in a patient with Chiari type 1 malformation (Dobkin 1978) only rather minor slow activity occurred, but the question of brainstem compression arises (see Chapter 10).

Central venous occlusion

Pampiglione and Waterston (1961) reported on EEG changes during operations for congenital heart disease without extracorporeal circulation. In conjunction with

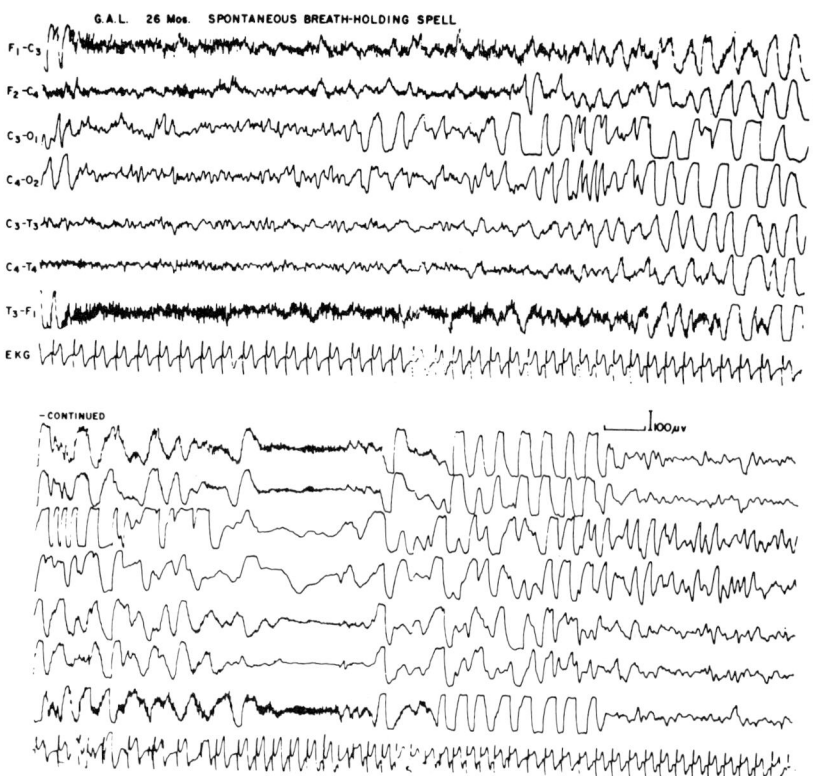

Fig. 7.7. Spontaneous breath-holding spell in 26-month-old girl. Note EEG flattening with tonic seizure but no significant bradycardia. (Maulsby and Kellaway 1964; reproduced by permission).

other studies they found that sudden occlusion of the aorta resulted in slow waves on the EEG in less than 10 seconds followed by generalized flattening in less than half a minute. They found a partial occlusion of the aortic flow was not followed by slow activity unless the fall in arterial pressure was marked and prolonged. More interesting were their findings in relation to main central venous occlusions. They found that clamping of the inferior vena cava on its own did not lead to any EEG change. Occlusion of the entire venous return to the heart led to slow activity and then complete loss of EEG activity with tonic seizures. However, of most importance they noted that if the superior vena cava was occluded for more than 10 seconds and the pressure rose toward arterial level, then recognizable EEG slowing was identified. They inferred, therefore, that EEG changes would occur when increased venous pressure prevented adequate arterial supply to the brain.

Breath-holding

The problem of 'breath-holding' will be discussed in Chapter 8. From the older literature it is not always clear whether the children described had been in a state of

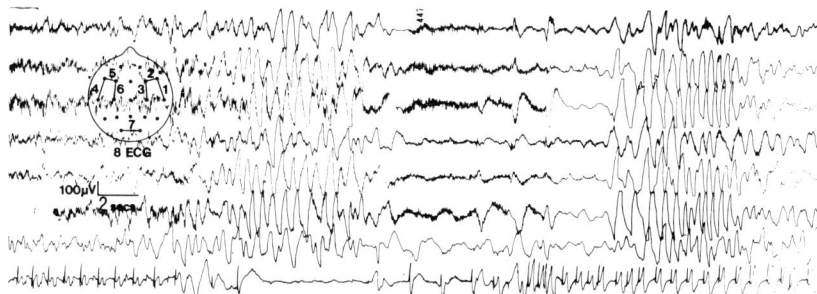

Fig. 7.8. Ambulatory cassette recording (seven-channel EEG, one-channel ECG) of breath-holding attack in 15-month-old girl. (Parents described the sequence as: held breath, went blue, got breath back, started crying, went to sleep.) Note eight-second asystole coinciding with onset of high-voltage one- to two-per-second delta activity, which lasted six seconds. The ECG 12 seconds previously had slowed from 180 to 100 per minute, with generalized muscle potentials in EEG channels. Loss of EEG signal (isoelectric, with baseline irregularity) lasted 12 seconds. In pure reflex asystole, EEG flattening of this duration would require around 17 seconds of cardiac standstill (A = 9 + 0.7F; see overleaf). In this example the 'breath-hold' presumably accounted for the additional hypoxic-ischaemic insult.

prolonged expiratory apnoea with or without Valsalva manoeuvre (Gauk *et al.* 1963), Maulsby and Kellaway 1964, Lombroso and Lerman 1967, Gastaut 1968, Gastaut and Broughton 1972) or experiencing sobbing syncopes (Gastaut 1968, 1974). At any rate, considerable variability in the EEG appearances is apparent.

A 'classical' anoxic appearance of the EEG in cyanotic breath-holding is clearly recorded in Figure 7.7 (reproduced from Maulsby and Kellaway 1964). EEG slowing occurs about 15 seconds after expiratory apnoea, and the loss of EEG signal occurs without cardiac asystole. Most other recordings in the literature demonstrate only EEG slowing, and in two examples of breath-holding in young children (Gastaut 1968, 1974) the illustrations appear to indicate tonic extension without appreciable EEG change. No explanation for this has been proposed.

In 'mixed' breath-holding there is a combination of apnoea with cyanosis and vagocardiac inhibition not explicable by post-Valsalva rebound. An example of this is given in Figure 7.8.

Anoxic-epileptic sequence
In a number of studies the typical anoxic appearance of the EEG has been concluded by spike and wave of an epileptic nature, irrespective of the mechanism of anoxia (Meyer and Waltz 1961; Gastaut *et al.* 1961*a*, 1987; Ossentjuk *et al.* 1966; Stephenson 1983*a*; Aicardi *et al.* 1988; Battaglia *et al.* 1989). This aspect is discussed further in Chapter 12.

Summary of qualitative anoxic EEG evidence
The evidence seems to suggest that, irrespective of age, abrupt total interruption of cerebral oxygenation leads to 'classical' EEG changes. However, there clearly are difficulties particularly with respect to certain sorts of 'breath-holding', in particular

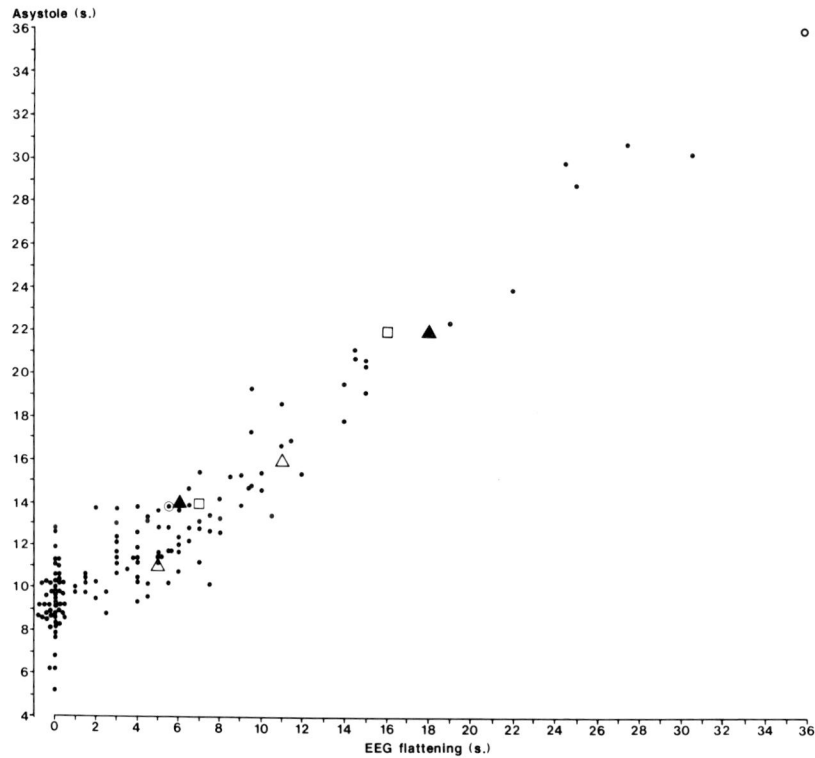

Fig. 7.9. Duration of loss of EEG signal (flattening) *vs.* length of asystole. Each symbol represents one observation.

Small filled circles. 144 children who had motor anoxic seizures induced by ocular compression when supine. (*Double circle* indicates child who had ambulatory cassette monitoring—Case 9.29, p. 102.)

Open circle. Ocular compression effect in patient of Manson (*personal communication*).

Solid triangles. Seizures induced by head bumps recorded by ambulatory cassette monitoring (Case 9.29).

Open triangles. Seizures induced by needle insertion (Braham, *personal communication*) and venepuncture (Roddy *et al.* 1983).

Open squares. Spontaneous asystoles in the supine position: 14 seconds (Case 8.10, pp. 81–82); and 22 seconds (Lombroso and Lerman 1967).

'sobbing spasms', and with respect to ventricular tachyarrhythmias. Further studies need to be done to elucidate the processes involved, and meanwhile caution must be exercised in interpreting the significance of the EEG appearance when these mechanisms may be involved. Nonetheless, there are no valid EEG data to contradict the proposition that anoxic seizures are non-epileptic. EEG changes vary from minimal slowing to marked slowing, to the 'classic' slow–flat–slow. The special case of 'anoxic-epileptic' seizures is discussed in Chapter 12.

Anoxic seizure threshold

The concept of an anoxic seizure threshold is quite different from that of an

TABLE 7.II

Derivation of anoxic seizure threshold

Asystole (seconds) = 9.7 + 0.7 flat EEG time
SD = 1.9; R^2 = 74.0 per cent
t = 21.8; df = 165; p<0.001
Threshold (seconds) = Asystole − 0.7 flat EEG time

epileptic seizure threshold. The anoxic seizure threshold may be regarded as the duration of cerebral anoxia/ischaemia necessary to lead to the clinical or EEG features of an anoxic seizure (Stephenson 1979*b*).

The data from which an anoxic seizure threshold can be derived come most easily from plotting the duration of asystole needed to induce EEG flattening (Stephenson 1979*b*). A recent alternative method is to plot the duration of the loss of consciousness against the duration of the ventricular tachyarrhythmia (Aminoff *et al.* 1988).

Figure 7.9 graphically displays the duration of EEG flattening for a large number of children in whom asystole was induced by ocular compression, plus some in whom it occurred spontaneously or was induced by stimuli such as head bump or venepuncture. From these data the relationship A = 9 + 0.7F derives, where A and F are the durations of asystole and EEG flattening respectively (correlation coefficient 0.94). Other published data fit with this formula: in the case of Moss and Rockoff (1981) asystole was about 27 seconds and EEG flattening 15.5 seconds; the longest asystole recorded by Gastaut *et al.* (1961*b*) (in a 21-year-old male) was 32 seconds, with 30 seconds EEG flattening.

From an earlier sample of children the relationship A = 9.7 + 0.7F was calculated, giving an expression for the anoxic seizure threshold as described in Table 7.II. Plotting these values against age (Fig. 7.10), it can be seen that, at least in the childhood age-group, there is a strong relationship (Table 7.III), so that with older children a longer duration of asystole is necessary to flatten the EEG, as shown graphically in Figure 7.11. There is clearly considerable variability in that, at any age, a given degree of asystole can lead to a wide range of EEG flattening. There are few data avaliable on this age relationship in adults. However, an isolated observation by Stern and Tzivoni (1976) refers to a 19-second asystole without syncope in a 56-year-old man, an observation not known in childhood.

The recent studies of Aminoff *et al.* (1988*b*) have allowed the duration of induced ventricular tachyarrhythmia (ventricular tachycardia or fibrillation) to be plotted against duration of loss of consciousness. From the data in their Figure 1, a formula may be derived such that the duration of ventricular tachyarrhythmia (VT/VF) equals 11 + 0.76 LOC, where LOC is the duration of loss of consciousness. Thus, in their population the anoxic seizure threshold would be VT/VF − 0.76 LOC. This would imply that a longer duration of circulatory standstill is necessary, in older patients, to induce loss of consciousness, and presumably an even longer duration to induce EEG flattening. This is in keeping with the observations reported above.

55

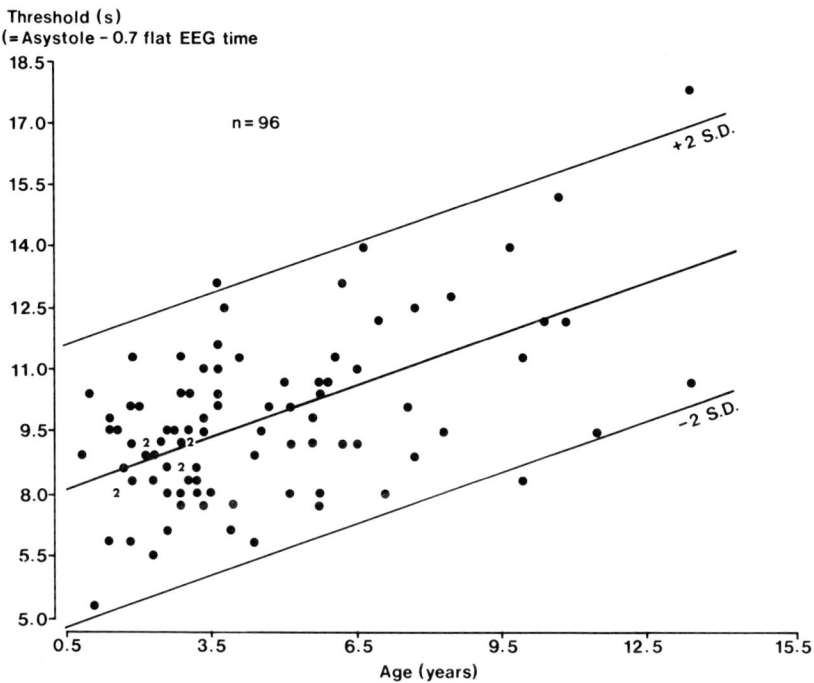

Fig. 7.10. Anoxic seizure threshold (calculated as A − 0.7F) *vs.* age in years at time of testing in 167 children. A significant increase in threshold occurs within the ages studied.

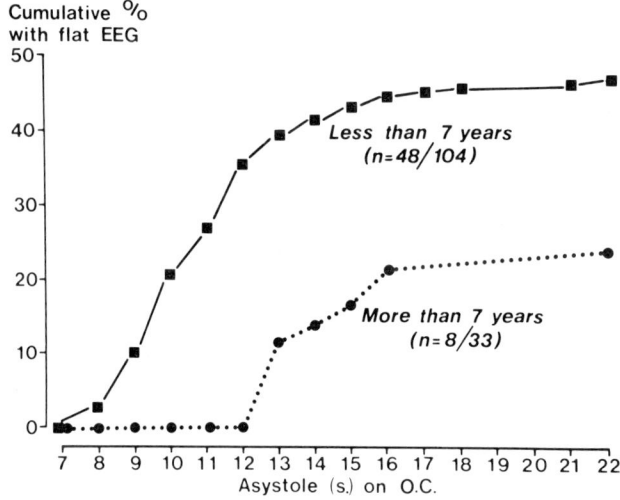

Fig. 7.11. Graphical representation of results of ocular compression in 137 children, comparing those above and below 7 years of age at time of testing. Substantially longer asystole is needed in the older children to induce EEG flattening.

TABLE 7.III

Anoxic seizure threshold and age

Threshold (seconds) = 8.2 + 0.3 age in years
SD = 1.6; R^2 = 28.0 per cent
t = 8.1; df = 165; p<0.001

Summary

In young persons, and in age-groups extending up to at least young adulthood, abrupt cessation of substrate for cerebral metabolism leads to classical EEG changes: diffuse slowing, interrupted by loss of cerebral activity if the syncope is sufficiently prolonged. How long this prolongation must be depends in part on age, such that the 'anoxic seizure threshold' is lowest in early childhood. Little information is available relating to early infancy or later adulthood. Some aspects are not understood, in particular the lack of apparent change in certain 'breath-holding' or 'sobbing' spells in infancy.

Case histories

CASE 7.1

A 21-month-old boy had frequent episodes of suddenly going pale, not breathing, becoming rigid and staring. The parents insisted that there were no precipitations whatever, definitely no stimulus.

Ocular compression induced an asystole of just under 29 seconds, with 20 seconds of flat EEG. Associated with this he had flexion, double extension, eyes deviating to the right, a snort, further extension, and then a gradual return of consciousness. The parents, who witnessed this anoxic seizure, said that the spontaneous attacks were identical in all respects to what they had just seen.

Three years later they wrote: 'His attacks continued without provocation for a short time after our visit and gradually decreased until they stopped completely about two years ago. After our visit to see you we were able to cope with the situation knowing that he would recover in his own time. I think before we saw you we were so scared . . . he means so much to us as we can't have any more children and we thought we would lose him. He has now started school and is very bright and clever and attends judo classes and loves all the rough sports.'

Comment. Knowledge of the detailed features of an anoxic seizure, coupled by its detailed reproduction after ocular compression, allowed the diagnosis of vagocardiac convulsive syncope despite the complete absence of any history of provoking factors.

CASE 7.2

The mother of a 13-year-old girl opened the conversation by saying 'I thought she was getting an EEG' (*i.e.* assuming epilepsy). Reflex anoxic seizures had occurred since early life under stimuli such as bumping her elbow, grazing her knee, going into a hot 'chippy' (fish and chip shop), or emotional stress, and more recently when she got up in the middle of the night to go to the toilet. The episodes had been preceded by dizziness or more recently vertigo, and if she had an episode in her room with several people around her, their voices would sound horrible. She would then flop, become unconscious and have brief jerking movements, and frequently would urinate and then wake up completely and then want to sleep for an hour. Pallor accompanied the episodes.

57

Comment. It is of course possible that this 13-year-old would have had a cardiac asystole as the EEG electrodes were being applied. On the other hand, some irrelevant EEG 'abnormality' might have been unearthed. The 'horrible voices' raised the spectre of temporal lobe epilepsy, but the setting, stimulus, aura, ictal course and immediate postictal state were all typical of a generalized anoxic seizure.

CASE 7.3

This 6-year-old boy had three attacks of unconsciousness in 18 months. In the first he was found unconscious in a high-walled lavatory, looking pale and grey. In the second, which occurred after a bout of influenza, he fell unconscious, rigid, recovering after a minute or two, pale and grey. On the third occasion he was on the floor playing an exciting game with his father when he lay back unconscious and wet himself; after about a minute he came to, flushing strongly.

Ocular compression induced an asystole of 27 seconds, with a typical anoxic seizure followed by a strong flush.

Comment. This boy would have satisfied the criteria for entry to the study of vagocardiac reflex anoxic seizures described in Chapter 9, had he presented during the study period.

8
SPECIFIC SYNCOPES AND ANOXIC SEIZURE TYPES

In this chapter I review the features of the better documented varieties of syncopes and anoxic seizures. It will be apparent that there are overlaps between certain of these categories. It will also be apparent that in several cases knowledge is less secure than it might seem on superficial inspection of the literature.

Breath-holding
The common breath-holding spell has been well known for centuries (Culpeper 1737). Every so often physicians are excited enough about the phenomenon to investigate its mechanism, but even now much is unknown and surprisingly little progress has been made in the past 50 years (Gordon 1987).

In mild breath-holding spells, the child 'becomes angry, afraid, or is injured. Two or three loud cries follow, after which he holds his breath in expiration and goes into a state of generalized tonic spasm which gives the impression of being induced voluntarily. An ominous silence accompanies the period of apnea. If this lasts only from five to ten seconds some cyanosis may be evident, but a feeble cry followed by more vigorous crying soon indicates that respiration has been resumed. For approximately one-half minute the child may appear confused and exhausted, but thereafter acts as well as ever' (Bridge *et al.* 1943). In the more severe attacks a 'convulsive' phase follows which may be accompanied by incontinence of urine and/or faeces, followed by a brief limp or atonic phase before consciousness is regained (Maulsby and Kellaway 1964). It is thus within the differential diagnosis of epilepsy that breath-holding attacks appear in most standard texts (Bridge 1949, Lennox and Lennox-Buchtal 1960, Gastaut 1968, Gastaut and Broughton 1972, Livingston 1972, Aicardi 1986). In any particular child, an obvious provocation is usual although not necessarily obvious. Frustration, annoyance or minor hurts are well-known factors. Peiper (1939) studied an infant who disliked banana sufficiently to 'breath-hold' whenever this was offered. He demonstrated clearly that, in an attack, respiratory arrest took place in full expiration, and he also observed repeated small movements of the diaphragm during the expiratory apnoea without change in the visible cyanosis.

Gauk *et al.* (1963) concluded that anoxic anoxia was the mechanism in two infants who were induced to have opisthotonic cyanotic breath-holding attacks by noxious stimuli. They observed arterial hypertension and a drop in the oxygen saturation to about 30 per cent. They also noted, although they did not comment upon, considerable heart-rate variations after the onset of the expiratory apnoea.

Those conclusions were criticized by Maulsby and Kellaway (1964) because the illustrated details appeared to show that consciousness was lost and EEG slowing began when oxygen saturation at the ear was close to 90 per cent. Maulsby and Kellaway made two contributions. One was that anoxic seizures in young children could be divided into two types. What they called Type I was the well-known breath-holding spell in which, after a painful or emotional stimulus, the child cries briefly and 'loses consciousness while maintaining the expiratory phase of the final cry. Often the child's face is flushed or sometimes noticeably cyanotic at the onset of loss of consciousness.' The Type II 'hypoxic crisis' which they described for the first time was 'precipitated almost exclusively by sudden unexpected painful stimuli such as a blow to the head. The child without crying, without any apparent conscious acknowledgement of the insult, suddenly falls limply unconscious. He may then quickly regain consciousness or have an opisthotonic and clonic seizure followed by another atonic phase before consciousness is regained. Usually there is no cyanosis. Although it is often not obvious to the observer, the child usually does not breathe during the initial phase of the attack, the respiration being arrested in the expiratory position.' Their Type II phenomenon was later classified by Lombroso and Lerman (1967) as the pallid type of breath-holding spell (pallid infantile syncope), and is now referred to as 'reflex anoxic seizure' (Stephenson 1978a). Maulsby and Kellaway (1964) demonstrated that in a Type I breath-holding spell the 'classical' anoxic EEG appearance with slow–flat–slow occurred, with a sustained tachycardia with only minor intercalated slowings (see Fig. 7.7, p. 52), whereas a Type II episode appeared to be related to cardiac asystole, could be reproduced by ocular compression and could be prevented by atropine. From the point of view of understanding the mechanism of breath-holding spells, an important contribution of Maulsby and Kellaway was to show that both the Type I cyanotic breath-holding attack and the Type II asystolic anoxic seizure might commonly occur at different times in the *same* child.

Lombroso and Lerman (1967) further established the distinction between what they called the cyanotic and the pallid types of breath-holding or infantile syncope, while also demonstrating that both types of episode could occur at different times in the same child. On the basis of their observations these authors inferred that a plausible combination of factors in the mechanism of the cyanotic breath-holding attack would be: (i) violent crying leading to hypocapnic cerebral ischaemia; (ii) apnoea leading to hypoxaemia; (iii) respiratory spasm (Valsalva) leading to increased intrathoracic pressure; (iv) reduced cardiac output; and (v) impaired cerebral circulation secondary to (i) and (iv).

In his ealier works Gastaut favoured a type of reflex vagal pneumo-inhibition as the mechanism in breath-holding attacks (*e.g.* Gastaut and Gastaut 1958). Later observations led him to suggest that the Valsalva manoeuvre was more important, with syncope occurring during the bradypnoea, and rebound bradycardia occurring at the conclusion of the breath-hold (Gastaut 1968, 1972; Gastaut and Broughton 1972). Illustrations in those publications show a slowing of the heart rate at the end of breath-holding, such as one would expect in the overshoot phase of a Valsalva manoeuvre, and also a delayed slowing of the EEG with clouding of consciousness some seconds later. In addition to recognizing cardio-inhibitory syncopes *which might also occur in a child with breath-holding spells*, Gastaut (1974) made the distinction between breath-holding spells and sobbing spasms or sobbing syncopes in which the child would 'sob intensely and intractably for a long period of time (1–3 minutes)'. A striking observation (Gastaut 1968, 1974) was that intense cyanosis, loss of consciousness, collapse and tonic spasm could occur *without any EEG change* in a multichannel recording (*e.g.* see Figs. 6 and 9 in Gastaut 1974).

Laxdal *et al.* (1969) felt that they could not contribute to the pathophysiology of breath-holding spells; however, in common with the authors mentioned above, they did clearly recognize that, while cyanotic and pallid syncopal attacks were quite distinct, nevertheless the same child could have cyanotic and pallid attacks on separate occasions. They also observed that the four patients in their study who had recurrent vasovagal syncope in adolescence and early adult life all had a previous history of *cyanotic* breath-holding.

Rendle-Short (1972) sought to explain the extreme rapidity of the onset of cyanosis by postulating a right–left shunt through a patent foramen ovale. However, recent studies using contrast echocardiography have not confirmed this (Southall *et al.* 1985, Southall and Talbot 1987).

In recent years, the subject has been reopened and what Southall calls 'prolonged expiratory apnoea' extensively documented (Southall *et al.* 1985, 1987*a,b,c,d*, 1988*b*; Southall and Talbot 1987; Southall 1988). The evidence of Southall's studies is that the mechanism is similar to that proposed by Gauk *et al.* (1963). In a somewhat small sample of patients Southall *et al.* (1985) showed continued expiratory activity at low lung volume with partial or complete glottic closure. The rapid development of arterial hypoxaemia is attributed to ventilatory/perfusion mismatch or intrapulmonary shunting (Southall *et al.* 1990), the anatomical basis of which has recently been reported (Wilkinson and Fagan 1990). The lack of a Valsalva type of manoeuvre (as suggested previously by Duvoisin 1962) is supported by the continuation of cyanotic spells after tracheostomy or tracheal intubation.

Critical review of all the available data confirms the complexity and heterogeneity of 'cyanotic' breath-holding spells. The role of vagal (Johnson 1985) or non-vagal (Blanc *et al.* 1988) pneumo-inhibition is uncertain, but the evidence that cardio-inhibitory syncopes may occur in the same child is compelling (an example of dual mechanism *in the same attack* has been illustrated in Fig. 7.8, p. 53). One suspects that the importance of Valsalva manoeuvres has been underplayed. Sobbing spasms have not been adequately investigated by modern methods. Most important, how may the EEG not alter despite cyanosis and unconsciousness and tonic spasm? Is localized hypoxia of the brainstem a feasible possibility?

The important question of prognosis will be discussed briefly in Chapter 16.

Obstructive apnoea
It is not proposed to discuss all explanations of apnoea, several of which are discussed elsewhere in this book. The important syndrome of awake apnoea associated with gastro-intestinal reflux (Spitzer *et al.* 1984) is described in Chapter 15 (see also Chapter 12).

A not uncommon clinical difficulty is establishing the basis of non-epileptic anoxic seizures where apnoea is the primary event and precipitations or triggers are not obvious. Such, for example, was the situation in Case 8.3. In that case there was uncertainty as to whether the degree of malacia of the tracheobronchial tree was more important or whether the mechanism resembled that discussed above as 'prolonged expiratory apnoea'.

In apnoea which appears to have an 'obstructive' basis but without visible mechanical obstruction, the question of epileptic apnoea may arise—this problem is discussed in Chapter 12.

Valsalva–Weber manoeuvre

For practical purposes the Valsalva manoeuvre and the Weber manoeuvre are the same. Forced expiration against a closed glottis impedes cardiac filling and increases cerebral venous pressure (Sharpey-Schafer 1953a,b; Duvoisin 1961, 1962; Picornell-Darder et al. 1978). The gross reduction in cardiac output is accompanied by tachycardia and often by a reduction in the amplitude of the ECG QRS complex (Aicardi et al. 1988). Of importance from the point of view of differential diagnosis is the pronounced vagal bradycardia, which may amount to junctional escape rhythm, appearing abruptly in response to the arterial pressure overshoot at the conclusion of the forced expiration (Duvoisin 1962).

Duvoisin (1962) took the opportunity to use the Valsalva manoeuvre to induce convulsive syncope in a large group of airforce recruits who had previous episodes of loss of consciousness. He confirmed previous studies (Duvoisin 1961, Gastaut et al. 1961c) in showing that preceding hyperventilation increased the likelihood of convulsive syncope. The 54 convulsive syncopes which he recorded were similar to each other and were pure anoxic seizures. The mildest episodes included several bilaterally synchronous coarse clonic jerks of the upper limbs immediately after the subject slumped unconscious. These movements were described as brief flexion and pronation of forearms, with adduction of the arms repeated four or five times while the hands remained open with the fingers semi-flexed in the resting position. The head might bob up and down but there was no general increase in muscle tone. In more severe convulsive episodes Duvoisin noted extensor thrusts of the lower extremities but no definite tonic phase, the jerks occurring against a background of hypotonia. In the most severe episodes there was an initial vacant stare followed by loss of postural tone, and then a moderate generalized increase in tone and a decerebrate posture without striking opisthotonus. Several convulsive jerks of arms and legs then occurred, the most violent jerks being the first with decreasing amplitude over five to 10 seconds. Autonomic manifestations included sweating, salivation and occasionally incontinence of urine during the unconscious phase. The face might be bluish but was pale afterwards. Recovery was very rapid with only a throbbing headache thereafter.

The contribution of Valsalva manoeuvres to natural syncopes and seizures has probably not been fully established. In particular, the contribution to 'breath-holding attacks' is uncertain (see previous section). More clear-cut are the syncopes and seizures induced by compulsive Valsalva manoeuvres in older children with autism and similar disorders, with or without mental impairment (Gastaut 1980; Gastaut *et al.* 1982, 1987; Aicardi *et al.* 1988). Self-induced episodes of this nature may be extremely frequent throughout the day and lead to blanks or falls with or without stiffening and one or two clonic jerks. Dramatic motor phenomena may be evident (see Case 8.4; Li *et al.* 1989), and it may be difficult on clinical grounds to distinguish between a Valsalva-induced pure anoxic seizure and a Valsalva-induced anoxic-epileptic seizure. Well-described instances of the latter have been published (Gastaut *et al.* 1987, Aicardi *et al.* 1988), with three-per-second spike and wave absence superimposed on syncope. It is likely in Rett syndrome, in which hyperventilation is prominent (Southall *et al.* 1988*a*), that the Valsalva mechanism is important in inducing seizures of one kind or another (see Gastaut *et al.* 1987, Cases 6 and 8). In 'stretch syncope' of adolescence (Pelekanos *et al.* 1990), neck extension compounds the effect of the Valsalva manoeuvre.

Suffocation
Self-asphyxia or strangulation as a cause of anoxic seizures is rare (Lai and Ziegler 1983), but the induction of anoxic seizures in an infant by the mother unfortunately is all too common. This is the 'active' form of Meadow syndrome (Meadow 1984), other aspects of which will be discussed in Chapter 13.

Characteristic histories are given in Cases 8.6 and 8.7. The episodes might be very frequent in an apparently well-loved baby. As detailed in Case 8.6, seizures are predominantly tonic, although they may be described by observers as 'grand mal' (Case 8.7). Cyanosis, pallor, bradycardia, sweating, 'collapse' and a 'moribund' appearance may give clues that severe syncope has occurred. A recording method which makes it clear whether the mother is present at the onset of each episode is essential. If the mother's method of suffocation involves pressing the baby's face into her bosom (Fig. 8.1), the hospital staff may easily be misled. A novel seizure chart, like that shown in Fig. 8.3 (p. 74), may help staff to realize the timing of the seizures.

The diagnosis has been confirmed in a number of cases by covert video surveillance (Rosen *et al.* 1983, Southall *et al.* 1987*c*), but this can prove difficult (Williams and Bevan 1988). The publication by Rosen *et al.* (1983) of an EEG/polygraph with time-coded videotape information (Fig. 8.2) has facilitated the use of diagnostic monitoring in the absence of covert video surveillance. Recordings made in two personal cases (8.6, 8.7) are shown on pages 76–77 and 79. The pattern of movement artefacts, heart-rate changes and anoxic EEG changes, together with the late stage at which the event button was pressed by the mother, combined to indicate the diagnosis. In the infant reported here as Case 8.5 (p. 73), suffocation should have been suspected from the data on her limited channel EEG recording, but at the time it was not considered because a recorded episode occurred within two metres of an attending nurse. The diagnosis was finally established by covert video surveillance.

In certain cases, acquired epileptic seizures may complicate the diagnosis (see Cases 16.2, 16.3). However, since death or brain damage may be the outcome, early identification of these patients is vital.

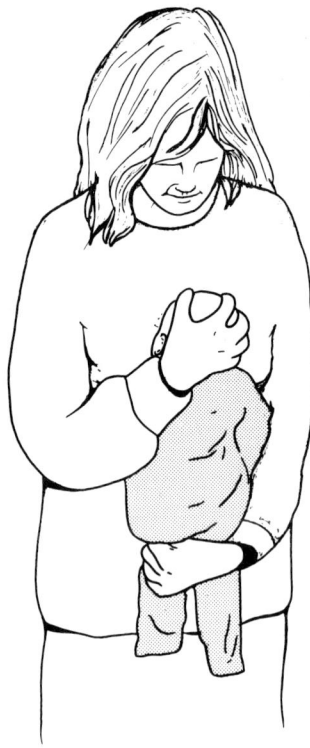

Fig. 8.1. Method used for suffocation of baby in Meadow syndrome (Cases 8.6, 8.7).

Fig. 8.2. *(Opposite.)* Continuous polygraphic recording of 7-month-old girl, suffocated by her mother. Each strip lasts 60 seconds. From the time-coded videotape, the mother's hand appears over the baby's face at the first arrow ('ON') at 19.48.03. Increased movement artefact occurs in the EEG and the respirations become out of phase until the baby is released at 19.49.35 (second arrow, 'OFF'), at which time the EEG becomes essentially flat, respiratory effort is minimal, and the ECG reaches a low of 50 per minute. The mother begins resuscitation efforts at 19.49.48 (at the beginning of the third strip) and closed-chest massage and bag and mask ventilation are evident at 19.50.15. The baby begins crying at 19.51.35 (fourth strip, right-hand section) and the heart rate reaches 165 per minute. (Reproduced by permission from Rosen *et al.* 1983.)

Cardiac disease

In most congenital heart disease the diagnosis of syncopal episodes of anoxic seizures is not a problem. For example, the presentation of aortic stenosis as exercise syncope is too well known to require further description. However, difficulty may arise in Fallot's tetralogy, in which seizures may present in infancy before the cyanosis which prompts the cardiac diagnosis has developed (Shinebourne *et al.* 1975). For many years it has been assumed that the episodic collapse or convulsions in this condition are anoxic seizures and this has been confirmed by telemetric EEG video monitoring (Daniels *et al.* 1987). Propranolol is commonly used preoperatively to palliate the cyanotic episodes in Fallot's tetralogy, but a

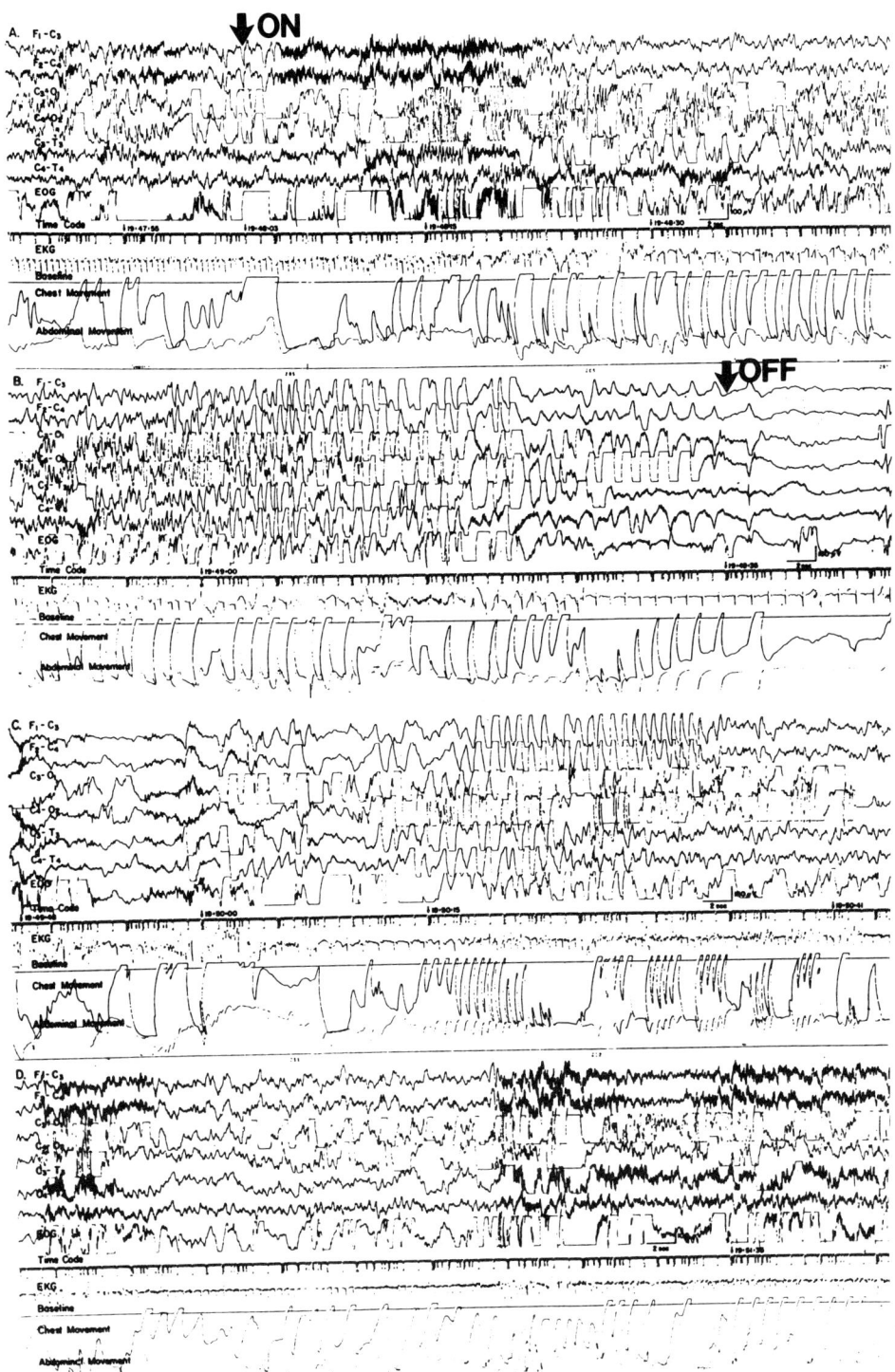

65

recent report suggests that in this situation the drug itself may induce syncope through sinus arrest (Clark *et al.* 1989).

Pulmonary hypertension
In 'congenital' heart disease, syncopes from intermittent exacerbation of pulmonary hypertension do not normally cause diagnostic difficulties. This may occur, however, and the clinical and EEG/ECG method of confirming an anoxic seizure in such a situation is illustrated in Case 8.8 and Figure 8.7 (p. 80).

Ventricular tachyarrhythmias and QT syndromes
The established teaching is that there are two separate genetic conditions with a prolonged QT interval on the ECG and paroxysmal ventricular fibrillation or tachycardia. One is the autosomal recessive disorder associated with congenital deafness as described by Jervell and Lange-Nielson (1957). The other is the Romano–Ward syndrome (Romano *et al.* 1964, Ward 1964) with autosomal dominant inheritance and normal hearing. O. Connor Ward (*personal communication*) has speculated that Morquio (1901) may have been the first to describe such a disorder, but although the descriptions of the epileptiform anoxic seizures are superb, the nature of the familial cardiac disorder cannot be established with certainty. Prolongation of the QT interval should be obvious on measurement and the use of the QTc allows prolongation to be detected at different heart rates.

Inevitably the reality is more complex (Moss *et al.* 1985). Evidently sporadic cases are common with or without deafness (Schwartz 1985). There is controversy as to whether the QT interval should be corrected (Ahnve 1985) or not (Ward and Camm 1988). The abnormal shape of the T waves has been stressed (Dean 1988). Most alarming for the clinician is the possibility that one might have a QT disorder, or at any rate something that is closely related, with a normal QT interval (McRae *et al.* 1974, Weiner and Stünkel 1982). Certainly those authors make a good case for the recognition of fainting fits due to paroxysmal ventricular tachyarrhythmia even when QT lengthening cannot be demonstrated, and certainly when QT shortening does not occur with increasing heart rate. To complicate matters, asystole (as well as ventricular tachyarrhythmia) may occur in QT disorders (Rennie and Arnold 1984).

Although it may sometimes be clear (Storstein 1949) that a patient's seizures are precipitated by tachyarrhythmia—ventricular fibrillation, ventricular tachycardia or *torsades de pointes* (prefibrillatory ventricular tachyarrhythmia with beat-to-beat alternating electrical polarity—Moss and Schwartz 1982)—differentiating these anoxic seizures from epileptic seizures may be difficult (Weiner and Stünkel 1982, Ballardie and Murphy 1983, Pignata *et al.* 1983). If there are clinical clues such as a family history, or a seizure or syncope induced by exercise, excitement, psychological stress or fright (Lown *et al.* 1976, Brodsky *et al.* 1987)—rather than the usual stimuli for vagal or vasovagal attacks—then Weiner and Stünkel (1982) have recommended cassette EEG/ECG in combination with exercise testing. Recent detailed studies in adults (Aminoff *et al.* 1988*b*) have shown that malignant ventricular arrhythmias do not necessarily induce the classical 'anoxic' EEG changes, but this difficulty should not arise in children (Wennevold *et al.* 1965, Driver and Selby 1977).

Summary
Anoxic seizures occurring on exercise or excitement (with or without sleep convulsions) suggest a tachyarrhythmia of the QT disorder associated type, requiring expert cardiological evaluation.

Sick sinus syndrome
Cardiac sinus node dysfunction with bradycardia and periods of asystole leading to syncope with or without motor anoxic seizures have long been well known (Laslett 1909, Pearson 1945). It is evident that syncopes can relate to both asystole and an intercurrent tachyarrhythmia, and such patients are included in many series of syncopes and convulsions (Schott *et al.* 1977; Luxon *et al.* 1980; Day *et al.* 1982; deBono *et al.* 1982; Kapoor *et al.* 1983, 1987). Of particular interest to this author is the relationship of autonomic dysfunction to what is called sick sinus syndrome. It certainly seems sensible to distinguish the condition in which a slow heart rate does not increase on exercise or on atropine (Scott *et al.* 1976) from what may be, for example, vagal bradycardia (Ector *et al.* 1983, 1984), using autonomic assessment (Dighton 1974) and evaluation of the intrinsic heart rate (Szatmáry *et al.* 1983). Difficulties arise in accepting a diagnosis of 'autonomic sinus node dysfunction' in patients with apparently no intrinsic involvement of the sino-atrial and atrioventricular nodes, but with episodes of sinus arrest and cardiac standstill (Caralis and Varghese 1976; Szatmáry *et al.* 1983, 1984; Szatmáry 1984). Since it has become fashionable (Lagergren 1988) to insert pacemakers even in the young (Duvernoy *et al.* 1980, Sapire *et al.* 1983, Ector *et al.* 1984), it may not matter whether the patient has an intrinsic disorder of the sinus node or hyperactive vagal reflexes. This is discussed in the section on vagal syncopes. It should be borne in mind, however, that bradycardia may be a normal effect of athletic training and due to a reduced intrinsic heart rate (Katona *et al.* 1982) rather than to the increase of vagal 'tone' as suggested by others (Rasmussen *et al.* 1978, McLaren *et al.* 1986).

Sick A-V node
Before leaving this difficult interface one should mention that although heart block from clear intrinsic heart disease is an ancient observation, such block may apparently be of vagal origin (Weiss and Ferris 1934). More recently the question of a selective hyper-responsiveness of the A-V node to vagal reflexes has been discussed (Strasburg *et al.* 1982).

'Fainting'
Although, as is repeatedly emphasized, syncope is what happens when cerebral metabolism suddenly stops, to many people syncope means 'fainting', or a swoon from the upright position with marked pallor and sweating thereafter. Within this ambit, therefore, are included both vasovagal and vasodepressor syncope, and those admittedly less well-understood syncopes of infancy, from those induced by

bathing (Sheldon 1952) to those related to pertussis immunization (Barraff *et al.* 1988). When the diagnosis and prognosis of 'syncope' is discussed in the literature, it is normally this type of pale limp fall which is in the author's mind or protocol, rather than an equally genuine syncope due, for instance, to respiratory obstruction or complicated by dramatic motor seizures (Fischer 1967, 1979; deBono *et al.* 1982; Kapoor *et al.* 1983; Kenny 1986; Vingerhoets and Schomaker 1988). An example would be: 'patients with tonic-clonic movements, post-ictal state or aura were excluded' (Kapoor *et al.* 1983).

The term 'vaso-vagal syncope' was coined by Lewis (1932) for the type of syncope which we understand as 'fainting'. Begging the question of whether there is one disorder or several, it may be said that a lot is known about the mechanism, but by no means all. Barcroft and others showed (Barcroft *et al.* 1944, Barcroft and Edholm 1945, Anderson *et al.* 1946) that similar mechanisms were involved in the fainting after oxygen lack or haemorrhage. In brief, first heart rate and muscle blood flow increase, then there is a marked further increase in muscle blood flow, with an abrupt fall in the heart rate and arterial pressure (the faint) but nevertheless an increase in the previously declining cardiac output. Some aspects of this sequence are explained, others are not. 'Vasovagal syncope', or at any rate hypotension bradycardia, has recently been demonstrated in a patient with denervated heart (Scherrer *et al.* 1990). The peripheral skin pallor is now generally agreed to be the result of vasopressin secretion. The increase in muscle blood flow was originally thought to be due to activation of sympathetic vasodilator nerves but the evidence now is that two mechanisms may be involved and that active vasodilation does not occur. Observations such as those of Wallin and Sundlöf (1982, 1984) indicate that sympathetic vasoconstrictor fibres (which are noradrenergic) cease to fire during fainting. Secondly, the observations of Robinson and Johnson (1988) indicate that plasma adrenaline levels *increase* consistently in fainting. These authors suggest that, in the presence of excessive vagal activity in bradycardia, this will contribute to arterial hypotension. Such may not be the only explanation, as illustrated by the case of Goldstein *et al.* (1982). Their patient, investigated at the age of 17, began having syncopes—occasionally convulsive—at the age of 2. They usually occurred with sitting or standing and sometimes with stress, and were associated with presyncopal symptoms of light-headedness and abdominal discomfort, and then pallor and sweating. An episode provoked by venepuncture led to a drop in blood pressure and marked decrease in heart rate with a few seconds of asystole. Profound hypotension persisted despite cardiac pacing. The key observation was a lack of noradrenaline response to the hypotension, and the girl was successfully treated with elastic stockings.

Whichever mechanism of vasodilation (or failure of compensatory vaso-constriction) occurs in an individual, an unsolved problem appears to be the mechanism of the vagal response (Hainsworth 1988). The vagal effect may be regarded as part of a 'syncopal reflex' (Gastaut 1974), and many publications have attempted to produce evidence in support of increased vagal 'tone' (Sapire *et al.* 1979, 1983; Lucet *et al.* 1984; Sapire and Casta 1985; McLaren *et al.* 1986). However, examination of respiratory sinus arrhythmia (O'Brien *et al.* 1986, Rawles *et al.* 1989) has not shown abnormalities in individuals with a tendency to emotional fainting (Steptoe and Wardle 1988). Such a negative finding would not be unexpected were it a vagal *phasic* reflex rather than vagal hypertonia which is involved (Katona *et al.* 1982, Dighton 1986). That there should be a sufficiently dominant vagal reaction to cause fainting in the supine position tends to cause surprise (Verrill and Aellig 1970, Weinstein 1982, Milam *et al.* 1986). The supine 'faints' described by those authors were not convulsive, and it is probably the rule that in this sort of syncope a motor anoxic seizure (*e.g.* Case 8.10) implies a substantial duration of asystole (two of the patients of Grossi *et al.* 1987, Table 9.IV, being apparent exceptions). The relationship between the delayed asystole, traditional vasovagal syncope and short latency 'reflex' asystole is discussed in Chapter 9 (see also Milstein *et al.* 1989). A brief account of reflex asystole follows.

Reflex anoxic seizures
The term 'reflex anoxic seizure' has been used for 'a particular type of fit which is neither epileptic nor due to breath-holding, but rather results from brief stoppage of the heart through excess activity of the vagus nerve' (Stephenson 1980, 1985*a*). The term has been criticized particularly in so far as 'seizure' may be interpreted as 'epileptic seizure' (Bower 1984), but it has been defended (Aicardi 1986) and employed by other authors (Roddy *et al.* 1983, Palm and Blennow 1985). A justification for the separate category is that often the latency between stimulus and seizure seems so short that it is comparable to that seen in carotid sinus and vagovagal syncopes (see below). The distinction between anoxic and anoxic-epileptic seizures is discussed in Chapter 11.

Various aspects of reflex anoxic seizures are illustrated in the many case histories included in this book (see especially those in Chapter 9).

The typical description of an episode in a toddler was given in an earlier paper by the present author (Stephenson 1978*a*):

In a typical case an unsteady toddler on his own trips and falls. His mother hears the bump but no succeeding cry and hurries to him. She finds her child lying deathly still with eyes fixed upwards, lips dusky. As she lifts him, he abruptly stiffens into rigid extension with jaw clenched and hands fisted, gives a few jerks, and after what seems an age (but in fact is less than half a minute) relaxes limply with an absent far-away look. Then he opens his eyes, at once recognises his mother, cries a little, and drifts off to sleep, his face distinctly pale.

Although this type of episode was clearly distinguished by Maulsby and Kellaway (1964), by Lombroso and Lerman (1967) and by Gastaut in various publications (*e.g.* 1968, 1974), it has tended to attract the inappropriate term 'breath-holding' (Lombroso and Lerman 1967, Laxdal *et al.* 1969). To a certain extent this is understandable in that clearly there are children who do have breath-holding episodes and something closely resembling or identical to reflex anoxic seizures (see section on breath-holding above). Further, the fact that the heart may be inaudible or the pulse imperceptible during an episode, with pallor seen thereafter, does not necessarily imply that asystole has occurred: the same features would be expected with a Valsalva manoeuvre (Duvoisin 1961, 1962). In his earlier papers, Gastaut (1968, 1974) posited that the artificial anoxic seizure induced in the EEG laboratory by ocular compression is purely an artificial syncope never occurring with such short latency in the natural world. Arguments and illustrations favouring short-latency vagal asystole will be given in Chapter 9, but the difference between an immediate response of one or two seconds and a 'tardive' response of 15 seconds may be difficult to judge in ordinary life. In older patients, with stimuli such as needle insertion (Lloyd-Smith and Tatlow 1958b, Tizes 1976, Nash and Horton 1978, Duvernoy et al. 1980, Braham et al. 1981, Roddy et al. 1983) or intrauterine device insertion (Acker et al. 1973, Faden et al. 1977), the effect is often prompt, but marked delay may occur particularly in blood phobia (blood-injury-illness phobia) (Hand and Schröder 1980).

Pale atonic attacks also occur quite commonly after head bumps in susceptible toddlers. Presumably in these children substantial asystole does not occur and the episodes might be expected to have a mechanism similar to that in more traditional vasovagal syncope. They are certainly candidates for the term 'pallid syncope' (Bower 1984).

Miscellaneous circulatory syncopes
Many other syncopal mechanisms are well known in older individuals (Ross 1989) but of considerable rarity in the very young.

Vagovagal syncope is well established as a purely cardio-inhibitory type of syncope in adults (Weiss and Ferris 1934). Similar syncopes may occur in children with mass lesions involving the vagus but may also occur as a 'functional' disorder. Woody and Kiel (1986) reported a girl who from the age of 18 months had frequent episodes of loss of consciousness without warning or episodes of dizziness (a total of 345 episodes were logged by the mother up to the age of 4 years!). It became apparent that there was a relation with swallowing, eating or the thought of food. ECG recordings during a meal revealed complete heart block with a ventricular rate of 37 per minute accompanied by loss of consciousness. Episodes were abolished by a permanent ventricular demand pacemaker (see also Case 15.41).

'Hypervagism' has been described by Coryllos et al. (1981, 1984) as a chronic or progressive condition in which neurologically abnormal infants have syncopes due to extreme bradycardia and indeed anoxic seizures thereby, this condition being to an extent resistant to atropine and needing denervation of the sino-atrial node for treatment. Further reports from other centres are needed to assess the generality of these findings. Certainly, at the Royal Hospital for Sick Children we have observed something akin to hypervagism in a young child, in whom profound bradycardia of the order of 40 per minute (but normal intrinsic heart rate) was associated with medullary involvement in haemolytic uraemic syndrome which proved fatal.

Carotid sinus disorders (Lewis 1932, Gastaut et al. 1961d) are not a problem of the young, but death secondary to occlusion of a carotid artery after sinus massage has been quoted as a danger of ocular compression! [Johnson et al. (1984, p. 169) stated, 'Pressure on the eyeballs has long been known to produce bradycardia, and has been used to bring an end to an attack of paroxysmal atrial tachycardia. Occasionally however it may cause such profound bradycardia that there is syncope or even death (Nelson and Mahru 1963)', the title of the Nelson and Mahru paper being 'Death following digital carotid artery occlusion'.]

It is worth drawing attention to studies on carotid sinus hypersensitivity in older individuals presenting with syncope (Davies *et al.* 1979). The evidence for carotid sinus sensitivity seems to me to be analogous to the evidence for ocular compression hyper-reactivity discussed elsewhere, and might indicate more a liability to excessive vagal reflexes than anything particularly amiss about the carotid or the carotid sinus. Indeed, in studies of elderly patients fulfilling established criteria for carotid sinus syndrome, enhanced vagal activity and normal arginine vasopressin response on tilt-testing closely resembled the findings in 'malignant' vasovagal syndrome and suggested a disorder of brainstem control (Kenny 1986, Kenny *et al.* 1987).

Glossopharyngeal neuralgia with asystolic or vasodepressor syncope is not a known problem of childhood, but the mechanism of *paroxysmal sympathetic withdrawal* (Wallin *et al.* 1984, Onrot *et al.* 1987) is another differential in the general diagnosis of vasodepressor syncopes.

Autonomic dysfunction
Some aspects of autonomic dysfunction have been alluded to in previous sections on 'fainting' and on the vagus and ventricular tachyarrhythmias. The general autonomic impairment of the Riley–Day syndrome is mentioned at the end of Chapter 15: anoxic seizures are frequent in this condition. The most common acute illness which may be complicated by syncopes or anoxic seizures from autonomic hypofunction is the Guillain–Barré syndrome (see Case 8.11). Head-up tilt testing is valuable in detecting autonomic dysfunction in unexplained syncopes (Abi-Samra *et al.* 1988).

Case histories
CASE 8.1
This 2-year-old girl had convulsions almost every day, and sometimes more than once a day. Some were precipitated by a bump by her sister, or having her mouth wiped, or hurting her finger, or not wanting her jumper put over her head, but many others had no obvious precipitation.

A typical episode was observed in hospital. Her mother had been cleaning her nose when she started catching her breath and became dark blue and the cyanosis became even deeper. She had a tonic extension and her eyes deviated upwards and there were superimposed repeated small-amplitude flexion jerks of her upper limbs totalling more than 10 while her eyes were still upwardly deviated, with general rigidity. It was two minutes before she gave a look of recognition and began to cry.

Attachment to a cassette EEG/ECG monitoring system inhibited the episodes completely for the duration of the recording!

Comment. This is an example of the severe type of 'blue' breath-holding attack. Although it was evident that the initiating mechanism was severe arterial hypoxaemia, it was not immediately apparent whether the severe convulsions represented pure anoxic seizures or whether an anoxic-epileptic seizure (see Chapter 11) had been induced. In the event, the ambulatory cassette recording designed to prove this point inhibited the episodes completely over several days.

CASE 8.2

A 2-year-old boy had what were described as breath-holding attacks, usually provoked by pain, since the age of 3 months. His father gave the sequence as: no sound; straight back; (falls over) holding breath; into a spasm; arms and legs back; starts twitching [he mimed a coarse tremble]; grey for four or five minutes and purple round the lips; sleeps afterwards.

On ocular compression under split-screen video control, he had an asystole of 11.8 seconds after no latency. He sobbed in expiration at about four to five sobs per second and the last sob was synchronous with the first return of the ECG complex (without a P wave). Flexion of the upper limbs and then trunk extension occurred at the onset of the isoelectric EEG. A large inspiratory gasp occurred after three seconds of flat EEG.

Abolition of episodes occurred as soon as he started atropine methonitrate.

Comment. Although in certain respects these episodes resembled breath-holding attacks, and although expiratory sobbing occurred during the induced attack, vagal asystole seems likely to have been a prominent component. The result of the administration of atropine supports this concept, although the previous case (8.1) illustrates how non-specific alterations in management may abort breath-holding spells.

CASE 8.3

An infant girl had her first blue spell at the age of 3 months. Although her birthweight was 2950g after a concealed pregnancy of unknown duration, thereafter she failed to thrive and was hypotonic and had a high-pitched cry. She had unusual looking facies, a large tongue and symmetrical swellings of the buccal mucosae. She also had a single kidney with crossed fused ectopia.

Cyanotic spells occurred in clusters, commonly without obvious provocation. In the milder episodes she was apnoeic with cyanosis and bradycardia, while in more severe episodes her pupils became small and she was atonic before stiffening with flexion of the upper limbs, extension of the neck and extension of the lower limbs. On occasion a few 'jerks' were reported. The heart rate increased from 140 to 190 at the onset of these tonic seizures and then fell to a minimum of 50 per minute. Breathing movements were not observed during these episodes but on occasion recovery coincided with the passage of an endotracheal tube.

In addition to the mild enlargement of the tongue, there was a dubious and certainly not gross degree of tracheobronchomalacia. She was always improved by a nasotracheal intubation with complete abolition of apnoeic attacks, with one exception. In this episode, which was recorded on cassette EEG/ECG, apnoea, cyanosis, oxygen saturation below 40 per cent and a seizure with tonic extension were accompanied by 'classical' EEG changes (slow, then four seconds flat, then slow) and tachycardia throughout. A cluster of right-sided spikes was documented in an interictal EEG at the age of 9 months, but no epileptic seizures were ever documented.

At the age of 9 months she was found to have developed a Wilms tumour in her single right kidney, and she had considerable neurodevelopmental delay. Her facial features bore a considerable resemblance to those of a patient with Perlman syndrome (Neri *et al.* 1984), in whom apnoeic seizures of probable anoxic type proved fatal.

Comment. Unprovoked anoxic seizures occurred in this infant from apnoea which may have been central or obstructive, but which decreased with time. The dramatic nature of these episodes often provoked attending doctors to administer diazepam, with worsening of the child's condition.

CASE 8.4

An 8-year-old boy from New England was said to have a 'seizure disorder', beginning at the age of 2½ years, for which he had seen 50 physicians. In fact, he had considerable mental impairment with a mental age of about 3 years, had walked first at age 2 on his toes, and then used to fall backwards when running. The seizures were said to be typical tonic-clonic seizures occurring 20 to 30 times a day and they had only remitted for short periods of a few days when he had had tonsillitis, when he had started a ketogenic diet, and when he had begun carbamazepine. All other anticonvulsant therapies had been ineffective.

In fact, all the seizures occurred after what was described as breath-holding. The breath-holding in this case was a Valsalva manoeuvre. He seemed addicted to this and got a 'high' when he did it. If he did three Valsalva manoeuvres in a row this flipped him into a seizure. The seizure was characterized by first a lolling of his head, after which the head rocked back and his eyes went up and his upper limbs flew outwards, abducted and extended. Then his fists clenched, his arms adducted tightly to his body and his elbows flexed. Then there were alternating fluttering movements of his feet and hands, with three or four shakes and then a pause of a few seconds, and then three or four more shakes and perhaps another pause, and then maybe three or four more shakes. Then he would become very flushed, his whole body would relax and he would get up, then want to go to sleep.

In the Valsalva manoeuvres it was not possible to detect his pulse or auscultate his heartbeat. However, the ECG continued during the episodes, although the amplitude of the QRS complexes were reduced by 50 per cent compared with before and after the breath-holding. After the end of the Valsalva the QRS complexes remained of low voltage for a further one or two seconds before increasing, and then the pulse was felt. Echo studies during these episodes suggested a marked decrease in carotid flux and variable aortic flow. Atropine had no effect except leading to tachycardia.

It seemed that when he had the tonsillitis and when he had the ketogenic diet, and probably when he started the carbamazepine, he was not doing his Valsalva manoeuvres so often, or at any rate so strongly. His mother noted that she could abort the seizure if she hugged him strongly before the final attempted Valsalva.

Comment. This autistic boy certainly had compulsive Valsalva manoeuvres and anoxic seizures induced thereby. It is possible, though unproved, that he also had anoxic-epileptic seizures, the Valsalva manoeuvre being followed by a true tonic epileptic seizure. Naltrexone, an oral opioid antagonist, was associated with marked improvement.

CASE 8.5
A 6-month-old infant was referred because of frequent episodes of cyanosis, floppiness, loss of consciousness, pallor and slowing of the pulse. Monitoring had revealed interference in the ECG channel followed by atrial arrest and nodal escape rhythm at the time of the clinical syncope. Two-channel EEG and ECG were recorded on cassette when the child was in a bed close to the nurses' station. One episode was recorded, again showing movement artefact on the ECG channel and on the EEG channel, with no EEG spikes, followed by slowing of both the EEG and ECG, with loss of P waves from the ECG.

Comment. Nearly 18 months later, covert video surveillance finally demonstrated that the episodes were caused by the mother smothering the baby (Southall *et al.* 1987c).

CASE 8.6
A 5-month-old first-born male baby was admitted as an emergency with a story of having become blue and stiff during a feed. There was a previous history of reflux and poor weight gain.

His mother was 24; her father had been violent towards his wife and had hanged himself when she was 2 years old. The mother herself was said to have been abused as an adolescent by a visitor to the home. She had been successful in school, was successful socially and taught

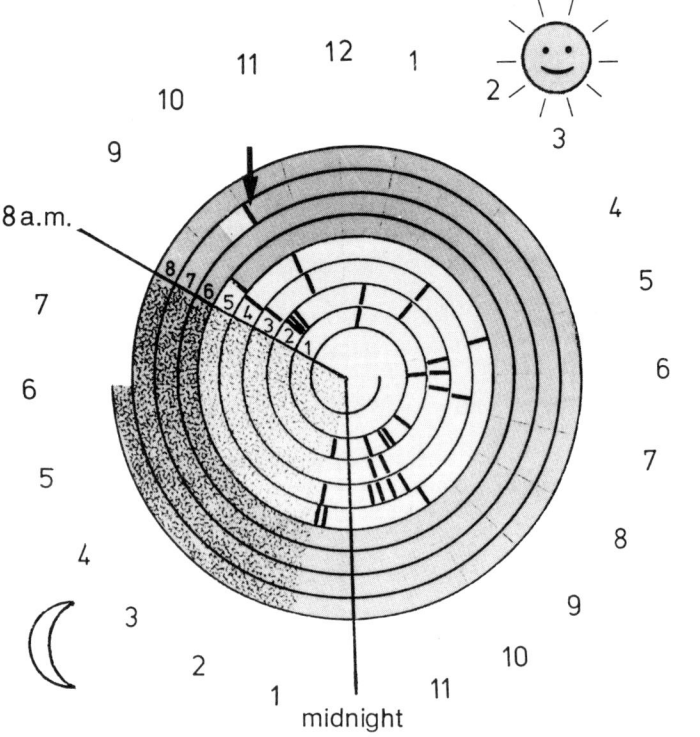

Fig. 8.3. Spiral seizure chart in case of Meadow syndrome (Case 8.6). Seizures are related to time and opportunity. On the 8 a.m. axis is the number of day of observation. A short radial black bar indicates a seizure. The dotted area indicates the time during which the mother was probably asleep. The shaded area of the spiral indicates the time during which EEG/ECG monitoring was undertaken with a nurse in constant attendance. The white part of the spiral shows the time during which this special monitoring was not undertaken. The vertical arrow indicates the seizure recorded after the mother had been unsupervised for half an hour, although with the EEG/ECG monitor still attached.

the clarinet. She married three years before the current admission. Her husband was violent to her. During her pregnancy she was depressed but this cleared. After delivery, the family doctor commented that his medical practice was 'like a little surrogate mother for her'. She had difficulties in feeding and settling the baby from the start.

During the first five days in hospital the baby had 33 episodes, 23 recorded as occurring in the presence of his mother. The features of the seizures which were recorded, with the number of episodes of each feature in brackets, included the following: cyanosis of the lips (28); stiffening of limbs or body, or back arching (20) (with a second stiffening observed on one occasion); apnoea (11) (not mentioned in the records until the 18th episode); pallor mostly after the attacks and sometimes with sweating (eight); grunting (five); twitching of some or all limbs, including more twitching of the right limbs (five) (not mentioned until the 20th episode); and slowing of the heart rate (four) (not mentioned before the 26th episode). Later analysis indicated that the mother was present at the onset of all these occasions, which clustered after breakfast and late in the evening and did not occur during the night, or at any

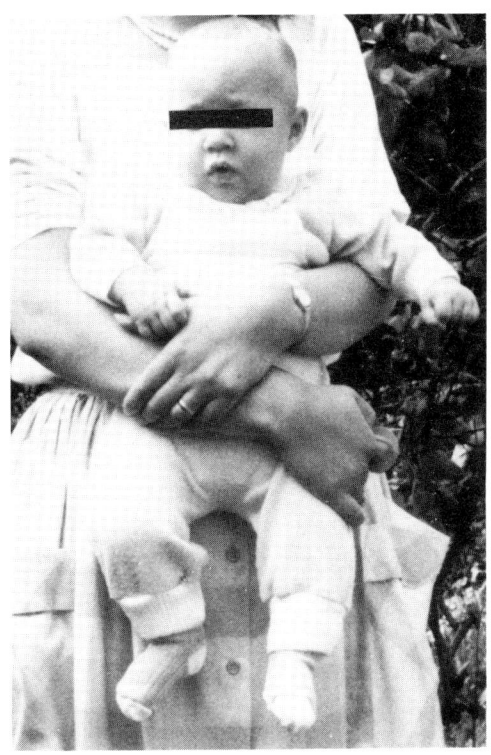

Fig. 8.4. Loving relationship with baby subjected to repeated suffocations, here held by mother (Case 8.6).

rate after 1am (Fig. 8.3). After helping to resuscitate the baby on one occasion, the registrar noted: 'Mother's reaction was very strange, she did not seem to be worried about it at all.' In between episodes the baby interacted happily (Fig. 8.4).

To record and define these anoxic seizures, the baby was connected to a seven-channel EEG, one-channel ECG cassette recorder (Oxford Medical Systems, Medilog 9000). For the first 48 hours a nurse was in constant attendance. The nurse was then called away and it was suggested that the mother might like to give the baby a cuddle. Within half an hour there was an episode of his going blue and stiff, the mother having been holding the baby in the open ward within a few metres of doctors and nurses on a ward round. The transcribed recording is shown in Figure 8.5. The detailed sequence is identical to that found by Rosen *et al.* (1983) who used simultaneous time-coded video recording, except that in the present case the asphyxia probably lasted for at least two minutes before the mother pressed the signal button.

Psychiatric involvement with both parents began before they were confronted with the evidence of the EEG/ECG monitoring. Later the mother admitted that she might have pressed the baby's face firmly to her bosom (as shown in Fig. 8.1, p. 64). Shortly afterwards she took a drug overdose and was admitted to an adult psychiatric ward. After several weeks she began to talk about her marriage and her baby: 'I was being hurt and I could not hit back so I hit at the baby.' Her personality resources were normal, she was intelligent, gifted at music, emotionally warm and attached to her son; she had no psychiatric illness. However, it could be said that there was a 'splitting' of her personality, with uncontrolled aggression finally expressed as repeated forcible suffocation.

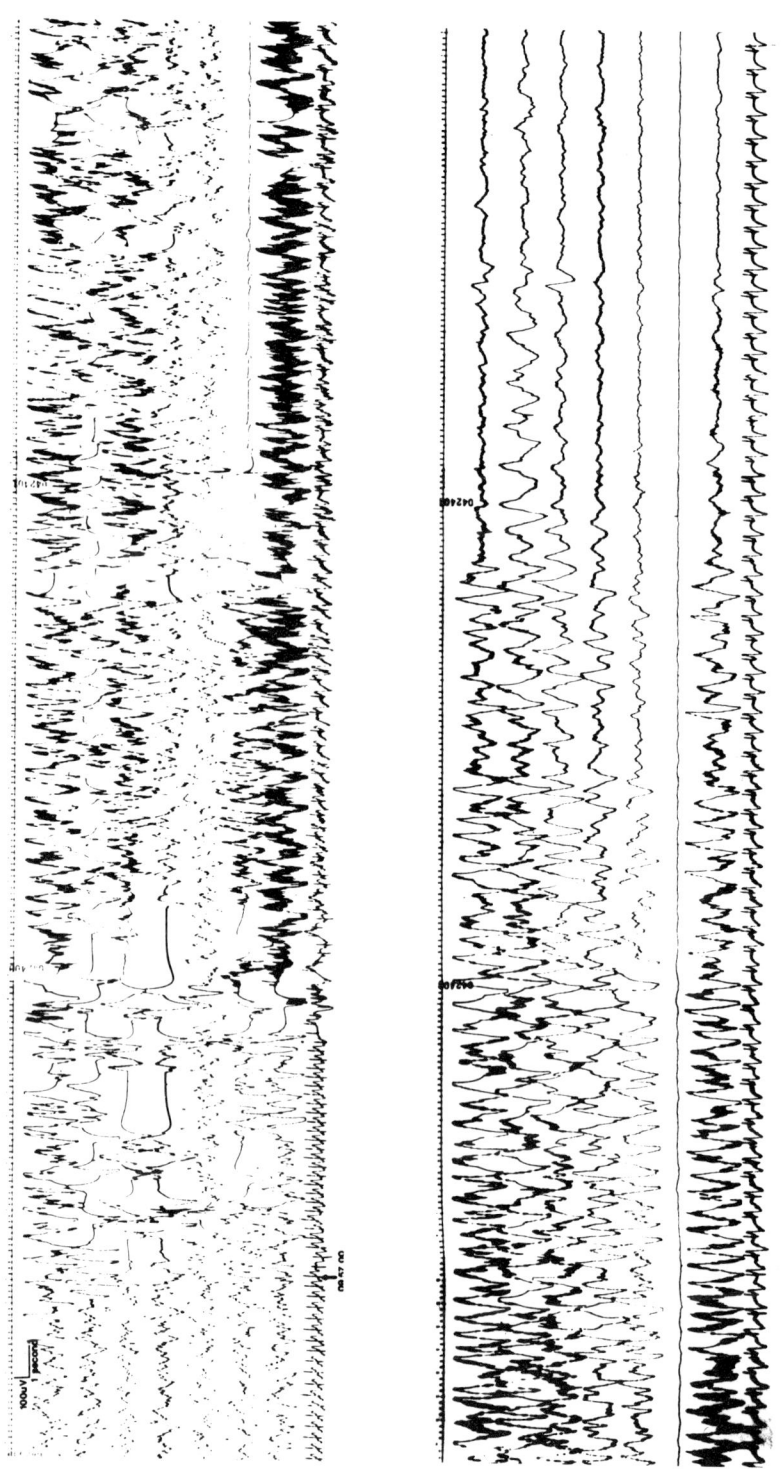

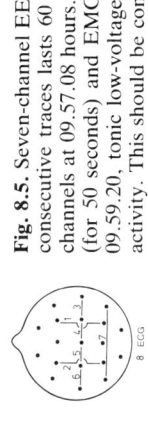

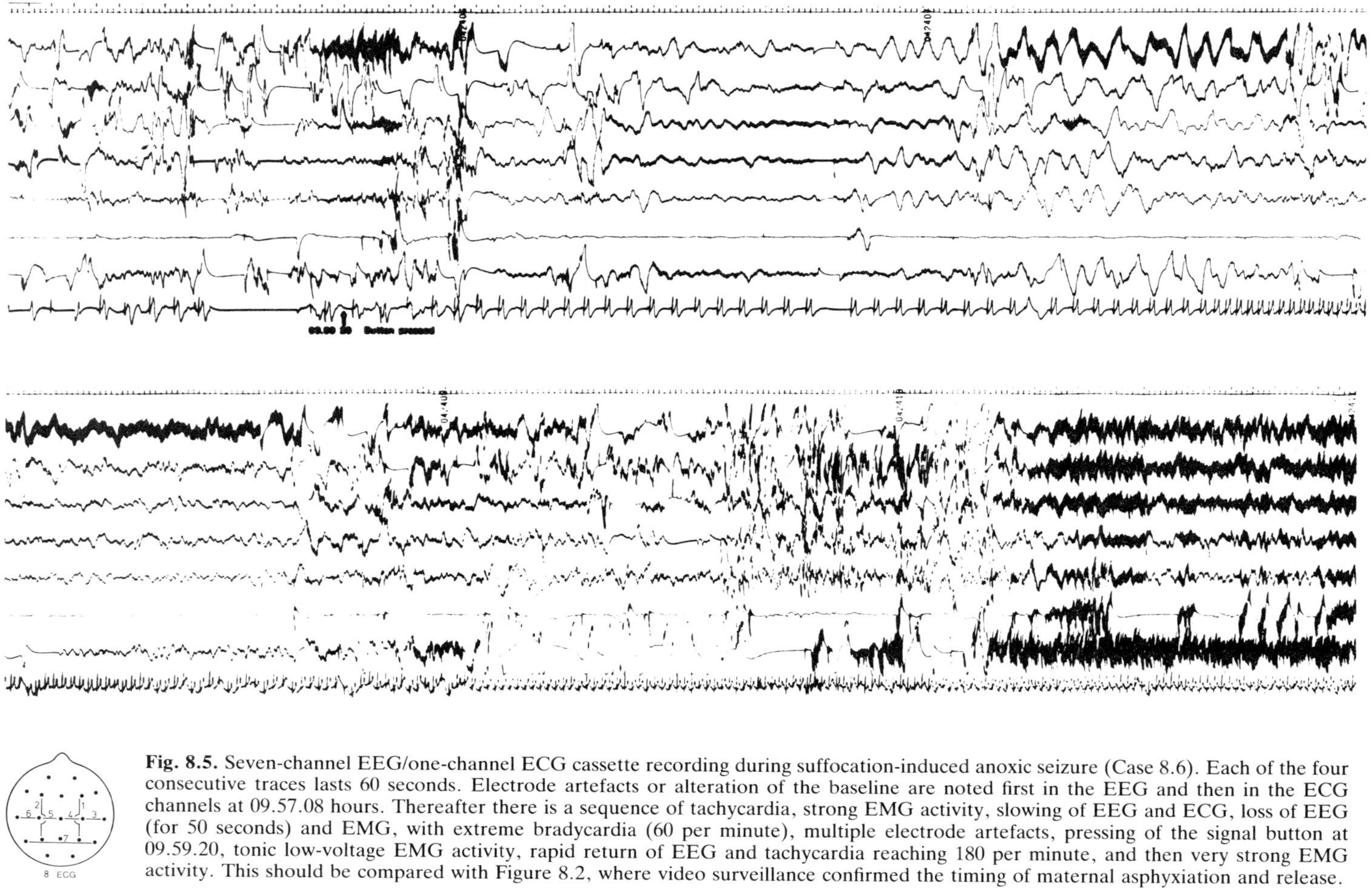

Fig. 8.5. Seven-channel EEG/one-channel ECG cassette recording during suffocation-induced anoxic seizure (Case 8.6). Each of the four consecutive traces lasts 60 seconds. Electrode artefacts or alteration of the baseline are noted first in the EEG and then in the ECG channels at 09.57.08 hours. Thereafter there is a sequence of tachycardia, strong EMG activity, slowing of EEG and ECG, loss of EEG (for 50 seconds) and EMG, with extreme bradycardia (60 per minute), multiple electrode artefacts, pressing of the signal button at 09.59.20, tonic low-voltage EMG activity, rapid return of EEG and tachycardia reaching 180 per minute, and then very strong EMG activity. This should be compared with Figure 8.2, where video surveillance confirmed the timing of maternal asphyxiation and release.

77

The baby himself appeared to have suffered no physical harm (that is, no brain damage) from the suffocations; no further episodes occurred after separation from the mother.

Comment.   This is a typical story of 'active Meadow syndrome', with what appears to be the typical EEG and ECG features of an attack.

CASE 8.7

This girl was 10 months old when cassette recording gave the diagnosis, but the denouement was delayed until she was 13 months. The mother described 11 episodes between the ages of 2 and 10 months, with two intervals of two months each in which no episodes occurred. Some of the mother's descriptions were as follows. 'I noticed her in her pram turning a bit blue and lifted her up; a neighbour hit her on the back to get her going again.' 'I just put her down to get changed, she turned blue and was violently sick and her bowels and bladder emptied.' 'She was irritable when sitting playing away on my knee and then she flopped back and went blue and her wee arms were jerking the whole time—three times—and then she went limp and a neighbour came and got her breathing again—and she was sleeping and in the middle of it she was violently sick and brought up blood that size [5cm] out of her stomach.' 'She was playing away—it always seems to happen in my arms—and then collapsed again—a wee touch of blue, jerking about four times, and then completely blue and then floppy, then she had the kiss of life.' 'She was playing away with my dress, and then completely flopped back into a faint and did a couple of twitchings and her wee hands were tight as fists and a wee bit blue—she had stopped breathing and was dead pale after.'

She was admitted to the District Hospital where a staff nurse observed the end of the 'grand mal fit' with twitching. EEG/ECG cassette recording was arranged. The episode recorded was described by her mother as: 'in my arms again trying to get to sleep, she threw her head back and went blue and her arms started jerking—four jerks—and then I got her back going in a minute. She was moaning in her fit, just a touch of blue round her lips—not dark blue, just a touch—and the rest of her pale and floppy. I pressed the button before the nurses arrived and she fell asleep right after it.' In fact, when the sister arrived the infant was grey, limp, apnoeic and looked moribund, gasping when sucked out. A review of the cassette recording (Fig. 8.6) showed that for about five minutes the recording varied between normal background EEG with ECG tachycardia, and a combination of slow waves on the EEG, bradycardia and movement artefact. This culminated in a short period of complete EEG flattening just before the mother pressed the event button.

One further episode occurred when the mother was alone with the child (as she had been in all previous episodes), this being similar except that the mother also said that she couldn't feel the baby's pulse, a lot of blood had come out of her nose, and the right side of her face had become puffy.

An unsuccessful attempt was made to capture an episode by covert video-recording, but thereafter the mother readily confessed that she had held her forcibly to her chest ('I held her too tight. I didn't mean to hurt her—I was jealous of her—I love her just too much.)' No further episodes occurred; the baby was fostered and the mother continued to receive strong psychiatric support.

Comment.   This was another typical case of 'active Meadow syndrome'. The final confrontation with the diagnosis was delayed because of a number of confusing factors, such as barium demonstration of sliding hiatus hernia, intermittent reduction of apparent cutaneous oxygen saturation when the mother was not present, and the observation by a staff nurse of a limp attack with supposed asystole again with the mother not present.

CASE 8.8

A girl with a history of tachypnoea and wheezy episodes in infancy began to have

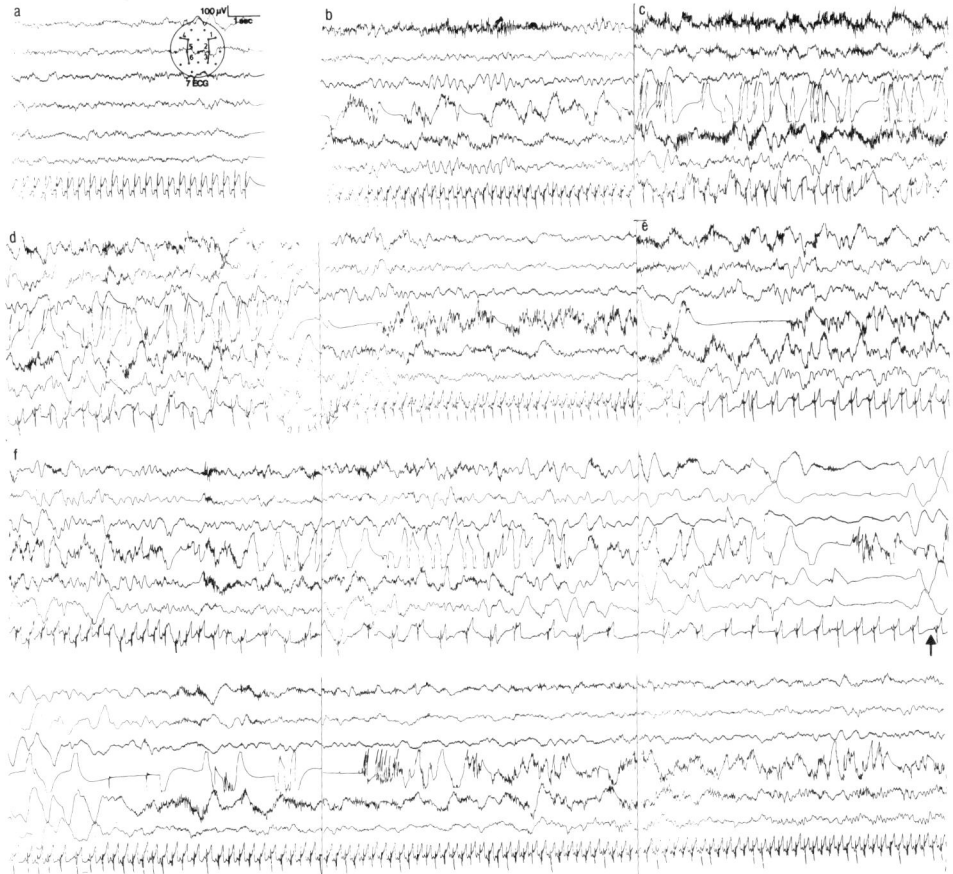

Fig. 8.6. Extracts from 24-hour cassette EEG/ECG recording of 10-month-old girl with apnoeic attacks and convulsions (Case 8.7): *(a)* sample of recording 12 hours before the event; *(b–f)* samples from the recording while the mother was suffocating the baby in the hospital ward, beginning four minutes before she pressed the event button and called the nurse—these five samples are at one-minute intervals. Fluctuating heart rate, intermittent EEG slowing, and superimposed movement artefact and muscle potentials are apparent. In *(f)* the EEG disappears completely for about four seconds before the event button is pressed (at the arrow), after which there is an almost immediate speeding of the heart rate to tachycardia and the EEG normalizes within five seconds.

stereotyped episodes at the age of 18 months. They were characterized by collapse with extreme pallor, rigidity, extension of upper and lower limbs, florid beetroot colour and recovery often with vomiting. She was found to have severe pulmonary hypertension, and a membrane of obscure pathology almost dividing her left ventricular cavity. After this was excised she was free of attacks for six months. Then they recurred in a typical episode at the age of 6, described by her parents as follows: 'She had been walking slowly along a street when she complained of a sore tummy. We stopped and let her rest. The pain didn't go away. I lifted her in my arms and during that time (about a minute and a half) she went

79

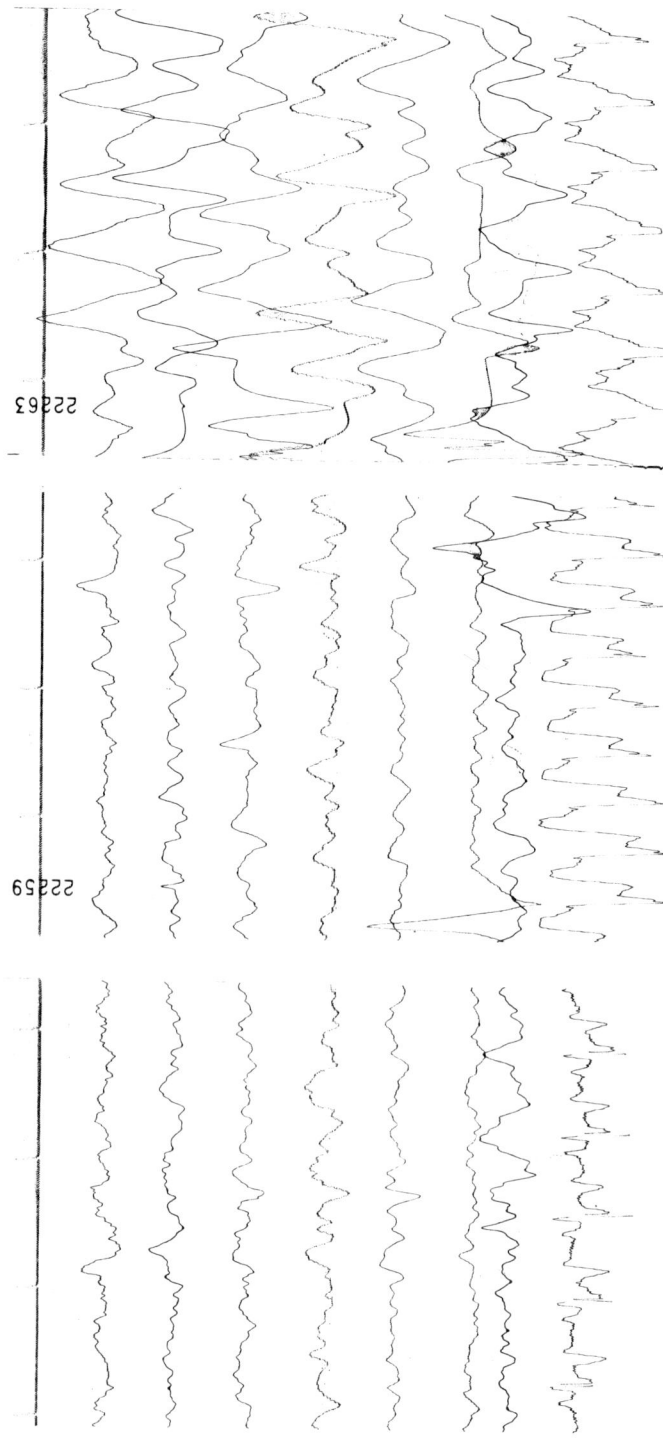

Fig. 8.7. Extracts from seven-channel EEG/ECG cassette recording of an anoxic seizure due to paroxysmal acute (on-chronic) pulmonary hypertension (Case 8.8). Time marker (upper trace) = 1 sec.

(*a*) One minute before episode. Abnormal ECG (lower trace) evident, rate 90 per minute. EEG normal.

(*b*) 30 seconds after acute alteration in ST segment of ECG, and 20 seconds after change to the ECG configuration shown. Heart rate 144 per minute. EEG has not yet slowed.

(*c*) 30 seconds after the end of (*b*). EEG began to slow 25 seconds previously and is now barely over one per second. QRST distortion is more prominent, rate 120 per minute.

Slow activity disappears from the EEG and the QRST complexes begin to revert to their previous form 10 to 15 seconds after the end of this tracing.

80

unconscious. She gave one kick with both legs to straighten them and her whole body went rigid. At this time she had no colour in her face but her lips were almost black. Then, still unconscious, she lost control of both bladder and bowel. After three or four minutes she started to come round and was then very tired.'

ECG rhythm did not change during episodes, but combined EEG/ECG ambulatory cassette monitoring revealed the sequence shown in Figure 8.7, with evidence of cardiac followed by cerebral ischaemia. It was interpreted that she was having repeated extreme paroxysmal pulmonary hypertension with cessation of cerebral circulation. She is on the waiting list for heart and lung transplantation at the time of writing.

Comment. Initially, scepticism greeted the proposal that this girl was having repeated anoxic seizures because the more common mechanisms had been excluded. Confidence that an anoxic mechanism must be acting motivated very long ambulatory cassette monitoring which allowed confirmation of the nature of the attacks.

CASE 8.9

This girl first presented at 3½ years with a story of numerous blackouts since the age of 6 months. The usual sequence was that following a minor injury she would cry, become bluish and unconscious, and have a tonic spasm of the arms and hands so that her arms went up and twisted; then after 60 seconds she would regain consciousness but remain lifeless for about 15 minutes afterwards, complaining of headache. Often she would wet herself in the episode. Her mother's mother had had fainting fits. An attack (with an asystole of 17 seconds) was reproduced by ocular compression, following which she was briefly disorientated and found to have been incontinent of urine.

Ten years later she was referred to the paediatric cardiologist because of ventricular ectopic beats. An ECG had been done by the paediatrician because of two recent abrupt syncopes following injuries to her hand and elbow. After these episodes she felt tired the whole day and complained of an unusual smell which no-one else noted. In the event, no cardiac abnormality was detected.

Comment. Reflex vagocardiac syncopes are by no means confined to early childhood. The anoxic seizures found in ventricular tachyarrhythmias and QT syndromes (see Chapter 8) do not have precisely the same provocations, albeit there is an overlap which still has to be explored.

CASE 8.10

A 9-year-old girl had fainting spells, or fainting fits, since the age of 5. They were usually after a knock, or falling over, having her throat examined, or some sort of injurious or stressful situation. She would know she was having it and feel something in her tummy beforehand and the sensation of a kind of shaking. One had occurred two years before when she was lying on her bed supine and her mother was trying to get a splinter out of her finger: she said she felt funny and her face was pale grey, her eyes went into the back of her head and she had tremors, and her arms bent stiffly. Some of the faints were ordinary faints rather than fainting fits, with a ratio of perhaps 3:2. The last one of these, said the mother, was a 'definite fit': she had knocked her elbow and came to tell her mother about it straight away. 'Then she said she felt funny, and looked grey as if she was going to faint, and then she slumped to the floor and started shaking, with her arms bent and tremoring and stiff for a matter of seconds, and she was foaming at the mouth and heavy breathing, spitting, and she made a sort of snort and then came to very tired and went to sleep.'

An EEG with an ECG channel in operation was carried out in the supine position (Fig. 7.6, p. 50). She was alert and cooperative, but apprehensive. After 30 seconds the ECG slowed from 84 beats per minute to 72, 60, 66, 54, and 48 in successive 10 seconds epochs.

Then, that is to say 80 seconds after the onset of the EEG, she said she was going to faint, went pale, and her left arm went up towards her head and she flexed stiffly. On the ECG channel there was an asystole of 14 seconds which began a few seconds before she said she was going to faint, and which was followed nine seconds later by diffuse EEG slowing and then by seven seconds of EEG flattening before return of EEG slowing and then the recovery of the EEG to normal. The colour gradually returned to her face and she said that before the episode she had had a funny feeling in her tummy.

Comment. This is an excellent example of a vagocardiac syncope such as is discussed in Chapter 9. With the clear-cut history the EEG was not necessary, but had been arranged on the basis of the referring letter. In the event, there was a rare capture of a common phenomenon.

CASE 8.11
Two adult patients were described to me in 1982 by Dr Fred Plum of the New York Hospital—Cornell Medical Center (*personal communication*). He wrote: 'Personal observations were both made on patients with polyneuropathy of the Guillain–Barré type and associated respiratory failure. Each had profound anxiety related to his helplessness, both having many years before been Jewish prisoners in a German concentration camp. The crucial issue in both instances was that of strange attendants briefly interrupting the action of a body (tank-type) respirator and in seconds, the patients being found pulseless, unconscious, and clinically asystolic. The onset of unconsciousness in the supine position was much too short to be explained by simple hypotension and the return of cardiac action with quickly administered chest CPR [cardiopulmonary resuscitation] was associated with striking auscultatory arrhythmia for subsequent 5–10 minutes. I published neither case because in the absence of monitoring (the patients were cared for several years ago), I reasoned that I probably could never convince skeptics that this wasn't simply profound vasodepressor syncope. My reasons for not thinking so, of course, were the very rapid onset of unconsciousness, the lack of parasympathetic systemic responses, and the rhythm irregularities during recovery.'

Comment. Professor Plum regarded these cases as examples of vagally mediated reflex cardiac asystole. He thought that the matter was clinically most important but that information was 'almost impossible to document'. In this book some attempt has been made to remedy this, especially in the following chapter.

9
VAGOCARDIAC SYNCOPE AND REFLEX ANOXIC SEIZURES

There are two reasons for devoting a separate chapter to the subject of anoxic seizures resulting from cardiac asystole of vagal origin but not involving vagovagal reflexes. The first lies in the importance (both in the English sense of being of significance and concern and in the French quantitative sense of considerable number) of such seizures in the differential diagnosis of epilepsy at all ages. The second is that precise diagnosis may allow not simply reassurance but also appropriate management of these dramatic syncopes (Fitzpatrick and Sutton 1989, Milstein *et al.* 1989).

Vagal-mediated asystole, not involving vagovagal reflexes, has been frequently documented (Table 9.I; see also Table 9.IV). In this chapter I will outline the artificial induction of asystole by ocular compression and by head-up tilt-testing, and then describe a series of 41 patients in whom the evidence for vagal cardio-inhibitory anoxic seizures seems strong (McWilliam and Stephenson, *unpublished data*).

Ocular compression
In the world of fits and faints ocular compression has been used to elicit the oculocardiac reflex in the study of vagal syncopes and as part of their management (Stephenson 1980).

The oculocardiac reflex was discovered independently by Aschner (1908) and Dagnini (1908). It is a brainstem reflex with the afferent limb being the ophthalmic division of the fifth nerve and the efferent path the vagus. The cell bodies of the cardio-inhibitory vagal neurons lie in the nucleus ambiguus (Chen and Chai 1976). An injection of bicuculline into the nucleus ambiguus leads to sinus arrest, which is reversed by the GABA* agonist muscinol (diMicco *et al.* 1979), and it is evident that the reflex 'fires' by disinhibition at this site. Although for practical purposes the reflex is regarded as being mediated by vagal acetylcholine, full atropinization does not inhibit it completely (Stephenson 1979a), the residual slowing being mediated by inhibition of cardiac accelerator fibres (Gandevia *et al.* 1978).

Normal responses
Although the evolutionary significance of the oculocardiac reflex is not clear, it is part of normal physiology and is used, for example, in the intensive care unit (Born *et al.* 1985) as one of the tests of the integrity of the brainstem. The limited amount of normative data available is shown in Table 9.II. The response is normally gauged

*GABA: γ-aminobutyric acid.

TABLE 9.I

Documented convulsive vagal asystole in patients with apparently normal hearts (excluding asystoles induced by specific internal or external vagal reflexes or by head-up tilt)

Author(s)	Sex	Age (yrs.)	Age at onset (yrs.)	Provocation	Posture	Duration of asystole (secs.)	Specific treatment
Symonds (1950)	M	Young adult	?	Examination by doctor	?Sitting	45	—
Greenfield (1951)	M	19	19	Patient made to drink blood he had just seen withdrawn from another person's arm	Sitting	11*	—
Lombroso and Lerman (1967)	F	2⁶/₁₂	?	EEG (?attempt to give sedative)	Supine	22***	—
Duvernoy et al. (1980)	F	21	'long ago'	Venepuncture	?	16*	Pacemaker
	F	19	19	Venepuncture	?	11*	Pacemaker
Hand and Schröder (1980)	M	19	7	Venepuncture	?	27*	Psychological (deconditioning)
Braham et al. (1981)	M	21	12	Needle into muscle	?Supine	58***†	Atropine
Gordon (1982)	F	12	—	Sight of scalp drip	Fell down	14***	—
Roddy et al. (1983)	F	11	3	Venepuncture	Supine	16***	—
Stephenson (1983a)	M	2⁶/₁₂	⁹/₁₂	Head bump	Fell down	22***‡	Atropine
Stephenson (unpublished)	F	9	5	EEG	Supine	14**	—
Ector et al. (1984)	M	23	?	Sport	?	30*	Pacemaker

*ECG recorded; **ECG and EEG recorded; ***ECG and EEG published.
†Also 11 secs. (*unpublished*); ‡ also 14 secs. (*unpublished*).

TABLE 9.II
Ocular compression: normative data for asystole in the supine position

Study	Population	Total sample	Asystole >4 secs. N	(%)
Lombroso and Lerman (1967)	Children (well 33, epilepsy 21, retardation or behaviour problems 13, non-neurological diseases 16)	83	0	(—)
Stephenson (1978*d*)	Children (miscellaneous disorders, excluding epilepsy, reflex anoxic seizures and febrile convulsions)	93	1	(1.1)
Kahn *et al.* (1983)	Infants aged 2–3 months (69 normal, 76 siblings of SIDS victims, 35 'near miss' infants)	180	4	(2.2)
Ramet *et al.* (1988)	Healthy preterm and full-term neonates during REM sleep	33	0	(—)

as the maximum duration of 'asystole', this being the maximum R-R interval induced during or after the compression. In their studies Lombroso and Lerman (1967) attempted to use a constant pressure, and more recently Ramet *et al.* (1988) have attempted to measure the pressure exerted. In the study of Kahn *et al.* (1983) the operator was blind to the diagnosis.

Method
The procedure used in ocular compression was detailed in an appendix to Stephenson (1980). It may be helpful here to restate those numbered points, amended in the light of further experience.

In the first place the operator should be satisfied that the procedure is justified. Justification would normally be either the reproduction of an unusual episode for diagnostic purposes, or the reproduction of a standard asystolic anoxic seizure in the presence of a parent as an aid to management.

(1) Preceding examination and history to exclude serious heart or ocular disease is wise practice but not of proven relevance.

(2) The test should always be carried out by a physician in the EEG department with telephone connection to other hospital departments, but no *additional* precautions need be taken with regard to potential resuscitation.

(3) The child (in this description little modification is necessary for adults) lies supine on a non-slip table with a thin mattress and firm head-rest. Preparations are made for the EEG and ECG recording. The child is laid on a sheet in case wrapping is needed for initial restraint.

(4) EEG electrodes are placed in the usual manner. Usually eight channels are used. A smaller number increases the chance of contamination of the recording by movement artefact in a seizure.

(5) ECG electrodes are attached, preferably to the chest, and two channels of ECG are recorded simultaneously on the same paper as the EEG.

(6) Meanwhile, the history is retaken from both the patient if old enough and the parent or witness.

(7) Standard EEG is performed with hyperventilation if possible and stroboscopic activation, but it is possible to omit this step if the test is solely for management purposes.

(8) The parent (or attendant) and the patient are told, in terms which they can understand, that the last part of the test is to press the eyes for 10 seconds and to see the effect on the recording, and that the test is harmless though it may look and feel unpleasant. In some cases it has been possible to induce rapid hypnosis with analgesia and amnesia (Case 9.44).

(9) Crying which includes hyperventilation appears to inhibit the oculocardiac reflex, presumably by raising the blood pH and inhibiting the depressant action of acetylcholine on the heart (Gesell *et al.* 1944). Therefore if the child cannot be quietened we use a two litre paper bag (such as is used to hold disposable aluminium trays), holding it over the child's nose and mouth to allow rebreathing for two minutes, guessing that the pCO_2 level will by then have risen towards normal (see also Blanc *et al.* 1983).

(10) Occasionally a child will vomit, so we always have a disposable 'potty' handy for use.

(11) The doctor performing the ocular compression (the operator) stands on a low non-slip stool *behind* the child's head and adjusts his or her watch so that the second hand will be visible during the compression.

(12) The operator asks the technician if s/he is ready yet: if so, s/he begins to make an audible signal of the heartbeat by tapping a ball pen on the flat metal section of the EEG machine in time with the ECG complexes.

(13) The operator places the palmar aspects of his/her fingers on either side of the patient's face and head, and the thumbs gently over the closed eyelids, speaking reassuringly.

(14) The operator again asks if the technician is ready.

(15) Noting the position of the second hand of the watch and saying 'now', the operator presses the eyes (under the closed eyelids, below the supra-orbital ridges) firmly backwards (towards the floor), using sufficient pressure to blanch the thumb nail beds for two millimetres. The pressure is maintained for exactly 10 seconds.

(16) During the compression an assistant either holds the patient or uses the sheet as a wrap to reduce ECG electrode disturbance. If an anoxic seizure (from cardiac asystole) or an anoxic-epileptic seizure is induced, the child is no longer held or restrained.

(17) Formerly, if the child had an anoxic or anoxic-epileptic seizure the operator would give a running commentary of what was happening and the technician would rapidly transcribe this onto the EEG paper so that the events could later be correlated. Split-screen video recording now makes much of this unnecessary. The operator does not look concerned or touch the patient and, aside from describing the fits, awaits recovery. S/he is helped in this relaxed attitude by getting an audible signal of the heartbeat restarting tapped by the technician while the seizure is still continuing. While asystole persists, the operator is reassured by the knowledge that the heart will start

automatically.

(18) The patient and witnesses are then strongly reassured.

(19) If an asystole-mediated anoxic seizure has been induced in the child, the operator immediately shows the mother the combined EEG and ECG recording (both being printed out simultaneously on the same piece of paper) and demonstrates that the heart was beating again when the seizure was manifest. This demonstration that the child is actually recovering or has recovered while still in the seizure is in itself reassuring. (If the patient is an adult this demonstration is given later.) If an anoxic-epileptic seizure has been induced, more complicated explanations are indicated. If a split-screen video recording has been undertaken then seizures can be replayed to the parents or patient.

(20) (Instead of and supplementary to 20–22 in the previous appendix) The parent or other witness is questioned closely as to the difference or similarity between the induced seizure and the child's natural attacks, both with respect to details and in terms of 'severity'.

Complications

When used in the awake child for the purposes described (excluding its use in the treatment of supraventricular tachycardia and accidental evocation during ophthalmic surgery), the test has been without complication in many thousands of patients (Bridge *et al.* 1943; Gastaut and Fischer-Williams 1957; Gastaut and Gastaut 1957, 1958; Fildisevski 1961; Gastaut *et al.* 1961*b*, Maulsby and Kellaway 1964; Lombroso and Lerman 1967; Gastaut 1968, 1974; Stephenson 1978*a,b*; Lehovský *et al.* 1979; Stephenson and Ounsted 1982; Kahn *et al.* 1983; Lucet *et al.* 1984; Ramet *et al.* 1988).

Concern about ocular trauma has been voiced. Lombroso and Lerman (1967) did not recommend ocular compression in high myopia, and Bower (1984) remarked, 'Eyeball compression may seem repugnant, even punitive, and damage to the eyes, perhaps in the long-term, cannot be excluded.' So far as I know, the only documented evidence of ocular damage was a case of rupture of the globe in an 81-year-old woman (Mathis *et al.* 1982): in this case the ocular compression was being undertaken to terminate a paroxysmal tachycardia and, as it happened, vision recovered adequately. There seems to be no theoretical reason for concern about duration of asystole in the awake oxygenated patient. The maximum elicited is about 36 seconds (Manson, *personal communication*), which is well below the peak figures for asystole after injection (Braham *et al.* 1981—see Table 9.I) or after head-up tilt (Abi-Samra *et al.* 1988—see Table 9.IV). Ventricular fibrillation has been described after ocular compression, but only in a case of paroxysmal supraventricular tachycardia (Landman and Ehrenfeld 1952). In theory it would be possible for a ventricular tachyarrhythmia to be induced in a patient with such a tendency (see pp. 66–67), but this would be a non-specific effect and examination of the throat would be equally disastrous (McKinlay, *personal communication*). The concerns of Mallinson and Coombes (1960) about death from ocular compression appear to be unsubstantiated.

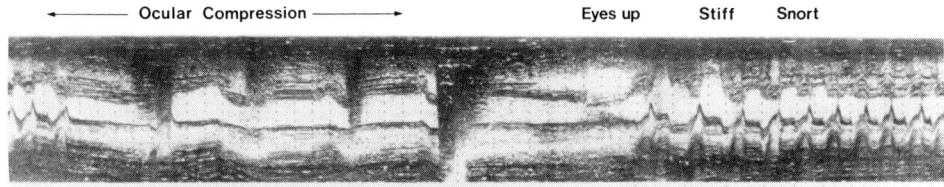

Fig. 9.1. Echocardiogram during ocular compression. Vertical dotted lines are time markers at intervals of 0.5 secs. The large, dark, downward deflexions from the top of the trace are related to respiration. The upward-pointing notches relate to mitral valve movement and correspond to the ECG signals in the bottom line. Note the different slope of the second and third deflexions. This trace was taken simultaneously with the EEG and ECG shown in Figure 9.2.

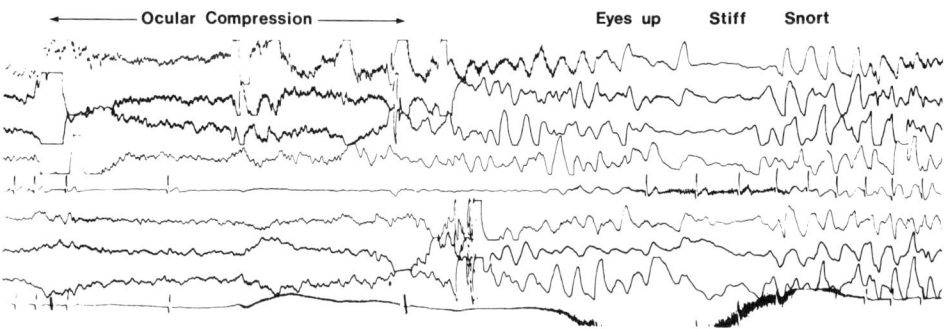

Fig. 9.2. EEG and ECG responses to ocular compression in the child whose echocardiogram is shown in Figure 9.1 (Stephenson 1978*a*).

Controlled gentle ocular compression

Ramet *et al.* (1988) have advanced the scientific and humanitarian aspects of ocular compression studies. Ramet's technique involves the use of disc-shaped, water-filled pressure sensors of external diameter 18mm, which are gently placed on the infant's eyelids and manually pressed abruptly to a pressure of around 100mmHg (103±9) for 10 seconds. Thus a square-wave stimulus is applied. This does not cause distress nor alert sleeping infants. It is necessary to correct a minor mis-understanding which led Aicardi (1986) to suggest that ocular compression 'may not be without danger'. This refers to a young child who had an asystole of somewhat over 20 seconds and an anoxic seizure after ocular compression by the technique described. Actually, the parents regarded the episode as *less* severe than the child's natural attacks (Ramet, *personal communication*).

'Abnormal' results

As indicated above, only a few publications give normative data: these are summarized in Table 9.II. (Quantitative data relating to the ophthalmic induction of the oculocardiac reflex—Blanc *et al.* 1983—are not relevant in this connection.) Normative data for the *oculorespiratory* reflex (Gastaut and Gastaut 1958, Blanc *et al.* 1988) with ocular compression as the stimulus are not available. Discussion will therefore be confined to the cardiac effect. Different authors have suggested different durations of asystole as 'abnormal', but with regard to differential diagnostic power, less arbitrariness is involved if a receiver operating characteristic (ROC) curve is constructed. In one such study, detailed later in this chapter (pp. 92–95), an ROC curve is constructed plotting the sensitivity of different cut-off levels of asystole duration against 1-specificity*, comparing 39 children with vagocardiac anoxic seizures against 102 children with febrile seizures of epileptic mechanism previously reported by Stephenson and Ounsted (1982) and Stephenson (1983*a*). It will be seen that the inflection in the curve is sharpest at about six to seven seconds, which would therefore become the level of diagnostic abnormality.

An example of a 10-second ocular compression, with its effect on mitral valve movement as shown by echocardiography, is shown in Figure 9.1. The electrical correlates are shown in Figure 9.2, with the ECG, EEG and superimposed EMG most obvious on the lower ECG channel.

Duplicate ocular compression results on the same patient at different times are illustrated in Figure 9.3. Included in this figure are data on three monozygotic twin pairs, all showing markedly excessive responses. In one of these pairs only one twin had been affected by reflex anoxic seizures at the time of the compression, but the second twin had naturally induced attacks soon after. Familial hyper-reactivity of the oculocardiac reflex is a matter of interest to ophthalmologists (Arnold *et al.* 1988).

Response latency
In the series of Ramet *et al.* (1988), latency of response (defined as the time between the application of ocular pressure and the first measurable R-R interval increase, compared to the mean control R-R + one standard deviation) varied from 433 to 5200 milliseconds, approximately two-thirds being over 1600 milliseconds. In my series of induced anoxic seizures, the latency was much less, 58 per cent having no more than one systole before asystole after the onset of ocular compression (Table 9.III).

Reproduction of anoxic seizures
The prime clinical value of ocular compression has been the induction of asystolic seizures of unusual characteristics and determining whether they are identical to those occurring naturally in that patient. This aspect is illustrated in many case histories in this book (see especially Case 4.9) and has been particularly helpful in the case of anoxic-epileptic seizures (see Chapter 11).

Tilt testing
Although the specificity has been questioned (deMay and Enterling 1986), head-up

*For definition, see Stephenson and King (1989, p. 229).

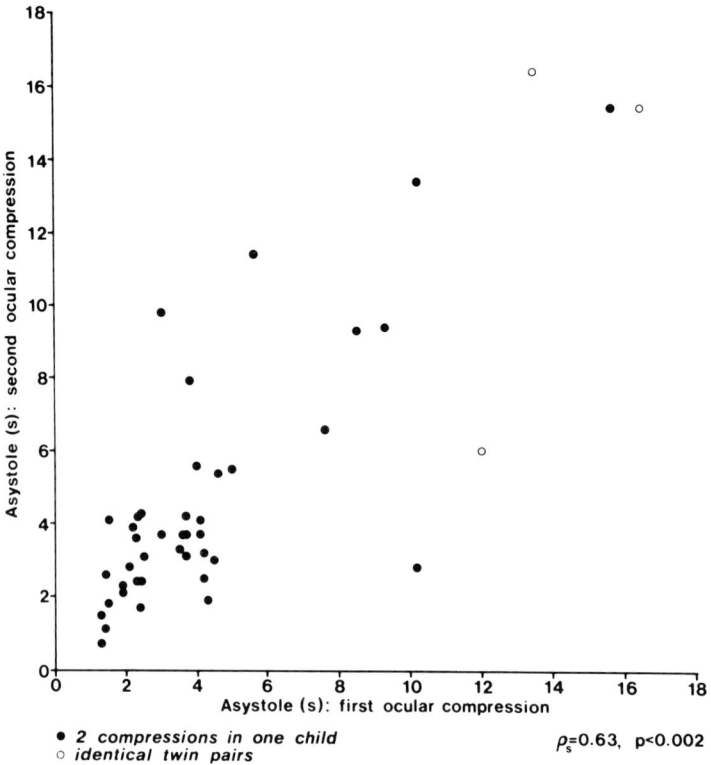

Fig. 9.3. Results of repeating ocular compression (OC) on a second occasion in 41 children, together with results of single determinations in three pairs of monozygotic twins (*i.e.* in each pair, first OC in one twin, second OC in other twin).

tilt is increasingly being studied in the evaluation of syncope (Kenny 1986; Kenny *et al.* 1986*a,b*, 1987; Grossi *et al.* 1987; Abi-Samra *et al.* 1988; Fitzpatrick and Sutton 1989). Results from the latter three studies are shown in Table 9.IV. The test has been used up to old age but one can see that older children also are being studied. From the cardiovascular response, patients have been classified as having autonomic dysfunction, vasodepressor syncope or vasovagal syncope. It is not always clear from the available publications what proportion of those who appear to have vasovagal syncope—that is, have bradycardia on head-up tilt—have significant asystole. The percentage seems quite low, although very long values have been published, in particular the 73-second asystole after 60° tilt recorded by Maloney *et al.* (1988). The comparatively low (from my point of view) proportion of asystolic responses may reflect the nature of the patients entering these studies. Tilt testing is often carried out in cardiological or cardiovascular laboratories with an entry criterion of unexplained syncope. One may speculate as to how many patients with anoxic motor seizure (convulsive syncope) will not have been studied

TABLE 9.III

Latency of asystole after onset of ocular compression in 296
induced anoxic seizures

Asystole latency*	Anoxic seizures N	% (cumulative)
0	65	22.0
1	107	58.1
2	74	83.1
3	35	94.9
4–7	14	99.7
11 ('tardive')	1	100.0

*See text for definition.

TABLE 9.IV

Asystole on tilt testing (without drug infusion*): three published series

Study	Degree of tilt	Age of patients (yrs.) Mean	SD	Syncopal on tilt N	Asystole N	%	Duration (secs.)	Symptoms
Grossi et al. (1987)	70°	24.6 (range 10–48)	11	28	8	28.6	2.2–11.7 (mean 6.3, SD 3.5)	Convulsive syncope in eight (without sinus arrest in two)
Abi-Samra et al. (1988)	60°	56	13.4	63	7	11.1	5–73	Not stated (syncopes)[1]
Fitzpatrick and Sutton (1989)	60°	68	10	53	5[2]	9.4	10–25	'. . twitching of head and arms at about 2Hz; arms may flail about rather alarmingly'; longest asystole accompanied by 'slight twitching motions in the limbs'[3]

*In the Minnesota tilt-test series of Almquist et al. (1989) and Milstein et al. (1989), isoprenaline (USA—isoproterenol) infusion was used (see text).
[1]The 39-year-old man who had 73 secs. asystole induced by tilt is described in a separate publication (Maloney et al. 1988) as having brief myoclonic jerks during the first few seconds of unconsciousness. His natural attacks had begun in *early childhood*.
[2]Only asystoles over 10 secs. listed.
[3]Fitzpatrick, *personal communication*.

because of a prior assumption that epilepsy was the diagnosis. It is of interest that the highest proportion of asystoles in reported convulsive syncopes came from a neurological department (Grossi *et al.* 1987).

The Minneapolis school has employed isoprenaline (USA—isoproterenol) infusion as an adjunct to tilt testing to increase the probability of ('paradoxically') inducing bradycardia in vagally mediated syncope (Almquist *et al.* 1989, Milstein *et al.* 1989). Of particular significance is the finding that patients with evidence of spontaneous (including exercise-induced) syncope behaved on tilt testing (with or

TABLE 9.V

Selection criteria for study of vagocardiac reflex anoxic seizures

1. Precipitations include head bump, pain, fright or surprise.
2. History is of convulsive syncope (anoxic seizure).
3. Cyanotic breath-holding excluded by one or more of:
   a) age of onset over 3½ years;
   b) persistence after 8 years;
   c) specifically no breath-holding;
   d) abolition by atropine.
4. Vasovagal syncope excluded by one or more of:
   a) lack of conspicuous pallor;
   b) abrupt onset;
   c) occurrence supine.

without isoprenaline infusion) in the same manner as those with conventional 'fainting' (vasovagal syncope, 'neurally mediated hypotension-bradycardia') (Milstein *et al.* 1989).

As yet there are few published data on tilt testing in children. Grossi *et al.* (1987) gave an illustration of the EEG/ECG and respiration of a 10-year-old girl who had 8.4 seconds asystole with sinus arrest and about 10 seconds high-voltage slow activity on the EEG in her syncope. Jaeger *et al.* (1990), using a positive ocular compression test (three seconds or more, mean five seconds) to select older children (mean 14 years) for head-up tilt, found that 11 of 16 with recurrent unexplained loss of consciousness reproduced their episodes, two of them with asystole and convulsive syncope.

Although it must be admitted that there is a lot to learn about the sensitivity and specificity of this test, and the effect of age (it may be unsuitable under the age of 10), it has the potential for repeated non-invasive within-patient studies, particularly to look at the effect of therapy (*e.g.* scopolamine—Abi-Samra *et al.* 1988; pacemakers—Kenny *et al.* 1986*a,b*; Fitzpatrick and Sutton 1989).

Clinical study of vagocardiac anoxic seizures

In 1983 Dr Robert McWilliam and I presented a paper to the British Paediatric Neurology Association entitled 'Reflex arrest of the heart as a cause of non-epileptic seizures: cardiovagal not vasovagal convulsive syncope.' The study population comprised those children attending the EEG department of the Royal Hospital for Sick Children, Glasgow, during the preceding five years, and their parents. Data were collected prospectively, but the study itself was retrospective. Over the five years covered, 41 patients had been seen who satisfied the entry criteria listed in Table 9.V—that is, they had a clinical history suggesting convulsive syncope after specific precipitating stimuli, but the story of their convulsive syncope was neither typical of breath-holding attacks nor of vasovagal attacks ('fainting'). Potted case histories of all 41 are to be found at the end of this chapter (Cases 9.1 to 9.41) and readers may judge whether they think that the mechanism is as postulated.

TABLE 9.VI

Evidence of asystole in 11 of 41 patients with clinical vagocardiac reflex anoxic seizures

Atropine effective: criterion	5
finding	2
No pulse in attack	3
No heartbeat in attack	2
No ECG in attack	2
Flat EEG in attack	2
Atropine evidence only	5
Other evidence	6

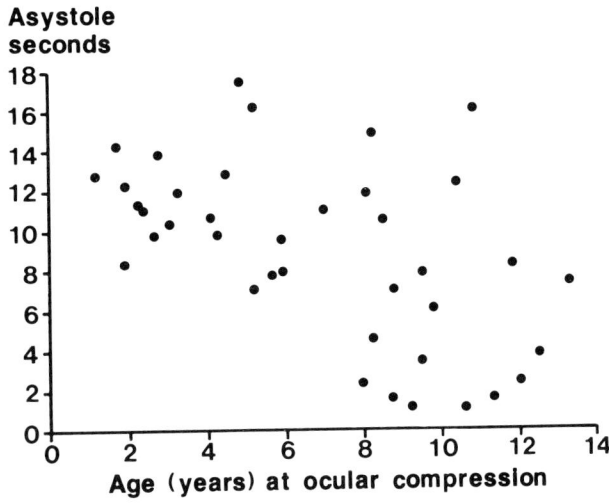

Fig. 9.4. Duration of ocular compression induced asystole in 39 children who had a clinical diagnosis of vagocardiac reflex anoxic seizures. (The two adults in the series did not have ocular compression.)

More direct evidence that cardiac asystole was involved in these anoxic seizures is outlined in Table 9.VI, relating to 11 patients. In some, more than one piece of evidence applied. It should be noted that abolition of attacks by atropine was a criterion for entry to the study but in two patients it was additional evidence after entry.

Ocular compression was carried out on all the 39 children in this study (ages 20 months to 13 years). The individual asystole values are shown in Figure 9.4. It is evident that as a group these children showed markedly excessive responses to ocular compression, consistently so before the age of 8 years. It must be

93

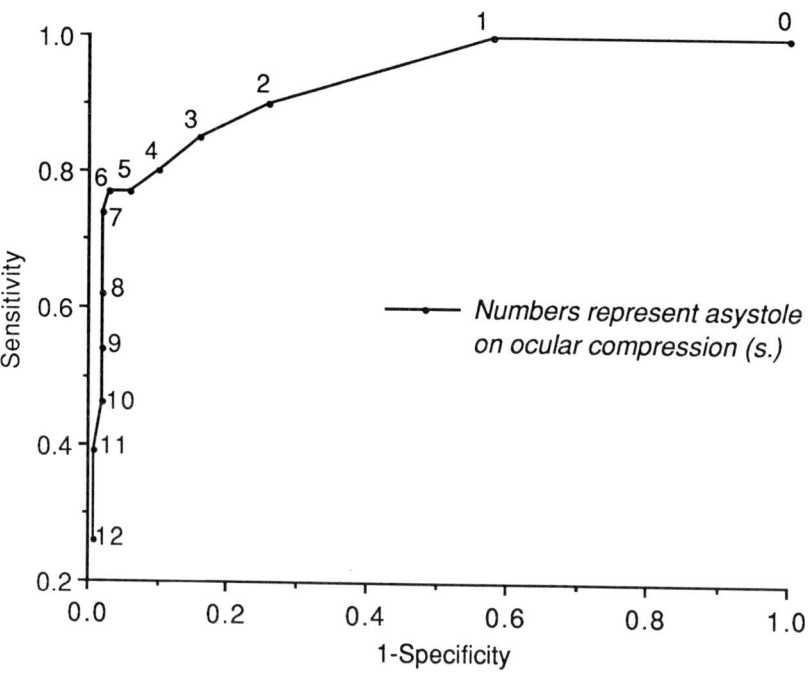

RECEIVER OPERATING CHARACTERISTIC (ROC)

Fig. 9.5. Receiver operating characteristic (ROC) curve constructed to discover what is an 'abnormal' duration of asystole in response to ocular compression. 'Sensitivity' is a measure of the true positive rate of the test and 'one minus specificity' is a measure of the false positive rate (see Stephenson and King 1989 for further details). To construct the curve a group of 39 children with cardiovagal syncope (see text) has been compared with a group of 102 children (those with epileptic febrile convulsions shown in Fig. 15.2, p. 171) thought *not* to have cardiovagal syncope. It can be seen that with a cut-off level of 2 seconds asystole there is a substantial proportion of false positives, whereas with a 10-second cut-off false negatives predominate (*i.e.* most of the children with cardiovagal syncope would be classed as having a negative ocular compression result). The cut-off of 6 seconds at the inflexion of the curve best minimizes false positives and false negatives and is thus the derived 'abnormal' value.

emphasized that this was a *finding* of the study and not a criterion for entry. The method of plotting a receiver operating characteristic curve (Fig. 9.5) allows one to see that if one wishes to use ocular compression as a diagnostic test then an induced asystole of 6 seconds duration or more is most efficient at maximizing the true positive rate (sensitivity) and minimizing false positives (1-specificity). All the children under 8 years in this study had an abnormal ocular compression result using this derived cut-off figure of 6 seconds asystole.

We would propose that the clinical and investigative evidence strongly suggests that short-latency vagal-mediated cardiac asystole was the mechanism of the anoxic seizures in these patients. Whether this should be regarded as a form of 'malignant' vasovagal syncope of cardio-inhibitory type (Fitzpatrick and Sutton 1989) or

TABLE 9.VII

**Aberrant management* in 23 patients with
vagocardiac reflex anoxic seizures**

Treated for epilepsy	12†
Epilepsy diagnosed (but not treated)	6‡
'Head injury'	2
Cardiac arrest treatment	2
Intensive care unit	1
Elective surgery postponed	1‡

*Paediatrician, general practitioner, neurologist, general physician, anaesthetist, paediatric surgeon, urologist or obstetrician.
†One to four anti-epileptic drugs, median two per patient; duration one to nine years, median four.
‡One child had epilepsy diagnosed *and* had elective surgery postponed.

'neurally mediated hypotension-bradycardia' (Milstein *et al.* 1989) is open to debate. Further explanation of the mechanism is in order, but whatever its precise nature, clinical and epidemiological studies of seizures should now recognize that this is an established entity, not confined to a particular age-group (see Case 9.42) and frequently mismanaged (Table 9.VII; Case 9.43).

Case histories
Cases 9.1 to 9.41 are those included in the five-year study of vagocardiac reflex anoxic seizures reported above. The remaining cases refer to other patients seen outside this time-frame. Comments are confined to those cases in which it is felt a particular point deserves special emphasis.

CASE 9.1
The 26-year-old father of an 8-year-old boy with reflex syncope commented: 'I wonder if this is anything to do with it? All my life, whenever I bump myself or have nothing to eat I flake out. Once, when lying in bed, feeling a bit sick, I felt it coming on, passed out and wet myself. Last month I was lying down for this IVP [intravenous pyelogram]—they injected the drug into the vein. The doctor said: "Take deep breaths, you'll probably feel sick." I could feel the sickness coming on and the next thing I knew I had woken up and they were banging on my chest. The doctor said that he had felt for the pulse and that there was nothing there. The next thing the cardiac team were all around me. The doctor said: ". . . convulsed there." I heard this as I came out, when they were about to put a needle into my heart.' The urologist confirmed the father's story.

Comment. Something akin to dominant inheritance is common in these cases but has not been examined in detail.

CASE 9.2
A 4-year-old girl had many tonic seizures induced by passing constipated stools since infancy. Marked bradycardia was documented when her anus and rectum were examined under anaesthetic. Similar episodes were precipitated by being put in a bath, having her hair washed, and fever.

CASE 9.3

A 4-year-old girl had five tonic seizures, sometimes with urination, in the previous year. All were precipitated by bumps to the back of her head. Urination occurred during the asystole induced by ocular compression.

CASE 9.4

A girl aged 2½ years had a history of holding her breath without crying immediately after every painful stimulus since infancy. Her father had been similarly affected. After a bath she bumped herself, took a breath, went limp and glazed and white, with eyes rolling and large pupils. She then went stiff straight out in her mother's arms and 'jerked across'. After this, and just as her eyes were beginning to follow, she vomited and then stopped breathing and became limp and motionless. Her mother, who was a trained nurse, put her onto the floor on her side, sucked and then breathed into her mouth. She thought the child was already dead. When the ambulance arrived an airway was put in and both mother and child were taken to the intensive care unit. Then the child cried and spoke to her mother.

Two days later, ocular compression supine induced an asystole of about 10 seconds with an anoxic seizure. After coming round she was pale and slept for four hours. Her mother insisted that she be given atropine and that ocular compression studies be used to confirm protection against future attacks.

Comment. Details of this case have previously been reported by Stephenson (1979a) and Stephenson and Ounsted (1982). For commercial reasons, atropine methonitrate is no longer available; the best alternative medication for the very young has not yet been established.

CASE 9.5

A 5-year-old boy had three episodes of going stiff and incontinent of urine after bumping his head. On the most recent occasion he was walking along in a field after having been jokingly talked out of a row with his cousin. He tripped over a projection on the ground and fell. He cried a single scream, like temper, and as his mother pulled him up his back arched and she let him fall supine onto the ground. His head rocked, he made an 'ah-ah' noise and his eyes darted quickly. He was incontinent of urine and then came to and said, 'Where am I?' He had a headache and his eyes looked bloodshot.

CASE 9.6

This 8-year-old boy had had about 20 tonic seizures with his head back and an ashen white appearance. Most were precipitated by bumps to the head, others by falls, and he had also had one in church (see also Case 9.27 and pp. 159–160).

CASE 9.7

A 5-year-old girl had her worst episode when watching something unpleasant on the television. She felt strange, stood up and fell to the ground stiff, becoming white, followed by some cyanosis and then recovery. Similar episodes were induced by a head bump, getting a skelf (splinter) stuck in her hand, and having a plaster taken off an injury. The anoxic seizure on ocular compression was identical to the episodes witnessed by her mother.

CASE 9.8

A 13-year-old girl presented with a story of having had her first episode of unconsciousness at the age of 10 years. While dressing she had fallen down and become stiff with her arms and legs straight back and her eyes rolling, white in colour. Almost all episodes were preceded by accidental self-injury such as bumping her knee.

CASE 9.9
This 5-year-old girl had been treated for epilepsy in the preceding year. The first episode occurred at the age of 1½ years. She came over and said to her mother, 'My tummy. . !' and fell down. Her mother thought she had fainted but then she turned blue. The mother ran to her neighbours with the child in her arms and, thinking she was dead because she was not breathing and her eyes were 'empty', gave her the kiss of life. Further episodes were tonic, but admission to another hospital was prompted by a second-hand description of the supposed tonic-clonic seizure witnessed by her grandmother. She then had four episodes in hospital. One was described thus: '. . was wakened by father and talking to him for a few minutes when she suddenly fell backwards, became rigid and looked pale. It lasted two minutes.' On another occasion in hospital it was noted that 'her eyes became glazed, and she became unresponsive and fell to the ground, limbs rigid out but no twitching noticed by nursing staff.' A further episode occurred while she was sitting having blood taken from her. She fell backwards with back arched, and was pale, this lasting about one minute. Two minutes later, the pulse rate was 68 per minute. In fact, she said that whenever she saw a needle or saw blood she had 'this' in her head and that was what made her faint.

CASE 9.10
This 5-year-old boy was admitted to a surgical ward as a head injury case, having had two episodes of extensor spasm after bumping his right forehead falling off a swing. In fact he had had several episodes since the age of 6 months, precipitated by falling or particularly by bumping his head, in which he would become unconscious and go stiff and the colour would drain from his face, although he never looked as if he held his breath. The mother panicked on every occasion, but was much reassured after the reproduction of an anoxic seizure by ocular compression.

CASE 9.11
A 2½-year-old girl had been treated for epilepsy for the previous year, with several admissions to hospital. From the age of 14 months she had had more than 10 episodes in which she had fallen and become stiff and unresponsive, followed by irritability and diminished responsiveness for 20 minutes before a full recovery. At times the episodes had suggested myoclonic seizures to the paediatrician, while on other occasions a series of rhythmic symmetrical movements of arms and legs had been noted. No breath-holding had ever been noted either by her mother or by the attending doctors. In fact, all but two of the first 11 episodes were associated with minor head injury, such as falling over and bumping her head, and the more recent episodes were induced by other painful stimuli such as catching her finger in a door. Her mother recollected that she herself used to have similar episodes from around the age of 5 or 6 years, passing out when she hurt herself, for example by bumping her knee, but she had not told the consultant about this.

CASE 9.12
An 8-year-old boy had episodes of increasing frequency from the age of 4—evidently, up to 10 or 20 in the preceding year. In fact they were all precipitated by falling and bumping his head, almost exclusively after bumps to the occiput. After a 10-second delay he would become stiff and white, then fall unconscious with a few twitching movements, recovering fully within about five minutes.

CASE 9.13
A 10-year-old girl had been treated for epilepsy for several years, supposedly having grand mal seizures following original febrile convulsions. The evidence that one fit had been precipitated by panic after being chased by a dog and the statement that she had been found

by her mother in a toilet 'grey-blue' in colour prompted further investigation of the history. In fact all her seizures were tonic and predominantly induced by bumps on her head, hurts and falls.

CASE 9.14

A 23-year-old mother was standing over her 3-year-old daughter while the girl had an anoxic seizure induced by ocular compression. The mother's eyes became glazed, and she fell to the floor, pulseless, with eyes deviated upwards. Small jerks of her limbs followed. She woke after one minute, yellow in colour, with no retrograde amnesia. She had been under treatment on valproate for 'post-traumatic epilepsy'. Evidently her seizures began after a minor bump to the head when she was pregnant and they all occurred when she was standing up.

Comment. Patients with reflex cardiac standstill do not necessarily change colour at all, but often go first pale and then red as in classical Stokes–Adams attacks. When there is pallor, it may seem to the observer as a greenish tinge to the skin or, as in this case, a yellow appearance.

CASE 9.15

A 2-year-old girl had a story of nine seizures with falling to the ground, head going back, eyes going up, no cry, going stiff, noisy breathing, face bluish then white, seeming to come to and then falling asleep. On one occasion, when she was stuck under a cot, the episode seemed to come and go for 20 minutes until she came round fully. In fact all the episodes were induced by bumps to the back of her head, and the episode under the cot was regarded as an instance of status syncopus.

CASE 9.16

The physician from the adult teaching hospital wrote: 'This nine year old boy was referred to the Chest clinic because of a history of bronchial asthma since infancy. Following the skin tests for asthma he had a short lived grand mal seizure starting with an aura followed by a cry. He then arched his back and fell unconscious to the ground. He then had generalised tonic clonic movements of his limbs. He was not incontinent of urine and did not bite his tongue. The whole episode lasted approximately one minute. There were no neurological sequelae. Further history from his mother yielded the information that the boy had been subject to these seizures as an infant up to the age of two years. They were usually preceded by some noxious stimulus such as falling down and hurting himself, but the present fit was the first he had had since the age of two. I have arranged an out patient EEG and would be grateful if you would see this young boy and advise us as to whether long-term anticonvulsant treatment is indicated in this case.'

The boy's mother said that the present episode looked just like an epileptic fit which she had seen. However, what she did see was as follows. He had had eight skin tests and was waiting for the results. He looked a bit unwell and a bit pale. He said he felt sick. Then his back arched completely and he fell to the ground and he let out a grunting cry, his arms went rigid and made five or six flexion movements, then he went limp. Then he slept briefly and awoke with a headache and feeling sweaty.

Comment. 'Anticonvulsant' is a dangerous word, as it does not force the speaker or writer to distinguish between epileptic and anoxic seizures. Obviously anti-epileptic drugs were inappropriate for this boy with anoxic convulsions.

CASE 9.17

A 6-year-old girl had two tonic seizures with no breath-holding after pain. She was due for eye surgery and the ophthalmologists were informed of her hyperactive vagal reflexes.

Comment. Ophthalmic surgeons are rightly concerned about preventing excessive cardiac standstill under hypoxic conditions through activation of the oculocardiac reflex in strabismus surgery. One might suspect that patients who in other circumstances had been shown to have exaggerated vagocardiac reflexes would be more at risk for this complication during ophthalmic surgery, but confirmatory data are not available.

CASE 9.18

The initial referral letter from a family doctor when this girl was aged 9 years read: 'During the past two years this little girl has had four blackouts. On two occasions she was having dental treatment, lost consciousness, twitched slightly and recovered within a few seconds. On the third occasion she was having attention to a knee abrasion and passed out again with some arm twitching. Recently she had a further attack while at home in bed with a mild respiratory infection. She was unconscious for about 10 to 20 seconds, both arms twitching noticeably. I feel this girl may be having mild epileptiform attacks, but would be grateful if you would investigate her further. In the meantime I have treated her with phenobarbitone twice daily.'

Despite the clues in this letter, the paediatrician replied that: 'Over the past two years she has had five episodes of what sounds like generalised tonic clonic seizures lasting around 20 seconds. She has recently been started on phenobarbitone by you and rather surprisingly for an intelligent girl her parents have found her to be taking the phenobarbitone tablets secretly to the extent that she has become ataxic. From her history she appears to have idiopathic epilepsy and I have arranged for an EEG to be carried out. She should continue with the phenobarbitone twice daily in the meantime.'

In fact, the episodes—in which she went white (possibly with her tongue going out) and stiffened for several seconds with her eyes deviated upwards—were all precipitated by some sort of stimulus such as attention to an injury, 'tweaking' of a loose tooth, excitement, being at the dentist, having an injection, and on one occasion supine with fever accompanying a respiratory infection. Her father's sister used to become unconscious at the sight of blood.

Comment. The diagnosis of idiopathic epilepsy in the form of diurnal tonic-clonic seizures (daytime grand mal) should be regarded with considerable suspicion. Either the seizures are manifestations of some other type of epilepsy, or, commonly, are non-epileptic anoxic episodes as in this case.

CASE 9.19

A 12-year-old girl had three identical episodes, after falling off her bicycle, when bitten by a hamster, and when playing on a wall (there were no witnesses to the provocation in the last of these). After the hamster bite she passed out, growled in her throat, went very tense and rigid with slight body spasms (a few jerks), then came round talking gibberish, a horrible white colour. Later she said that she had had a dream about firemen spraying blood out of a hose. Her mother also appeared in the dream, which resembled the hallucinations reported after cardiac defibrillation.

Comment. Some sort of dream-like state at the end of an anoxic seizure of whatever mechanism seems to be not uncommon but the phenomenon has not been systematically studied.

CASE 9.20

This 3-year-old girl had episodes of staring, rigidity and twitching, all precipitated by bangs to the head. During the episodes she became pale. Ocular compression induced an identical episode.

CASE 9.21

The mother of a 2-year-old boy articulated the questions of many others. He had had several episodes of falling and bumping his head and then rolling his eyes, becoming rigid and unconscious. Each time he had been taken to Casualty and X-rayed as a 'head injury' case. Ocular compression induced 14 seconds of asystole and an anoxic seizure. The mother asked: 'Should he be X-rayed every time he bangs his head? Does it mean concussion? Should I go to Casualty every time? Is it epilepsy? Will he have epilepsy later? Do the fits cause damage? Is it febrile convulsions? Should he be treated for shock? Does he need any treatment? What do I do if he has another? Will he grow out of it?' And then, 'Oh, the vagus! My husband has that—he blacks out due to stress. Why don't the doctors know about this?'

Comment. The answers to the mother's questions are as follows: (1)–(9) no; (10) nothing; (11) yes; and (12) because they had not read this book[!].

CASE 9.22

A young girl had a story of fainting in her cot a few times before the age of 2 years. Later if she cut her finger, or if her sister had a tooth out, she would faint and be stiff. Recently when she was off school with a minor cold, sitting doing the dishes at the sink she fell from the chair onto the floor and went stiff and her arms moved about briefly before she woke up. Her mother stated that she herself whenever she got a cut would 'drop like a stone'.

Comment. There is always concern when a syncope with an anoxic seizure occurs without any apparent provocation. If similar episodes have occurred with typical provocation the diagnosis is likely to be correct.

CASE 9.23

An 8-year-old girl previously had breath-holding attacks with stiffness and twitching from age 1 to 2½ years. Recently she had episodes induced by pain such as falling or banging her nose, with apnoea, some cyanosis, eyes rolling, arms jerking and stiff, after which she would suddenly be awake and talking, pure white in colour. Phenobarbitone was discontinued.

CASE 9.24

A 9-year-old boy had had several episodes provoked by minor injury such as a knocked elbow or cut finger in the past few months. He would give a slight lurch, then his eyes would stare and he would go rigid with his arms coming forward, part flexed, and his legs extended, and turn white and cold. As he recovered his face would turn a beetroot colour and he would sweat, sometimes feeling sick and faint. On the first occasion, when he was aged 7 years, the parents found him in his room pale and sweating and he said he had just knocked himself. Another time he sat heavily on his bottom and a second or two later exclaimed, 'It's there . .!' Before the last one he had time to say, 'Oh, my eyes!' and then he was rigid. Afterwards he said his eyes had been 'prickly and trying to burst out', his sight going pitch black and blurry.

Ocular compression induced an asystole of about 15 seconds. After seven seconds asystole there was diffuse slowing of the EEG for five seconds and then eight seconds relative electrical silence in which his eyes deviated upwards, his eyes jerked, his arms flexed and he snorted. As the diffuse EEG slowing returned he flushed strongly. Later on he had only very minor pallor around the mouth. He said he felt fine afterwards and did not mind the ocular compression. He said his eyes felt blurry before going out like they did in his natural attacks. His father, however, looked very pale and felt awful and said that he always went like that with injections, having felt awful for two hours after a smallpox vaccination. The father emphasized that the ocular compression induced anoxic seizure was identical in all respects to the natural attacks.

CASE 9.25

This girl was born in September 1965. At the age of 3 years she split her chin, and when the stitches came out she 'had a faint' and wet herself. At 3½, when unwell with a fever and feeling sick, she fell down and became very stiff. She had a total of three such episodes with fever before the age of 5 and also two similar episodes when her mother was brushing her hair. They were all about the same. When she began school at 5 the school doctor referred her to hospital; she was given an EEG and put on phenobarbitone. Since then she had had occasional 'turns' about once every nine months. Most had been precipitated by emotional situations, such as going to a doctor or dentist, but one apparently occurred in the night, her mother finding the stair-carpet damp for no apparent reason. The general sequence of events was that the child would feel sweaty, with her head 'going funny and dizzy, and feeling sleepy', and she would 'go out' with eyes rolling, rigidity and incontinence of urine, and then afterwards she would grab her mother and want to sleep, being a 'terrible colour', grey and staying that way for half an hour afterwards.

In September 1976 she 'took a turn' in the doctor's consulting room and also in the EEG department, where there was tonic rigidity and an apparent 30-second cardiac arrest, the EEG being flat for about that duration (see Fig. 7.3, p. 46). Later that month she felt unwell in the hospital waiting room, was taken outside and sat on a wall, and then 'went out' with rigidity, foaming, eyes rolling, incontinence and 'twitching in the middle', regarded by her parents as a 'definite convulsion'. Afterwards her pulse was said by the consultant to be 'very low'.

In December 1976, when standing at a bus stop she said, 'Mum, I'm not feeling very well.' She then 'went right down', twitching, incontinent and stiff, 'just like a convulsion'. She had been treated with phenobarbitone, and was not allowed to go to the swimming baths because she was on these tablets for her 'epilepsy'. In fact almost all her episodes were associated with some definable situation or stimulus, either noxious or emotional—for example, when she was having stitches taken out or her hair brushed.

On the occasion when she had the 30 seconds of flat EEG, her father on entering the EEG room went white at the sight of the EEG paper and sat down and sweated. He remarked, 'I have been fighting this all my life, it is awfully embarrassing.' He said that if he got over-excited, or went to the doctor or hospital he used to faint, but now he can get it when standing and sometimes feels dizzy when getting up from sitting. However, he was pleased to note that his fainting was much less prominent than it was when he was a young child.

CASE 9.26

A 7-year-old boy had two episodes of loss of consciousness with pallor and 'tetanic spasms'. His sister was said to have febrile convulsions and his father epilepsy.

The boy's mother gave the story that when he was a toddler, if he had a knock on the head, in particular the back of the head, he would go completely rigid and quiet with some grunting; when he recovered he was a grey colour and didn't know where he was. At 4 years, after being hit on the chin in his nursery the same thing happened. A recent episode occurred in church on a Sunday morning after being unwell with a fever the night before. He was sitting in the pew and then fell over completely rigid, while his skin took on a green tinge, his eyes went up to the top of his head and his hands turned in like claws. After five minutes he started to come round, completely dazed and not knowing where he was. His mother said that his sister had exactly the same type of attacks, brought on by knocks, the last being at the age of 5 after bumping the back of her head falling off a couch. She added that her husband, who was treated for epilepsy with phenobarbitone, had actually only had two episodes, once when he got up quickly to see his daughter being sick in the night-time, and the other at a stag-night. She described the episodes as fainting with a 'snort'.

CASE 9.27

A 10-year-old boy had had six attacks since the age of 5 years, all with abrupt onset and precipitated by venepuncture, fever, being in church and being in school assembly. In all cases he suddenly became stiff, ashen white, and fell to the ground, recovering in 30 to 60 seconds.

CASE 9.28

A 10-year-old girl had a history of having fainting fits when hurt since the age of 2½ years. The most recent episode, precipitated by a bump to the elbow, consisted of staring and abrupt rigidity, this occurring during a febrile illness.

CASE 9.29

A 2-year-old boy had increasingly frequent episodes of loss of consciousness with rigidity, beginning at age 9 months. Although the onset was not always witnessed, all those which were began after he bumped his head or face. He would give a brief cry and then go rigid, with back arched, head back and arms twisted, and with leg tremors but no breath-holding. His teeth seemed to be clenched very hard. He had begun to wet himself during each attack. Most often he was a ghastly pale colour afterwards. The frequency was now at least once a day. Postictal somnolence or sleep disrupted family life. His 5-year-old sister also had recent fainting fits, and is included here as Case 9.30.

Ocular compression produced an asystole of just under 14 seconds with six seconds of EEG flattening, and an accompanying anoxic seizure characterized by much extension and some flushing afterwards, with mild pallor thereafter.

Twenty-four hour ambulatory cassette EEG/ECG recording was undertaken to confirm the nature of the naturally occurring attacks. For the first 48 hours, perhaps conscious of the recording apparatus, he had no bumps and no seizures. In the following 48 hours he had two seizures. The first occurred when he bumped his head and started to cry. Then his arms extended, his fists clenched, his legs bent up, his head went back and his back arched. He was unconscious for two or three minutes, then came round very tired and very pale. A replay of the tape showed an asystole of 14 seconds preceded by four seconds of relative bradycardia and followed by six seconds of electrical silence on EEG (Fig. 9.6a). The second episode was similar, except that he released his bladder on this occasion. The recording showed an asystole of just over 22 seconds following no more than three seconds of bradycardia. There was EEG suppression for about 18 seconds, the ECG showing prolonged bradycardia, with absent P waves thereafter (Fig. 9.6b).

Atropine methonitrate (three doses per day of 200µg/kg) reduced the number of episodes to one per month. He relapsed when the medication was briefly withdrawn and responded in the same manner when the atropine was reintroduced (McWilliam and Stephenson 1984a, Case 6).

Comment. This was the first case in which short-latency asystole as the mechanism of reflex anoxic seizures after head bump was confirmed by direct recording.

CASE 9.30

The 5-year-old sister of the previous case had two episodes in the preceding months. In one her mother had smacked her and she keeled over flat out, quite stiff and unconscious for about two minutes. She then came to and lay down and went to sleep. In the second she had banged the bridge of her nose. Her eyes glazed, she fell forward and while on the floor had some small twitches of arms and legs. She then got up and went on playing. No colour changes were recollected by her parents.

A minor anoxic seizure consisting only of downward eye jerks accompanied the seven seconds of asystole induced by ocular compression.

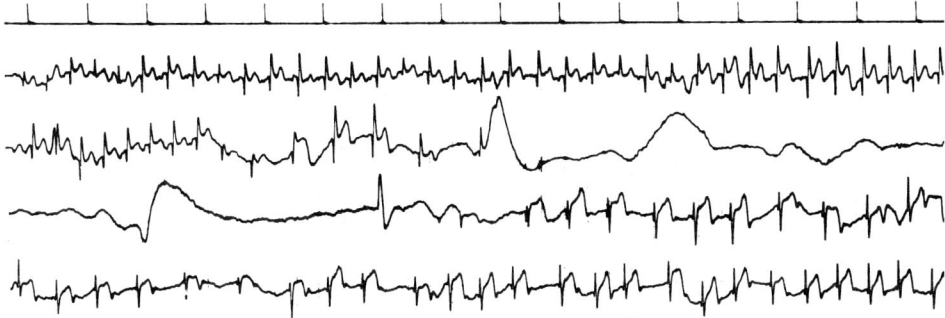

Fig. 9.6. *(a)* Continuous ambulatory ECG recording during seizure induced by head bump in 2-year-old boy (Case 9.29). The upper trace is a time-marker (in seconds); consecutive 16-second epochs follow. The asystole of 14 seconds is preceded by three seconds of relative bradycardia. The simultaneous EEG trace (not illustrated) showed six to seven seconds of electrical silence. (Stephenson 1983*a*.)

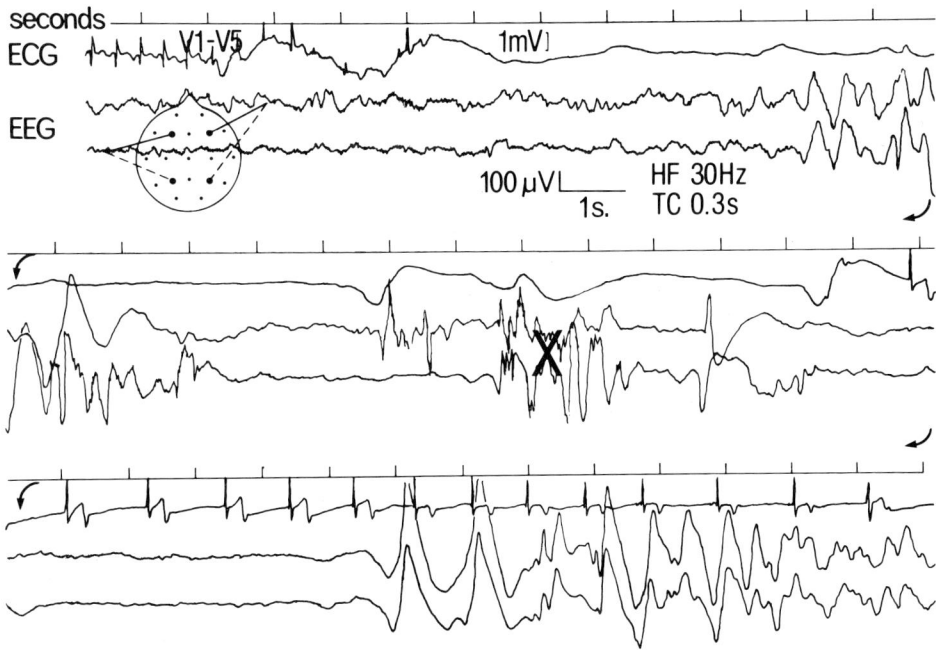

Fig. 9.6. *(b)* Cassette EEG/ECG recording of tonic seizure precipitated by head bump (Case 9.29). The onset of asystole is preceded by approximately two seconds of relative bradycardia and after 20 seconds of standstill is followed by a nodal escape rhythm. EEG flattening lasts for 18 seconds before abrupt return of cerebral activity occurring six seconds after restoration of the ECG. There is no 'epileptic' spiking.

103

CASE 9.31

A 9-year-old girl had had a number of episodes in the previous two years, precipitated by bumps or injuries such as tripping on the stairs and falling off the swing at the park. In each case there was an abrupt loss of consciousness with some pallor and cyanosis of the lips and small jerkings of clenched arms, with recovery within a couple of minutes.

CASE 9.32

This 7-year-old girl began having episodes of stiffness and rigidity precipitated by head bumps at the age of 5 years. More recently she had had similar episodes without any obvious precipitation, for example, when sitting playing cards. She would say 'Oh, mum . . !' and apparently feel funny, and then would become rigid and bluish and might vomit thereafter. Atropine sulphate by mouth was effective in markedly reducing the frequency of attacks. Treatment was complicated by atropine poisoning on one occasion, due to a dispensing error by the pharmacist.

CASE 9.33

A 9-year-old girl with a haematological problem had been admitted for dental extraction and was given an intramuscular injection of premedication ('Omnopon') into her left thigh. Within 30 seconds she suddenly turned pale, her eyes rolled up and her whole body stiffened. Her upper limbs started to jerk. The doctor who had been called urgently by the nurse witnessed a 'myoclonic phase' for a few seconds before spontaneous recovery. The child then told the doctor that she remembered receiving the injection and then becoming dizzy. She felt very drowsy and slept for an hour. The attending medical staff diagnosed this as an epileptic-type grand mal seizure, postponed her dental extraction and ordered an EEG.

Comment. As this girl had a bleeding disorder one might question the intramuscular premedication, but the other three errors were of course the diagnosis of an epileptic seizure, postponement of the dental extraction and the ordering of the EEG.

CASE 9.34

A 9-year-old girl had been treated for epilepsy for three years, and indeed her mother believed that phenytoin made her school-work better. However, all the seizures were characterized by upward deviation of the eyes, flexing of the upper limbs and general stiffness, and were precipitated by bumps and hurts. Her brother had the same tendency to reflex convulsive syncope.

Comment. Some families become quite attached to the false diagnosis of epilepsy, which the passage of years makes difficult to reverse.

CASE 9.35

A 4-year-old boy had two episodes after bumping his head and bumping the side of his face. The description given by the referring doctor was of short generalized convulsions characterized by first being rigid and then shaking all over. However, the parents' description was of snorts, sniffs, being dazed, some jerks and a stare. They were sure that his colour did not change.

On ocular compression the asystole of about 13 seconds was accompanied by an anoxic seizure characterized by snorting at the onset of the EEG flattening; he was then stiff, dazed, had a few jerks and stared for two seconds. No colour change was noted.

CASE 9.36

A 2-year-old girl with Down syndrome and congenital heart disease had a habit of going stiff and appearing dead after fright or temper. Her mother knew that her heart stopped because it was normally so easily felt because of the congenital malformation.

Ocular compression induced an asystole of about 12 seconds with flexion and extension, snorting and sighing, and pallor afterwards, but her mother said that the natural attacks were distinctly worse and longer and with more after-effects.

Comment. See also Case 15.47, and the section on Down syndrome (p. 176–177).

CASE 9.37

A 9-year-old girl had had a number of episodes since the age of 2. With no warning, her head would go back, her eyes become wide, she would make an 'uh-uh' noise, her eyes would close, she would be limp, and then she would go very stiff, and then within a minute she would be sitting up again looking very white with her lips a slightly blue colour. Precipitation had included being punched in the stomach, having her ears examined by the family doctor, waiting for a taxi, and having her school tie fixed before going off in the morning. One had occurred just after coming out of the bath while being dried. The family doctor who observed the episode induced by auroscopic examination described it thus: '. . she had what appeared to be a short-lasting grand mal seizure. She had been quite well until this happened and collapsed onto the floor and had fine tremor-like movements of her arms and legs while in an unconscious state. Her eyes were open and staring during the fit. The entire episode lasted about two minutes, followed by a postictal period of perhaps 10 to 15 minutes.'

CASE 9.38

An 11-year-old girl had had two recent episodes. In one, she bumped her knee and then fell with some jerking, becoming very pale. The other was associated with a visit to the dentist in which she fell and jerked, her eyes rolled and she was again white in colour. From age 9 months to 7 years whenever she had a fever she had seizures characterized by throwing herself back from a sitting position, jerking for a few seconds, rolling her eyes, and being very white thereafter.

Comment. See also the section in Chapter 15 on fever and febrile illness (pp. 169–175).

CASE 9.39

A 1-year-old girl had a history of white or mixed breath-holding attacks since the age of 4 weeks. The frequency had increased until it was three times per day. Initially the provocations were not obvious: for instance, she might have an episode when breaking wind. More recently it was apparent that a hurt, fright or excitement would precipitate an attack. The episodes were characterized by a cry, breath-holding, going from blue to pure white, going stiff with arched back, eyes rolling and bulging, and limbs making rhythmic movements.

The parents insisted on atropine therapy, and this was successful (McWilliam and Stephenson 1984a, Case 3). The dose of atropine methonitrate was at first titrated using further ocular compressions, which in the unprotected state induced asystole of 12 or 13 seconds.

Comment. See comment on Case 9.4.

CASE 9.40

This girl presented as a head injury patient at the age of 3 years. She fell off her bicycle in the house onto the floor and hit the left side of her head. She got up and staggered, and then fell backwards, her eyes rolling and all four limbs jerking, and thereafter was drowsy. She was found to have a fracture of the left parietal bone. In fact she had had many other episodes in which she went stiff and threw back her head, went blue and then white, and was thereafter very groggy, all precipitated by bumps to the head. Similarly triggered episodes occurred after the hospital admission with the fractured skull.

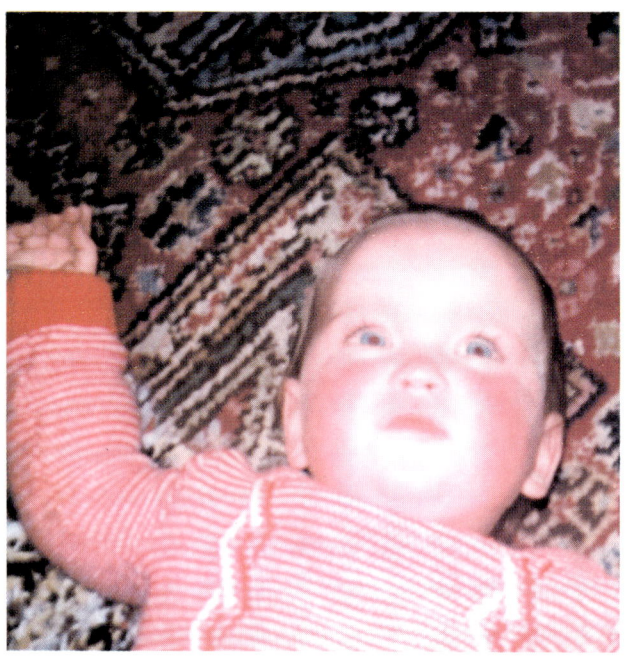

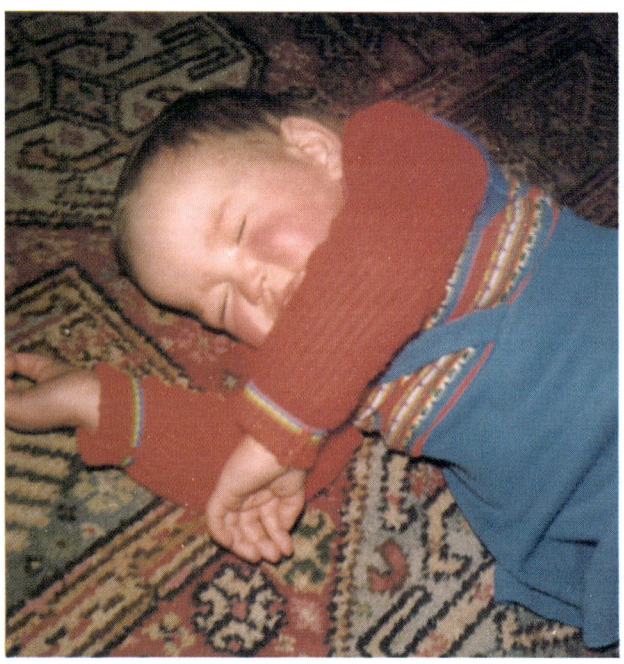

Fig. 9.7. 'White' *(a)* and 'blue' *(b)* anoxic seizures in the same child, abolished by atropine (Case 9.41).

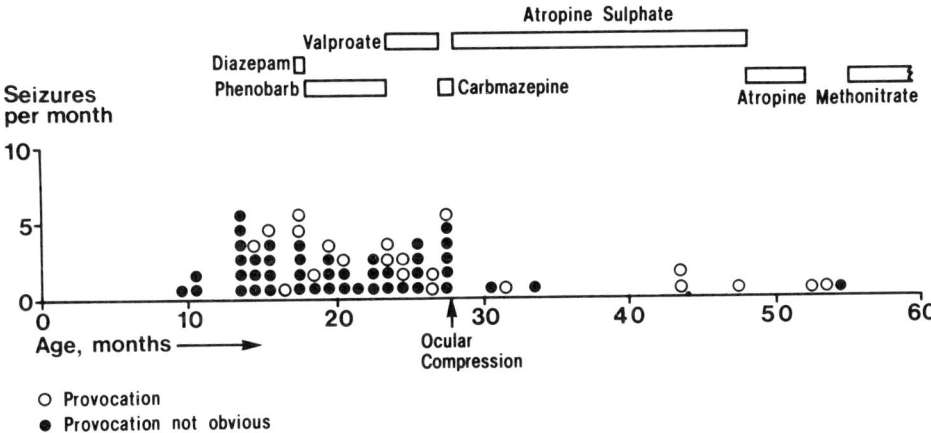

Fig. 9.8. Lack of effect of 'anticonvulsants' and good effect of atropine preparations in child with frequent reflex anoxic seizures (Case 9.41). (Note that provocations were not obvious to her otherwise perceptive parents before the majority of episodes.)

CASE 9.41

A 5-year-old girl had experienced 'white' and 'blue' attacks (Figs. 9.7a,b) since infancy unless protected by atropine. Her mother, a nurse, described the latest episode as follows: 'She stumbled through the door curtain and collapsed into my arms, not having made a sound. Her face was a purplish colour. I laid her on her side. She had no response when spoken to. I could not feel a radial pulse. Her eyes were wide and her pupils dilated and there were jerking movements of her eyes which appeared to be projected forward. She was slightly mucusy around the mouth. Her arms were bent up from the elbows and her fists were clenched, then relaxed, and then rigid again. There were jerking movements of both arms, definite steady jerks. She became limp. She looked at me for a moment with a terrified dazed look and then got up. She wanted to be cuddled. The colour gradually drained from her face leaving a greyish pallor. After a few minutes she went back to play with her friends. The pallor persisted for 20 minutes. The duration of the actual seizure was approximately two minutes. Apparently she had been playing, the younger boy gave her a slight push and she lost her balance, falling on the older boy's upturned foot, catching herself under the ribs and being winded.'

In fact, she had presented at the age of 2 years with a history of more than 60 convulsions since the age of 9 months. Although at least 50 per cent of these had no known noxious precipitation, and none of them occurred after any considerable crying, it was evident that many were precipitated by bumps or surprising pain. Because of the difficulty of the history she had been treated by a consultant paediatrician with a number of anti-epileptic drugs. Her subsequent excellent response to atropine sulphate and methonitrate was reported by McWilliam and Stephenson (1984a, Case 1), and her subsequent progress is shown in Figure 9.8.

Comment. The lack of obvious provocation in about half of this girl's seizures made the diagnosis particularly difficult.

CASE 9.42

A 13-year-old boy was referred as having had two generalized tonic-clonic seizures. In fact, he had had typical reflex anoxic seizures as a young child, with a prolonged asystole observed after ocular compression. The first of the two recent episodes occurred when he was fighting with his brother. He fell down grey, with his hands and legs shaking, and then recovered and wanted to sleep. The second occurred when he was playing ball and was 'winded' by the ball. He lay on the ground with 'eyes rolling and legs kicking and arms going', and then recovered promptly.

Brief ocular compression induced asystoles of no more than three seconds, but thereafter P waves disappeared from the ECG for 30 seconds.

Comment. Episodes in adolescence or adulthood have caused surprise in the past but no longer do so with the recognition of the 'malignant vagal syndrome' up to old age.

CASE 9.43

This 10-year-old boy was excluded from school because his faints were so frequent. They began at age 8, occurring when he was hurt or if he attended the dentist, but later they would also occur for no apparent reason, for instance, while sitting in the classroom reading. He said that he felt it coming on just for a very short time and then he would go white and stiff and grit his teeth and flop.

Ocular compression reproduced an anoxic seizure.

Comment. 'Reflex anoxic seizures', 'vagocardiac syncopes', the 'malignant vagal syndrome'—whatever label is attached to such episodes, it is important not only that the false diagnosis of epilepsy is avoided but also that appropriate treatment for the syncopes be devised. The therapeutic armamentarium for cases such as this is still far too limited— pacemaker implantation for selected adults, and generally nothing for a child.

CASE 9.44

A 10-year-old girl had five episodes of seizure. Some had occurred after stimuli such as changing a dressing over a graze, and on one occasion when putting a poultice on a poisoned finger, when 'she flaked out backwards, rigid, with eyes open and going back the way and jerking—more a tremble than a twitch.' Another time she was found unconscious at a fête. On Christmas Day, when standing up, she suddenly said, 'I am dizzy' and then was immediately 'out with her body stiff and a choking noise'. She then came round and didn't remember anything about it, but was speaking fine as soon as it was ended, although tired and pure white.

Ocular compression under brief deep hypnosis (using the imagery of sitting on a beach on a summer's day and then climbing via a kite to a spaceship high above the earth) induced prolonged asystole without recollection that her eyes had been pressed at all.

Comment. 'You will see stars', she was told—and she did!

10
BRAIN COMPRESSION

This short chapter serves to draw attention to non-epileptic seizures and syncopes which depend on increased pressure for their induction. In Chapter 7 syncope was described as the result of an abrupt failure of cerebral metabolism. Much the same mechanism must apply when cerebral perfusion drops not because of impaired cardiac output or oxygen input but primarily because of increased intracranial pressure. In this situation tonic seizures may be expected, due to brainstem release. This will of course be exacerbated if there is simultaneous reduction in cardiorespiratory function. On the other hand, if brainstem structures are directly compressed, activity resembling a motor seizure need not occur, but rather loss of consciousness with an atonic state resembling the common conception of syncope.

The 'Friday afternoon syndrome' is the telephone call to the neurosurgeon expressing great surprise that the young patient seems to be 'coning'. Often this seems to arise either because of a belief that papilloedema is a necessary sign of increased intracranial pressure, or a misinterpretation of 'convulsions' as epileptic seizures (e.g. Cases 10.1, 15.46).

Readers are referred to the sections on febrile convulsions (in Chapter 15), hydrocephalus (ibid.) and tonic seizures presenting as acute illness (Chapter 5) for further discussions of this important clinical area.

Brainstem malformations
'Syncope' may be the presenting feature of hindbrain herniation in syringomyelia (Hampton et al. 1982) and may be a prominent feature in the adult type of Chiari malformation (Dobkin 1976). In such episodes of unconsciousness, collapse may relate to differential pressure changes around the foramen magnum (Williams 1976), and EEG changes during the unconsciousness may be very slight with mild slowing. This is a situation where coughing (Larson et al. 1974) or sneezing (Corbett et al. 1976) may induce loss of consciousness and tone.

More dramatic motor manifestations may result when brainstem malformations coexist with hydrocephalus, as illustrated in Case 10.2.

Summary
Normally, patients with brainstem malformations have neurological signs, and those with increased supratentorial pressure have clinical features which suggest this probability. If there is a message for those new to this clinical situation, it is that *no papilloedema does not imply normal intracranial pressure*.

Case histories
CASE 10.1
A 21-month-old boy had been less active over the previous two months and had vomited

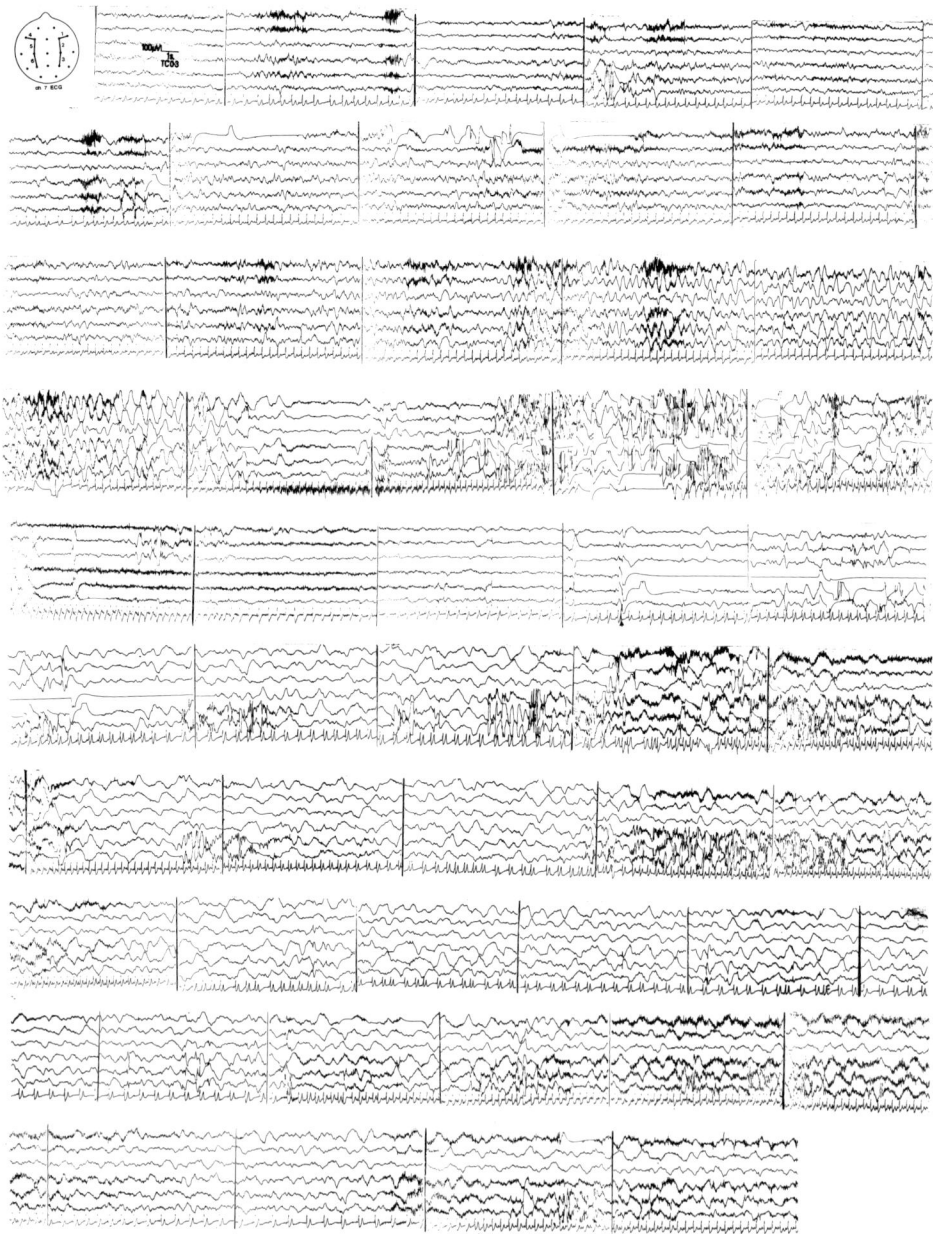

Fig. 10.1. Eight-minute EEG/ECG recording of non-epileptic tonic seizure in girl with meningomyelocele, hydrocephalus and brainstem malformation (Case 10.2). Each horizontal section represents 50 seconds. EEG slowing becomes obvious during the third row, and flattening occurs about 13 seconds after the onset of the fourth row with tachycardia and superimposed tonic EMG potential. There is then a lot of movement artefact but thereafter the EEG is not obvious for at least a minute, during which intermittent mild bradycardia is seen. There is then prolonged generalized EEG slowing with considerable heart-rate variability.

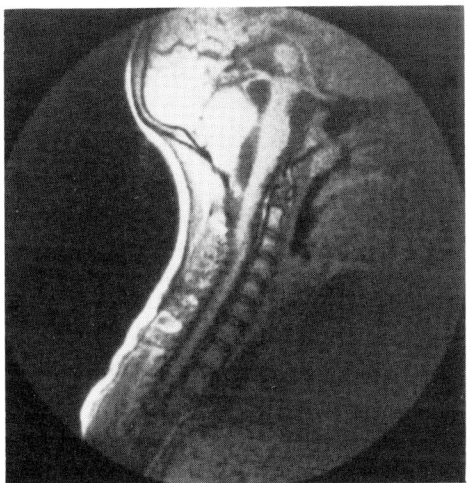

Fig. 10.2. Sagittal magnetic resonance image of girl with bouts of prolonged severe tonic seizures whose cassette EEG/ECG is illustrated in Figure 10.1. The findings were of a complex Chiari II malformation with slightly enlarged and elongated fourth ventricle and tonsillar herniation. Aqueduct stenosis was probable. Cysts were demonstrated just superior to the fourth ventricle and inferiorly in the herniated tonsil. No syrinx or cervical dysplasia was detected.

several times. On several occasions he had seemed blank and in the previous three weeks he had had three tonic seizures. Without any precipitation he had become stiff and arched and unaware for three to four minutes. One of these episodes occurred when he was in his mother's arms and was associated with a cry, but she could not remember at what stage. On questioning it was evident that his gait had been a little more unsteady over the period in question. On examination the boy played without ataxia but was irritable, and there was a distinct 'cracked pot' percussion note over the coronal sutures. CT scan demonstrated a large irregularly enhancing posterior fossa tumour with slight hydrocephalus and mild periventricular oedema.

Comment.   Such tonic 'cerebellar' fits have nothing in common with epileptic seizures and usually imply paroxysmal increase in the intracranial pressure as here.

CASE 10.2
A girl with meningomyelocele, shunted hydrocephalus and normal intelligence began to have seizures at the age of 11 years. At first there were 'absent' attacks in which she was unresponsive for up to three minutes, then she began to have bouts of tonic seizures. During these episodes she complained of pain in her head, neck and back. They were characterized by tonic extension, and her upper limbs were commonly raised, abducted and extended. During one attack which was said to have lasted up to five minutes her eyes were fixed, her pupils dilated and she salivated, although cyanosis was absent. Another episode was recorded on cassette tape and is shown as Figure 10.1. Complete loss of EEG of hypoxic-ischaemic appearance occurred with tachycardia rather than bradycardia, and without impairment of oxygen saturation. The anatomy of her deformed brainstem is illustrated in Figure 10.2.

Comment.   Unlike many patients who have tonic non-epileptic seizures from increased intracranial pressure, this girl was remarkably well in between attacks.

111

11
ANOXIC-EPILEPTIC SEIZURES

In the chapter on anoxic seizures (Chapter 7) and in many other parts of this book attention has been drawn to the mechanism, clinical features and EEG characteristics of anoxic seizures. It has been emphasized that convulsive syncope is not synonymous with anoxic seizure because there is another seizure, the anoxic-epileptic seizure, in which the convulsions after the syncope may be much more dramatic. This chapter is about these attacks. It is *not* about epileptic seizures secondary to brain lesions brought about by previous devastating syncopes (Aubourg *et al.* 1985, Constantinou *et al.* 1989).

Anoxic activation of the EEG
Meyer and Waltz (1961) and Gastaut *et al.* (1961*a*) summarized the evidence that hypoxia, through inhalation of nitrogen (or indirectly through the hypocapnia of hyperventilation) could activate epileptic discharges. Thus, petit mal absences with three-per-second spike and wave could be induced by inhaling nitrogen, as could, less clearly, some partial epileptic seizures (Gastaut *et al.* 1961*a*).

Notwithstanding these experimental observations in man, documented epileptic seizures succeeding documented syncopal or anoxic events were not recorded. Many comments in the literature (to be found scattered throughout this book) have suggested that it is common knowledge that severe anoxia induces epileptic convulsions; however, this belief was based almost entirely on a misperception of anoxic seizures, which even in their pure form may be startlingly dramatic. In fact, on published evidence and on personal experience, classical grand mal, that is to say generalized tonic-clonic epileptic seizure, has not been observed as a sequel to syncope of whatever hypoxic mechanism. However, epileptic seizures may definitely be triggered by syncopes, making the combinatory 'anoxic-epileptic seizure', and these seizures could easily be more common than is supposed. What is known about them now follows.

Epileptic seizures triggered by syncopes
In retrospect I believe that the seizure suffered by the patient of Ossentjuk *et al.* (1966) was the first documented example of an anoxic-epileptic seizure. This was a case of a man who had frequent headaches since childhood and episodes of unconsciousness preceded by 'a sensation of contraction in his stomach' since the age of 16: 'According to observers, he turns pale and falls backwards unconscious.' He had bilateral ptosis, acrocyanosis, clinodactyly, hypogonadism and mild mental impairment. The observations of note occurred in the EEG department. Photic stimulation, carried out with a stroboscope at 16 flashes per second, induced clonic twitchings of his scalp, and spike and wave complexes were seen on the EEG. About 30 seconds after the last train of flashes, on the first occasion, the EEG

changed and during the next 25 seconds showed complete electrical silence while the patient had an anoxic seizure. ECG was not recorded on this occasion. Another EEG was undertaken, this time with an ECG channel in addition (Fig. 11.1). Once again stroboscopic activation evoked spike and wave and clonic twitching of the scalp, during which the heart slowed (P waves are not visible in the illustration) and then stopped completely.

The patient looked pale, his head turned to the left and his eyes rotated upwards, the pupils being extremely wide. For about 10 sec after cardiac arrest onwards the EEG changed. Diffuse bilaterally synchronous waves at 2–2.5 c/sec and 200–250 µV occurred and lasted about 30 sec . . . In this period the patient showed tonic extension of the whole body, simulating a tonic postural fit. About 40 sec after the arrest cardiac activity returned, the heart quickly resumed its previous frequency . . . while the EEG changed and became irregular. The patient flushed and a clonic seizure lasting about 30 sec was observed, during which the EEG showed a delta rhythm synchronous with the clonic jerks.

My speculations are that this man had a mitochondrial cytopathy, photic stimulation triggered vagal asystole, and the prolonged vagal asystole led to both an anoxic seizure and a secondary epileptic seizure which was at first subcortical, until cardiac arrest ceased and allowed the cortical components of the epileptic seizure to be manifest at the scalp electrodes. Review of the cases next to be described will support this argument.

Stephenson and Ounsted (1982) postulated that an anoxic-epileptic seizure mechanism might determine some febrile convulsions. Part of the EEG and ECG of a child in whom an anoxic-epileptic seizure was induced by ocular compression has been published in Stephenson (1983a). Cases 11.1 and 11.2 give further details of two children who had clinical seizures with an anoxic syncopal component mediated by asystole followed by a prolonged clonic epileptic component. In each of these children the natural seizures were reproduced on ocular compression, and their appearance is shown in Figures 11.3 and 11.4. Other patients in whom similar histories were obtained are included as Cases 11.3–11.6 and 15.45. The latter case fulfilled the criteria for febrile seizures and was so diagnosed by the consultant paediatrician. None of these patients had separate unprovoked epileptic seizures or epilepsy, but I have known patients whose epileptic seizures were syncope-stimulated, and one patient with clonic or myoclonic epilepsy so triggered is included as Case 11.7.

Epileptic absences triggered by Valsalva-mediated syncopes were reported by Gastaut et al. (1987) and Aicardi et al. (1988). In these circumstances it could be shown that sodium valproate eliminated the epileptic absence while the Valsalva-mediated syncopal atonia remained unaffected.

The most recent and best-documented series of anoxic-epileptic seizures has been presented by Battaglia et al. (1989). These authors report three female children aged between 2½ and 11 years. Epileptic seizures were triggered by different types of syncopes. One of the three had spontaneous epileptic seizures and another had myoclonic jerks triggered by photic stimulation. Details of these episodes are given in Figures 11.2a–e (reproduced by permission from Battaglia et al. 1989).

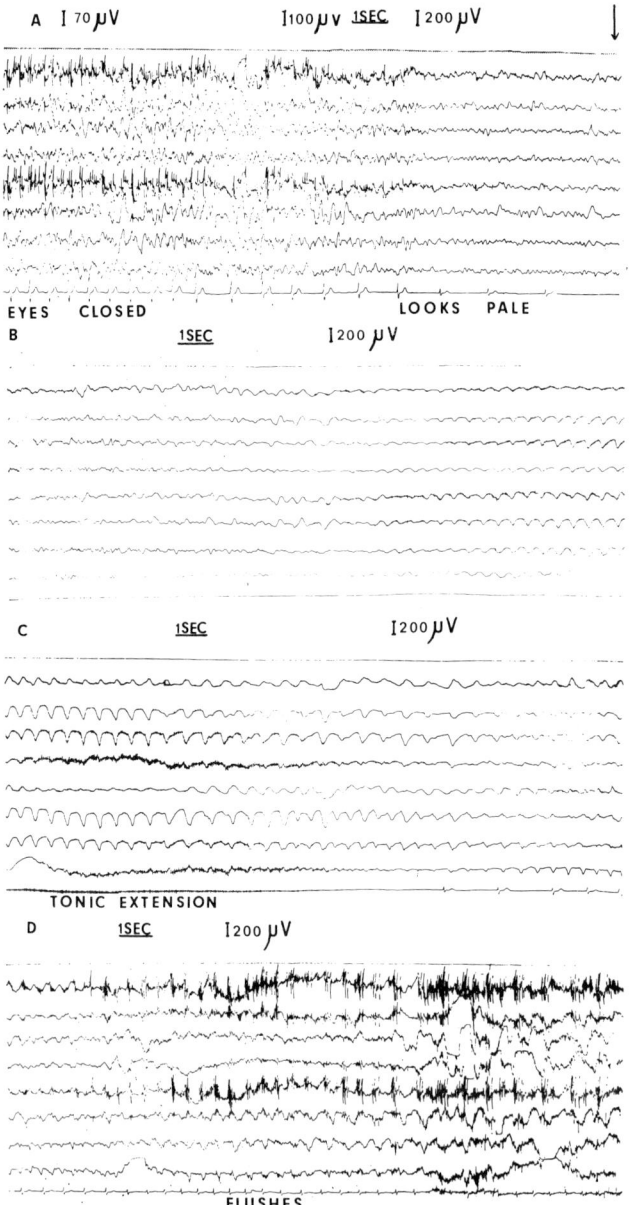

Fig. 11.1. Cardiac arrest induced by photic stimulation at 16–17 cycles/sec. in patient of Ossentjuk *et al.* (1966). *A*, *B*, *C*, and *D* represent a continuous recording. Time constant = 1 sec.; high frequency filter = 75Hz. The first channel records flashes which were stopped at the arrow. Channel 9 is ECG.

A. Provocation of irregular slow-wave activity and myoclonus of the scalp. Beginning of cardiac arrest. Amplification was decreased in the second part of the trace.

B. About 10 seconds after cardiac arrest, rhythmic waves at 2–2.5 cycles/sec. developed.

C. The amplitude of the 2–2.5 cycles/sec. activity increased and an anoxic tonic attack took place.

D. A few seconds after the heart resumed its activity the slow waves disappeared and subsequently an epileptic seizure occurred.

114

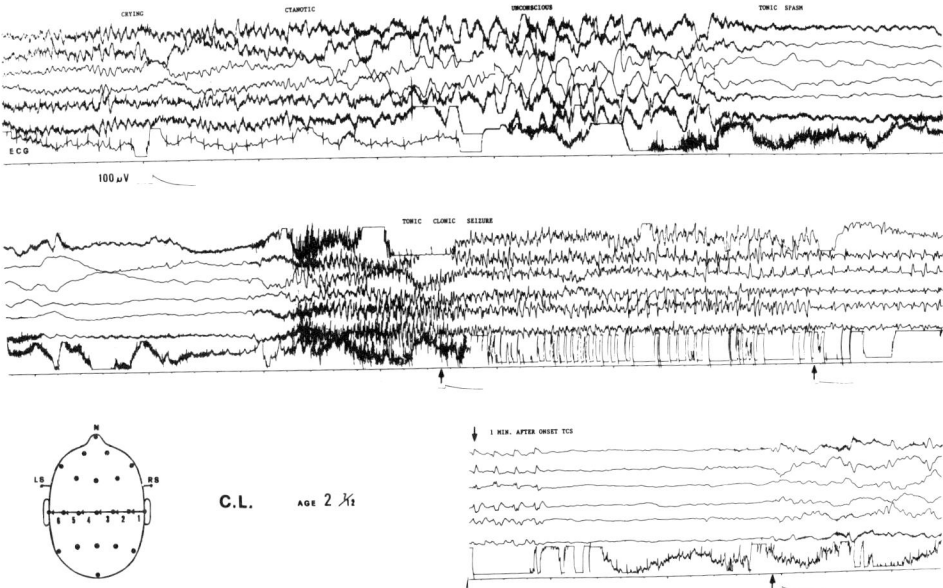

Fig. 11.2. *(a)* This 2½-year-old girl had breath-holding attacks since the age of 8 months, complicated by clonic features since the age of 18 months. An attack was induced by a frustrating experience and filmed with simultaneous EEG and ECG recording. Crying is followed by the rapid onset of apnoea and cyanosis. Note the minor bradycardia and EEG slowing in the upper trace, followed by loss of EEG signal for 20 seconds. In the second trace a clonic epileptic seizure develops, with repetitive spikes for 60 seconds, concluding with postictal suppression (in the third trace). (Battaglia *et al.* 1989.)

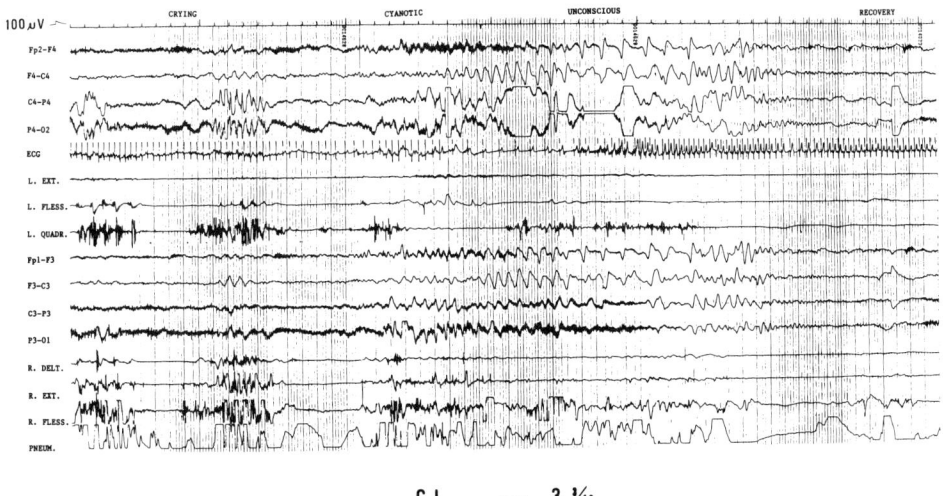

Fig. 11.2. *(b)* Breath-holding spell in the same child as in (*a*), now aged 3 years 3 months and on regular sodium valproate. Apnoea and bradycardia without asystole occur as previously, but no EEG spikes nor clonic epileptic seizure follow. (Battaglia *et al.* 1989.)

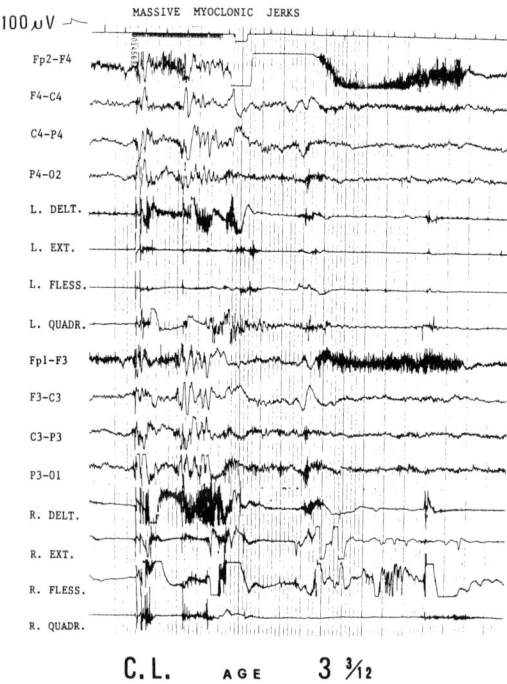

Fig. 11.2. *(c)* The same child as in *(a)* and *(b)*, during the same recording as *(b)*. Myoclonic jerks with spikes are induced by photic stimulation at 18 flashes per second. (Battaglia *et al.* 1989.)

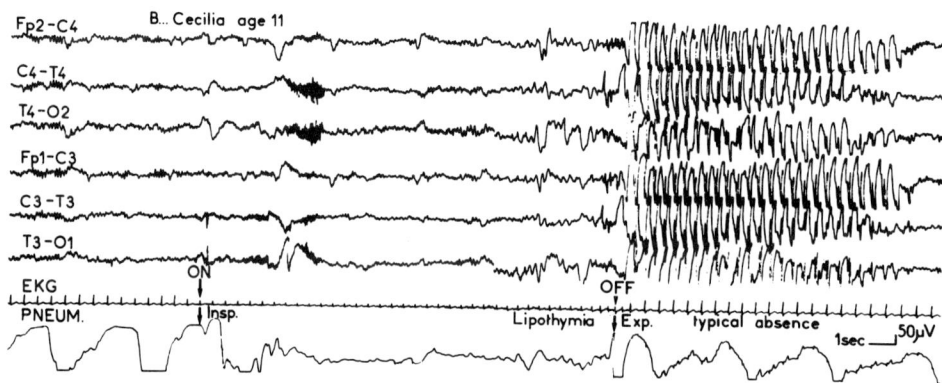

Fig. 11.2. *(d)* This 'withdrawn' 11-year-old girl had up to several daily faints or falls, eventually diagnosed as self-induced syncopes mediated by compulsive Valsalva manoeuvres. Later, these were complicated by typical epileptic absences. The trace shows the effect of forced expiration against a closed glottis. Note the reduction in the QRS signal during this apnoea, followed by generalized rhythmic three-per-second spike and wave of 11 seconds duration, accompanied by a typical absence.

Sodium valproate abolished the spike and wave and the accompanying absences, but the self-induced apnoea persisted. (Battaglia *et al.* 1989.)

116

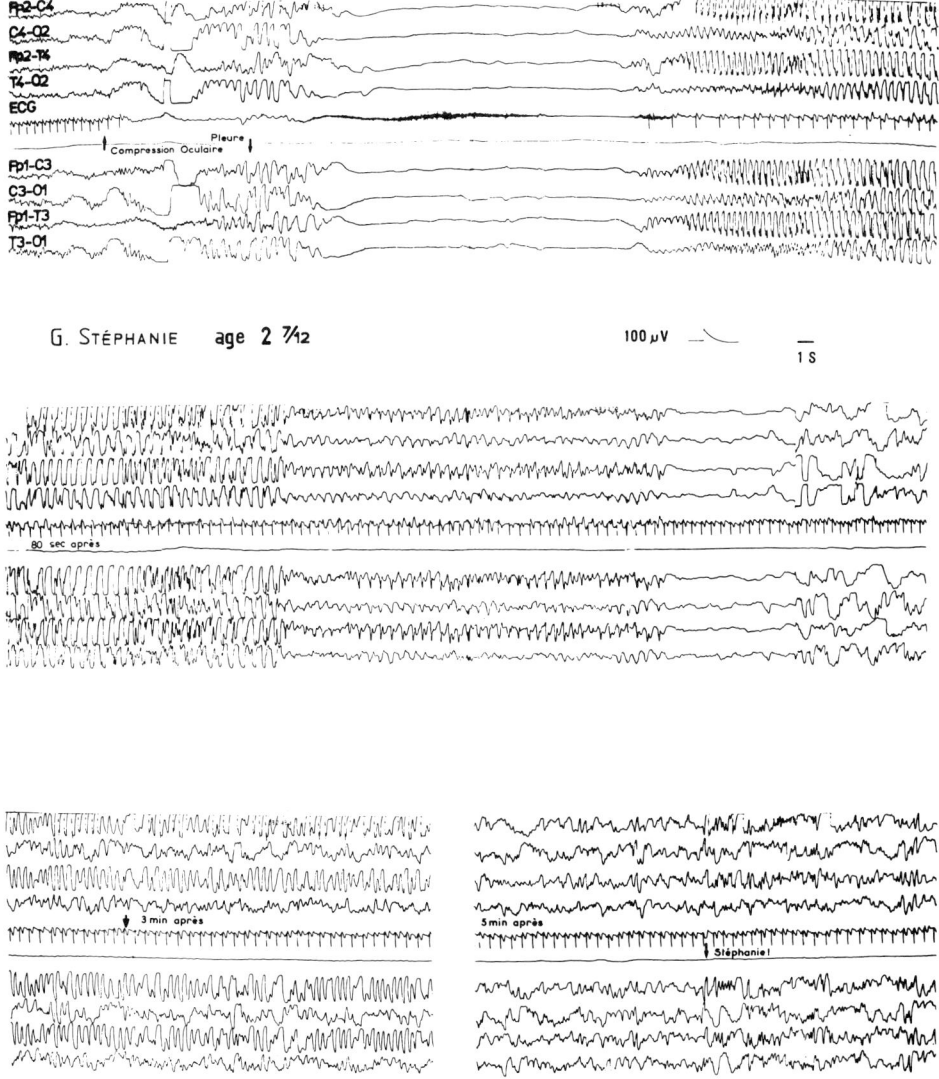

G. Stéphanie **age 2 7/12**   100 µV

Fig. 11.2. (e) This 2½-year-old girl had a history of going pale and losing consciousness for several minutes after anger or frustration. An episode was reproduced by ocular compression. In the upper trace there is cardiac asystole for 33 seconds. The EEG slows before 20 seconds of isoelectric EEG, accompanied by some brief jerks and opisthotonus. Thereafter, as the ECG signal returns, three-per-second rhythmic spike and wave discharges develop. Later (middle trace), these discharges slow and become irregular, before ending with EEG suppression 142 seconds after the onset of spike and wave. The lower trace illustrates the prolonged postictal EEG slowing with unresponsiveness. The child seemed back to normal after 15 to 20 minutes.

After sodium valproate, syncopal attacks still occurred but without accompanying epileptic absence status. (Battaglia *et al.* 1989.)

117

Summary

Anoxic-epileptic seizures are a special combination in which a syncope of one sort or another triggers an epileptic seizure. The epileptic seizure is likely to be an absence, or myoclonic or clonic, but other possibilities may exist and wait to be described. This type of combinatory seizure will not be recognized unless monitoring systems include not only EEG but also critical measures of cardiac and respiratory functions.

Case histories

CASE 11.1

A 15-month-old boy with a history of what was said to be breath-holding had been screaming with excitement and was kneeling on the bed bouncing up and down. His father gave him a 'wee skelp' (light smack) on his nappy. He threw himself down on the bed and held his breath. 'Then he went up the bed slightly to the right on his head and on his knees and slithered off the bed head first in slow motion. His head and shoulder hit the wall, not at all hard, on the way to the floor, which was about two feet below the bed.' When his father picked him up he was pale, his eyes had rolled back and his mouth was tight shut. He started jerking about 10 seconds later. He was still jerking and his eyes were still deviated upwards when he was in the car on the way to the hospital six or seven minutes later, but by then the jerking was not so frequent. About eight minutes from the start his eyes came down and he was groaning and pale. Within half an hour he was walking about again.

Two months later his EEG was normal awake and with photic stimulation. Ocular compression induced an asystole of 22 seconds with 16 seconds of EEG flattening during which he flexed his upper limbs and snorted. This was followed by generalized fast spiking on the EEG, and then spike waves slowing from two-and-a-half per second to one per second over nine-and-a-half minutes. During this time he had repetitive jerking of his face and upper limbs, and his eyes were deviated upwards, or slightly to the left. With the onset of generalized slow activity on the EEG his eyes came down and he was pale and asleep (Fig. 11.3). His father, who was present throughout, recognized the episode as identical to the natural attack. Five minutes later the boy still had extensor plantars, but after a further 20 minutes the plantar responses were flexor and he was able to stand briefly, albeit shakily.

Comment. At first it was thought that the father exaggerated the duration, but in the event his description was accurate in all respects. The anoxic seizure of a vagal attack stimulated a clonic epileptic seizure.

CASE 11.2

An 11½-month-old boy had begun to experience 'breath-holding' and limpness if hurt, for example after bumping his head, over the preceding months. He was sitting on the floor playing with gramophone records when he gave a wee scream. His mother presumed that he had hurt his lip biting a record. He then held his breath as if going to cry, stiffened himself with arms bent and eyes staring, and went blue but with his lips 'like stone' (grey/white); then he went limp and pale and not blinking for 20 minutes. When he came out of it he was very white and listless.

An EEG was recorded which was normal awake and during photic stimulation. Ocular compression induced prolonged asystole (Fig. 11.4). Artefact obscures the exact duration, but asystole was of at least 25 seconds and possibly over 30 seconds. The anoxic seizure consisted of flexion of the upper limbs and rapid down beat of nystagmus and extension. Then, jerks of limbs and face began with corresponding movement artefact on the EEG at about two per second for six seconds before fast spiking occurred. This was followed by spike waves slowing from three per second to one per second over 26 seconds. Jerking stopped with the transition from spike wave to EEG flattening. Generalized slow activity continued for eight minutes, during which the infant was unresponsive and very pale. His mother stated that this appearance was exactly the same as in his natural attack.

Comment. Presumably the attack at home was similar to that induced by ocular compression, that is, a vagocardiac syncope triggering a clonic epileptic seizure.

CASE 11.3

An 18-month-old boy had a history of blue breath-holding attacks since the age of 9 months. After playing or bumping himself he would normally 'catch his breath as if in a state of pain without crying and then go blue, dark blue, looking as if he was trying to get out of it', and pass out after 20 seconds or so, becoming rigid with back arched and fists clenched. Then he would go limp and regain his normal colour without pallor. These attacks declined in frequency from once a day to once a week. On four occasions the sequence was identical in all respects to that described above, except that after the limpness and just as his colour was beginning to return he started to jerk. The jerks were sharp and quite fast, mimed by the parents at about two to three per second in a regular manner. They lasted for about two minutes and were accompanied by his eyes flicking up into his head. When the jerks slowed down and stopped, he came round, cried a bit, then went to sleep without turning pale.

EEG awake and with photic stimulation was normal. Breath-holding with cyanosis occurred without EEG change. Ocular compression did not induce asystole nor EEG alteration.

His mother had a history of one or two simple breath-holding attacks with temper.

Comment. From the story given, this was a clear instance of cyanotic breath-holding ('prolonged expiratory apnoea') inducing clonic epileptic seizures. These could not be reproduced in the EEG laboratory, in contrast to the attacks in a young girl, reported by Battaglia *et al.* (1989), recorded at ages 2½ years (Fig. 11.2*a*) and 3 years 3 months (Figs. 11.2*b,c*).

CASE 11.4

A 16-month-old girl had a history of stopping breathing when she hurt herself. She gave one yell, didn't breathe in, went blue, rolled her eyes, fell, and was limp afterwards. In these 'breath-holding' attacks the onset was rapid and she did not become deeply cyanosed. Two additional episodes were described as convulsions. On the occasion of the first she jammed her finger in a drawer, not particularly hard, and held her breath. Then she took another breath (the parents thought she was recovering) but then began to convulse. This lasted for 10 to 15 minutes. During the first five minutes her eyes were rolling upwards, there was rasping breathing, salivation, a regular rhythmic croaking noise from her throat, and her legs and her arms were twitching. This twitching quietened down after five minutes. Then there was a fast tremble for about 10 minutes in which her eyes were still vacant but no longer deviated upwards. By this stage the family doctor had arrived and gave rectal diazepam.

On the second occasion her father had been playing with her in the bedroom in the evening. He was squeezing her between his knees in play. He squeezed her a few times and she laughed, then he squeezed her once more rather harder and she didn't like it. She started to cry, giving one cry expelling all the air, breath-holding until blue. She then took a gasping breath, her eyes became glazed and rhythmic twitching began, lasting four minutes. By this time the family doctor, who lived close by, had arrived. The twitching was calming down but the child then went into a shaking stage, with more rapid trembling and a moan and a fast quiver. Rectal diazepam was given and the child seemed to have recovered after about 20 minutes. After both these episodes she was very pale and miserable.

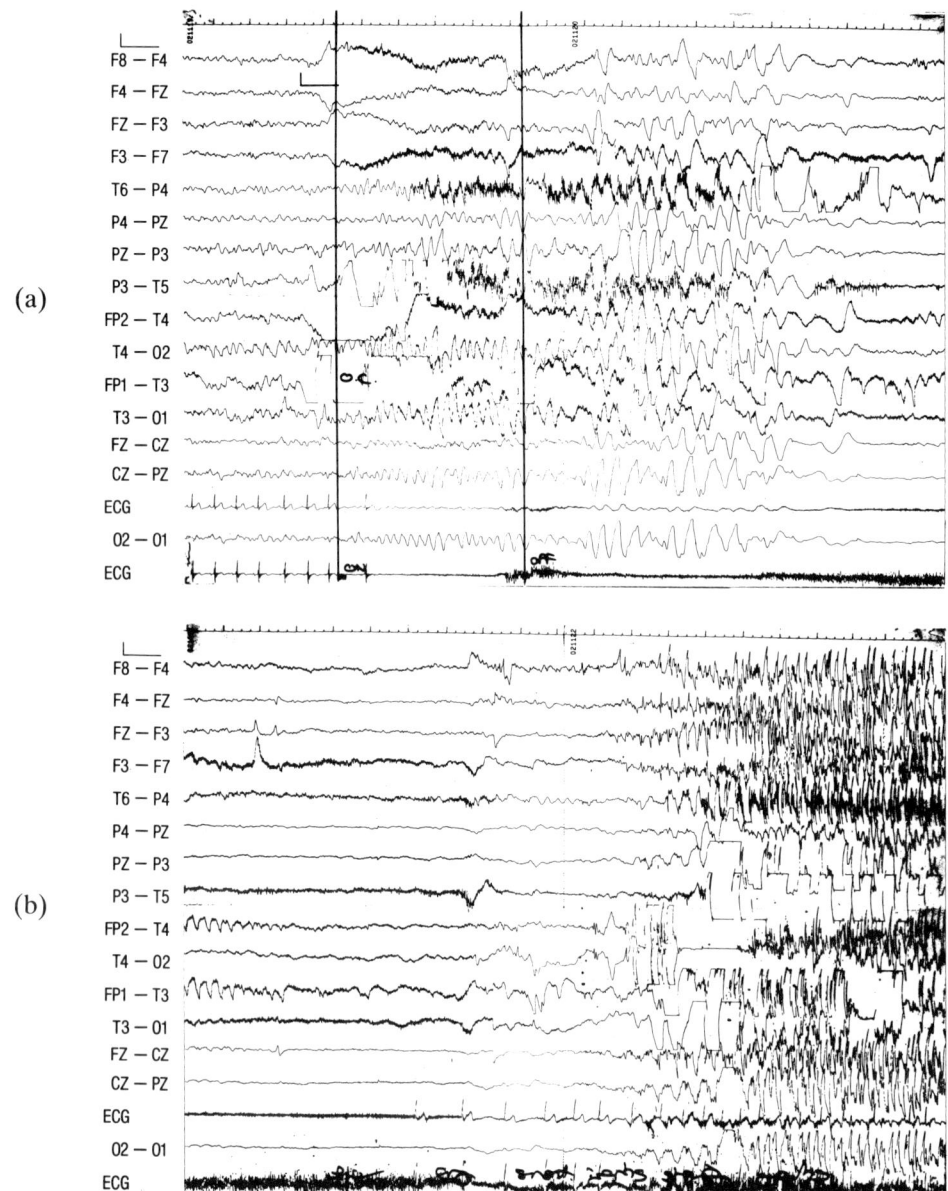

Fig. 11.3. Anoxic-epileptic seizure reproduced by ocular compression (performed for five seconds) (Case 11.1). The heart arrested after one systole. After a further 10 to 11 seconds, EEG flattening developed with tonic EMG on the ECG trace. Notchings in the ninth and 11th channels (FP2–T4 and FP1–T3) in (*b*) indicate downbeat nystagmus. At the conclusion of the EEG flattening, once the heart has restarted and there have been about eight QRS complexes, incrementing fast spikes are seen in the EEG trace, associated with fast repetitive jerks. In (*c*), these are seen to continue as regular high-voltage spike and wave complexes at about two per second with accompanying regular clonic jerks. (Calibration of EEG in (*a*) and (*b*) is 100μV, and in (*c*) 200μV = vertical bar. Horizontal bar is 1 sec.) (Adapted from Stephenson 1983*a*.)

120

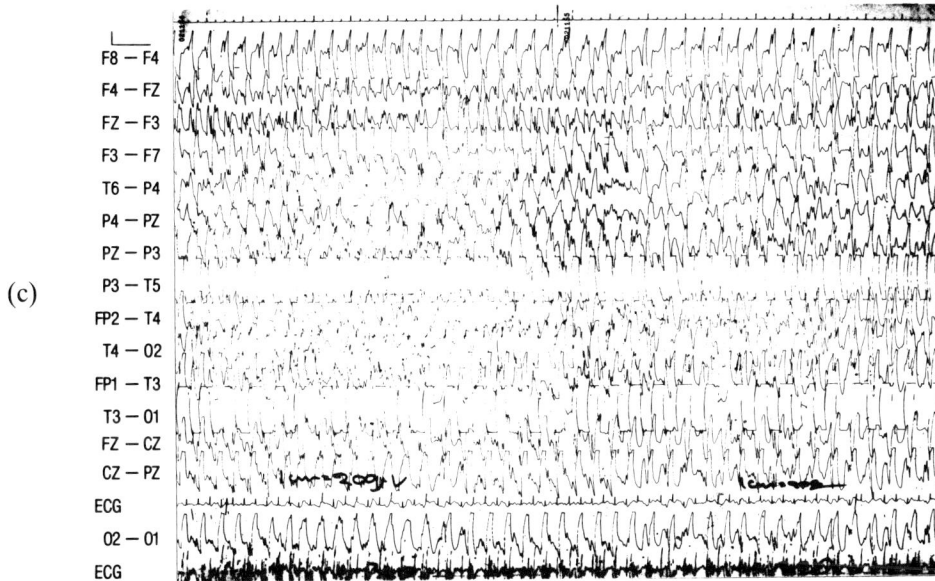

F8 — F4
F4 — FZ
FZ — F3
F3 — F7
T6 — P4
P4 — PZ
PZ — P3
P3 — T5
FP2 — T4
T4 — 02
FP1 — T3
T3 — 01
FZ — CZ
CZ — PZ
ECG
02 — 01
ECG

(c)

In the EEG department an anoxic seizure was induced by ocular compression, precipitated by an asystole of a maximum of 15 seconds with about five seconds EEG flattening, featuring extension, jerks and a stare. However, EEG spiking and rhythmic clonic twiching were not induced.

There is no family history of seizures of any kind, and no further clonic seizures have occurred during five years follow-up.

Comment. One may suppose that the anoxic or syncopal component of this girl's anoxic-epileptic seizures was a 'mixed' breath-holding attack, with both prolonged expiratory apnoea and vagal asystole. If a seizure, the setting, provocation and onset of which suggest an anoxic or syncopal mechanism, lasts long enough for it to be seen by the visiting doctor, then an anoxic-epileptic combination has to be presumed.

CASE 11.5
A 4-year-old girl had episodes from the age of 1 year in which, if she fell backwards, she would emit a tiny cry, then hold her breath and pass out with her eyes half-closed, become very tense in the face and jaw, and 'stiff as a board', then going completely limp and crying intermittently for half-an-hour, looking chalky white and exhausted. The parents' concern was accentuated because of an episode which occurred when she was being looked after by a neighbour. She tripped, fell backwards against a fireplace and passed out. The neighbour smacked her, thinking this was the way to bring back her breath. She started to jerk. The mother was there within a few minutes and got the family doctor. He reported that the appearance was that of the clonic stage of a fit. He said that she remained in that state, despite rectal diazepam, until she was admitted to hospital and given intravenous diazepam. The duration of the jerking was about 25 to 30 minutes. The parents emphasized that in these episodes she was always pale and never blue.

Comment. All but one of these episodes were reflex anoxic seizures (vagocardiac syncopes). One triggered a clonic epileptic seizure which, although rather long, presumably would have stopped spontaneously.

121

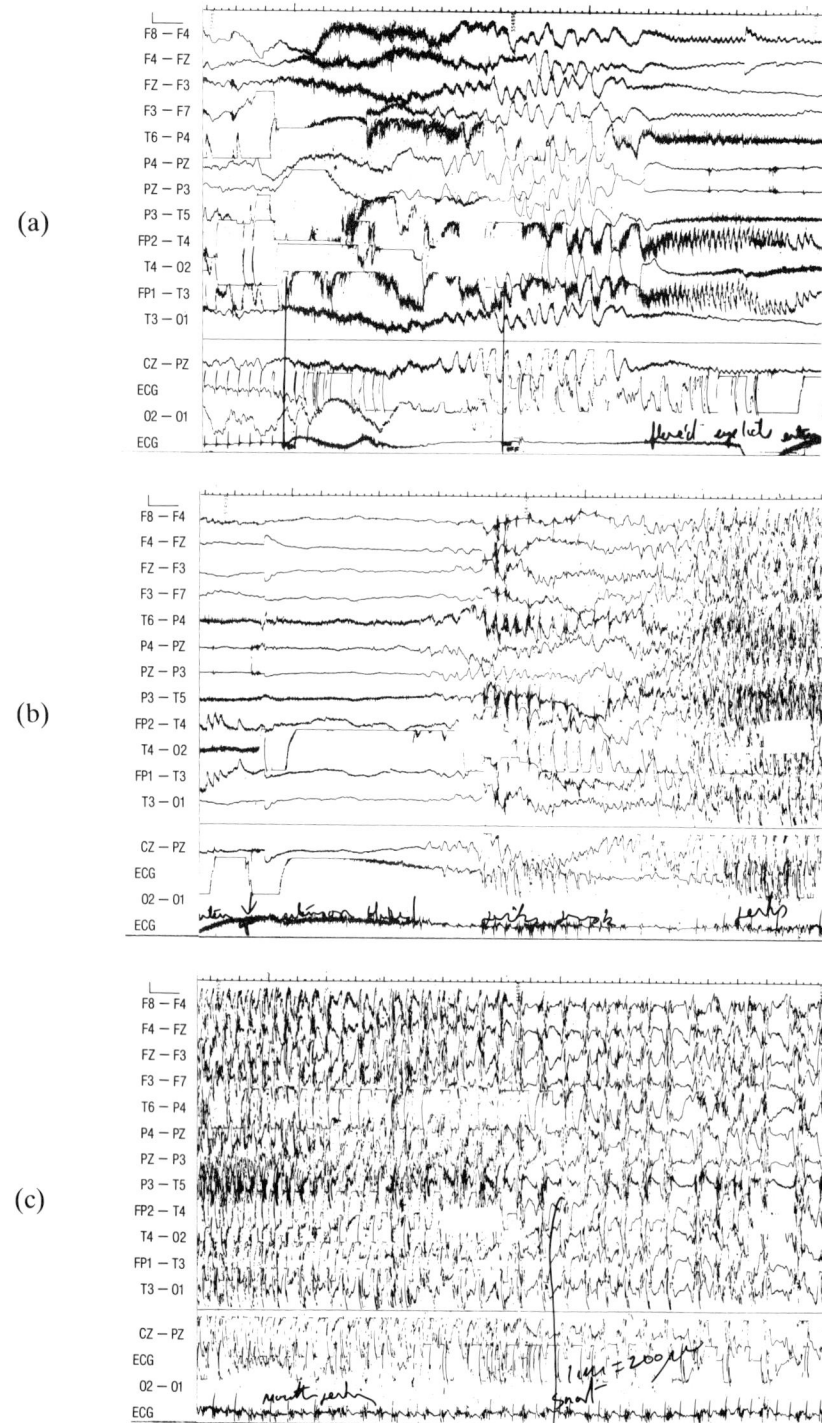

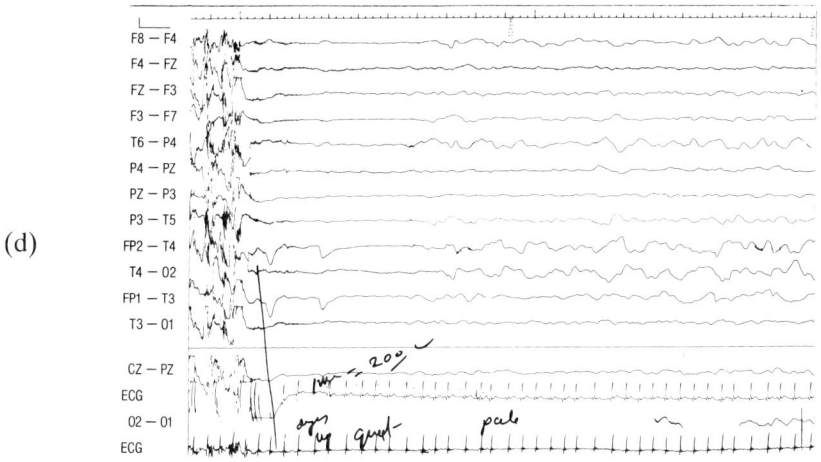

(d)

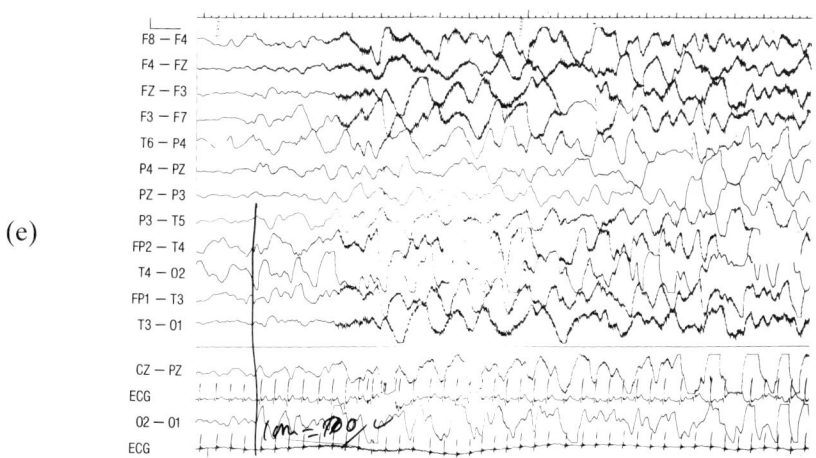

(e)

Fig. 11.4. Anoxic-epileptic seizure reproduced by ocular compression (Case 11.2). Cardiac arrest occurs within two systoles of the onset of ocular compression, which is carried out for about seven seconds. At the onset of EEG flattening a rapid notched appearance on the anterior EEG channels (channels 9 and 11, FP2–T4 and FP1–T3) indicates downbeat nystagmus. A tonic anoxic seizure including extensor thrust occurs during the flat EEG in the first part of (b). At the end of the EEG flattening, regular repetitive jerks occur with jerk movement artefact on the EEG followed by fast spiking toward the end of (b). In (c) this develops into regular high-voltage spike and wave associated with mouth and general rhythmic twitching, which slows in frequency. Close to the beginning of (d) the spike and wave abruptly concludes, and there is upward deviation of the eyes and general suppression of EEG activity associated with pallor. In (e) there is generalized postictal EEG slowing.

(Calibration of EEG is 100μV = vertical bar in (a) and (b), for the first 12 seconds. of (c), and for (e) after the first 2 seconds.; 200μV = vertical bar elsewhere. Horizontal bar is 1 sec.)

123

CASE 11.6

A boy began to have jerking episodes, which appeared to be clonic epileptic seizures, at the age of 7 months. They might last about a minute and were activated by drowsiness, but if they occurred when he was awake he would resume what he had been doing immediately on conclusion. He might remain sitting in a high chair during a seizure, with repetitive jerks at one to three per second, waxing and waning in amplitude. Video recordings confirmed that he might vocalize intentionally during times when the jerks were smaller, and the episodes could be described as myoclonic with variable absence. EEG during an episode showed three cycles per second spike and wave.

Later he developed a tendency to anoxic seizures after frustration or injury which were regarded as 'breath-holding'. In these episodes the initial tonic non-epileptic seizure was regularly followed, from the description, by regular clonic jerking for about a minute.

By age 4 the frequency of all types of episodes had markedly reduced, but he was diagnosed to have a mild mental impairment.

Comment.   This boy had a type of epilepsy blurring the distinction between myoclonic and clonic. When he also had anoxic seizures (it was not certain from the description whether these were breath-holding attacks, vagocardiac syncopes, or 'mixed' with a combination of these features), an epileptic addition was regularly triggered. This case may be exceptional: most cases of anoxic-epileptic seizures seem to occur in those without overt epilepsy. (See also Case 4.8, pp. 19–23.)

12
'EPILEPTIC-ANOXIC' SEIZURES

In the foregoing chapter I discussed those combinatory seizures in which a syncope triggers an epileptic seizure, and for which I coined the term 'anoxic-epileptic seizure' (Stephenson 1983a). In this chapter I discuss the converse phenomenon, in which epileptic seizures induce syncopal events, or at any rate alterations in cardiac and/or respiratory function which might be expected to contribute to cerebral anoxia. Such episodes may not be common (adequate population data are not available), but they do cause diagnostic confusion and they are frequently alarming for witnesses. Whether they contribute to mortality (Kelly *et al.* 1980, Katz *et al.* 1983) or to hypoxic brain damage (Aubourg *et al.* 1985, Constantinou *et al.* 1989) is speculative (Southall *et al.* 1987b), but in the case of secondary cardiac arrhythmias such a relationship does have experimental support (Mameli *et al.* 1988).

Epilepsy, respiration and cardiac action
Jackson (1899) described respiratory arrest during an epileptic seizure which, from its description, included temporal lobe involvement. Direct evidence of apnoea on electrical stimulation of the limbic system was obtained by Kaada and Jasper (1952) and by Nelson and Ray (1968). Apnoea is normal within generalized tonic-clonic epileptic seizures ('grand mal'), this being overshadowed by the motor manifestations. The observations alluded to, however, form a basis for epileptic seizures in which apnoea is a dominant component. The literature on the effects of the brain on the heart is larger, and has been reviewed by Natelson (1985) and Mameli *et al.* (1988). Monitoring studies have shown predominantly tachyarrhythmias in epileptic seizures with temporal lobe involvement (Blumhardt 1986, Blumhardt *et al.* 1986), without much evidence that such tachyarrhythmias might have a syncopal consequence. If ventricular tachyarrhythmias could be shown to have an epileptic genesis as well as asystole (Mameli *et al.* 1988), then this aspect would acquire considerable importance. Meanwhile I will confine discussion of epileptic seizures involving the heart to those with bradycardia or asystole, since the potential for cerebral anoxia thereby is obvious. For convenience, the clinical material will be discussed under three headings: (i) apnoea without bradycardia; (ii) apnoea with bradycardia; (iii) asystole or dominant bradycardia. The distinctiveness of the latter group may be somewhat artificial, since while positive data regarding the presence of apnoea (or absence of respiratory excursion) was a feature of the reports in the first two groups, in the third positive statements or evidence that there was normal respiration are not apparent.

Apnoea without bradycardia
Fenichel *et al.* (1980) suggested that absence of bradycardia was a feature of apnoeic attacks in infants which were 'convulsive' in origin, that is to say having an

epileptic mechanism. The seizures reported in this section are associated either with no change in heart rate or with tachycardia. Hooshmand (1972) reported episodes of expiratory crowing followed by apnoea beginning at about the age of 2 years in a developmentally delayed girl. The EEG was attenuated during what appears to have been a genuine epileptic seizure. This child's seizures were abolished by atropine alone and relapsed on two occasions when this was discontinued. Some of the patients with 'generalized electro-decremental event' described by Fariello *et al.* (1979) had apnoea without specified bradycardia, but the tonic seizures which these authors described included severe bradycardia in some and are described in the next section. Watanabe *et al.* (1982) described five young children with onset of epileptic seizures between 2 months and 2½ years, of which in many cases apnoea was the sole clinical feature. Rhythmic activities of various frequencies were illustrated in the EEGs; the majority did not have spikes. The two infants who also had tonic epileptic seizures were profoundly retarded at follow-up, but two other children were normal.

Clancy and Spitzer (1985) found epileptic apnoea in two of 173 neurologically intact children with near-miss sudden infant death syndrome (SIDS) and two infants with unexpected epileptic apnoea among 33 neurologically suspect infants with recurrent apnoea (they found no instances in siblings of SIDS victims). In these infants apnoea was virtually the sole feature of the seizures, but 'extremely subtle eye deviation' was sometimes noted. The EEG origin of these seizures was predominantly in one or other temporal region. Interictal EEGs all contained an excess of 'sharp EEG transients' (SETs), but more infants who did not have epileptic seizures had excess SETs than among those who did.

Monod *et al.* (1988) described a further five young infants, mostly neonates, with apnoeas (maximum 120 seconds). Rhythmic activity on the EEG during seizures was mainly temporal. One of their patients (Case 5 of their series) illustrated two types of apnoea. In the neonatal period this boy had onset of episodes of cyanosis with apnoea, bradycardia and hypotonia. 'Antral dyskinesia' was detected and antireflux treatment started. Later he had episodes of cyanosis, apnoea, ocular revulsion and hypotonia but *not* bradycardia, with an occipital alpha focus during the seizure and abolition on sodium valproate.

The relationship of apnoea to epileptic seizures and SIDs is discussed by Davis *et al.* (1986), and Oren *et al.* (1986), though neither study reported data on heart rates. Oren *et al.* studied 76 infants who had experienced unexplained sleep apnoea accompanied by a change in tone and colour, and who were unresponsive to repeated vigorous stimulation, the apnoea being terminated only after mouth-to-mouth resuscitation. 11 of these infants developed a 'seizure disorder' as evidenced by 'tonic-clonic activity'; of these, seven had further apnoeic episodes requiring either vigorous stimulation or resuscitation, of whom four died. The EEG was normal at the first presentation in all these infants but was subsequently 'abnormal' in six, although no details were given. Whether the initial apnoeas were epileptic cannot be determined from the evidence, but the mortality is alarming. From the description, these infants did not seem to have been seriously damaged by the 'near-miss' episode such that subsequent lesional epileptic seizures would be expected (Aubourg *et al.* 1985, Constantinou *et al.* 1989). Davis *et al.* (1986) reported two infants presenting with apnoeic episodes, one of which was regarded as 'near-miss' SIDs. In both, the administration of caffeine was followed by obvious epileptic seizures, tonic-clonic or myoclonic. These authors suggested that the caffeine might have 'unmasked' epilepsy or lowered the epileptic seizure threshold, but it is speculative whether the original apnoeas were also epileptic in mechanism.

The most controversial publication on this topic is that of Southall *et al.* (1987*b*). This report was of a boy aged somewhat over 4 years at the time of the study:

At nine months of age he was found in his cot severely cyanosed and unconscious. He recovered spontaneously, was found to have a high temperature and admitted to hospital, where a febrile convulsion was diagnosed.

At 18 months of age, while playing about 50 feet away from his parents, he started to walk toward them. He was pale, his eyes were staring and he became rapidly cyanosed. After about 30 seconds he fell down unconscious, and not breathing. Cyanosis appeared and became progressively more severe. His parents thought he was choking but could find no foreign body in his mouth. A nurse happened to be nearby and although she thought he was dead, she gave him mouth to mouth resuscitation and eventually he started to breathe.

On arrival at hospital he had a normal body temperature, and an eight-channel EEG was reported to be normal. From this time he underwent episodes every two or three weeks. Often the episodes would cluster, the onset of one being followed within 24 hours by four to six further episodes. On almost all occasions he became cyanosed, but in some attacks breathing would resume before *loss of consciousness* [my italics]. Some episodes began during sleep, when he would sit up, smack his lips, stare, then become cyanosed. He was rarely incontinent. When he was older he was able to describe an inability to draw breath during the cyanotic episodes. At the onset of some episodes he would point to his throat and try to speak . . . The episodes did not respond to sodium valproate, carbamazepine (with adequate serum levels) or phenytoin.

At three years of age he underwent a 16-channel EEG [which] showed that during sleep there was some evidence of a right temporal focus but when awake the record was normal. During one cyanotic episode at four years of age, an ambulatory four-channel EEG (Oxford Medical Systems) showed the following: 'multiple high-amplitude spikes, polyspikes and irregular spikes-and-waves appearing simultaneously in all leads and lasting for two minutes. The spikes were more continuous on the right side, whereas slow waves and spikes were of highest amplitude on the left side'. Computerised axial tomography showed no abnormalities.

Elaborate multi-channel recordings were then made over a period of two weeks, admittedly with great difficulties. Finally a series of episodes was documented.

Seven episodes were recorded, with the duration of physiological disturbances ranging from one to four minutes. In all cases the EEG was the first signal to alter. Desynchronised activity developed and was followed within two to five seconds by a sinus tachycardia. Breathing movements then ceased, with a latency of between five seconds and 3·5 minutes. The oxygen saturation began to fall approximately 15 seconds after cessation of breathing movements and remained below 50 per cent for between 30 seconds and one minute, staying at zero in some episodes for 10 to 20 seconds. When the seizure activity in the EEG gave way to a typically flattened postictal trace, breathing movements returned but recovery of oxygenation during some episodes did not reach normal levels for a further four minutes . .

127

Additional recordings were made, using a jacket plethysmograph to measure breathing movements (without simultaneous EEG). These recordings showed that apnoea began at end-expiration and that during a protracted recovery from hypoxaemia, each breathing movement was associated with a grossly prolonged expiratory phase, characteristic of expiratory braking (grunting) . .

Unfortunately the EEG information, including that in the printed figures, is from a single channel, does not show any convincing EEG spikes, and is wholly consistent with cerebral hypoxia. This child certainly had prolonged expiratory apnoea, but the authors (not clinical neurophysiologists) have not provided convincing evidence that this was an epileptic-anoxic seizure.

Apnoea with bradycardia
Although Fenichel *et al.* (1980) may be right that most apnoeas with bradycardia are not epileptic, some certainly are and the clinical picture may be dramatic. Several of the seizures described in that report began with a tonic epileptic seizure and concluded with an opisthotonic seizure, suggesting an anoxic seizure of syncopal mechanism. Mutani *et al.* (1970) described a patient with tonic seizures in whom the cardiac and respiratory alterations occurred at the onset of the epileptic EEG activity, which could be stopped immediately by the injection of barbiturate into the vertebral artery, whereas carotid injection was not effective (suggesting brainstem origin of these phenomena). Mutani *et al.* (1970, 1971) emphasized and illustrated bradycardia with junctional escape rhythm. When a similar epileptic seizure recurred after intravenous atropine, these cardiac changes did not occur, indicating a vagal mechanism. Fariello *et al.* (1979) reported epileptic seizures with generalized EEG suppression ('cortical electrodecremental event'). Their patients, who had static encephalopathies, manifested epileptic seizures with apnoea in which bradycardia might be severe, with escape rhythms developing when the rate dropped below 40 per minute. These authors found that when therapy was possible, phenytoin or methylphenidate might be effective.

The very young infant reported by Kelly *et al.* (1980) had episodes of eye rolling, 'clonic positioning', apnoea, cyanosis, limpness, and bradycardia down to 50 per minute. Later, cyanosis and brief staring were followed by limpness, unresponsiveness and an opisthotonic position. In such episodes the mother was unable to move the chest, and the authors visualized tightly adducted vocal cords and could not pass an endotracheal tube. In due course an ictal EEG was obtained which showed rhythmic generalized three-per-second to four-per-second high-voltage delta and sharp-wave activity in the left temporal area, becoming generalized. A left temporal gemistocytic astrocytoma was detected and removed, after which seizures became less frequent and less severe, consisting only of staring, cyanosis and irregular breathing without obstruction, and lasting no longer than 20 seconds.

The patient of Coulter (1984) presented with cyanotic episodes at the age of 3 months. At 8 months he was 'babbling and smiling responsively but also was microcephalic and unable to sit, crawl or stand'. At the age of 10 months, split-screen video–EEG monitoring allowed the recording of three typical seizures. Left temporal spike and sharp activity was associated with respiratory arrest. Severe bradycardia to the level of 40 per minute developed, with loss of P waves, and the EEG developed a suppression-burst pattern at which stage the infant was 'gasping, cyanotic, and arching his head and back in tonic contraction'. The duration of apnoea in the recorded seizures was from 55 to 80 seconds, and the authors gave cardiopulmonary resuscitation. Evidently phenobarbitone and carbamazepine controlled this boy's seizures except in febrile illnesses.

The most recent report of epileptic seizure with apnoea and vagal-mediated bradycardia is that of Navelet *et al.* (1989). This infant boy began to have episodes of 'respiratory obstruction with cyanosis, bradycardia and hyperactive movements of the upper limbs' at the age of 3 months. He was thought to have hyperactive vagal reflexes, in that a heart rate of 60 per minute was induced by ocular compression. Oesophagoscopy showed oesophagitis. Episodes appeared to be associated with meals or pain. One was recorded during a milk feed: its course is illustrated in Figure 12.1. In this epileptic seizure, in addition to respiratory arrest, vagal bradycardia with escape rhythm is clearly illustrated. Seizures from two similar patients are illustrated in Case 12.1 (Fig. 12.2) and Case 12.2 (Fig. 12.3).

Asystole or dominant bradycardia

As suggested above, there is not necessarily anything fundamentally different between the seizures in this section and those in that immediately preceding it. The first well-known case was that of Phizackerley *et al.* (1954). Although referring to a patient outside the 'paediatric age-group' (a woman of 71), the details are worth some attention for reasons which will become apparent. This woman gave a story of blackouts for six years, the first occurring at a picnic lunch when she suddenly lost consciousness for some minutes. She then had recurrent episodes in which she developed . .

. . an unpleasant feeling in the epigastrium which she was unable to describe at all clearly. This was accompanied by a feeling of intense apprehension, "as if I were going to die". . . Witnesses reported that at this stage she became pale and limp, but there were no convulsions or incontinence. She was out for less than half a minute, and on coming round always noticed a feeling of heat running to her extremities, "as if I were bathed in blood". This was a momentary phenomenon and was succeeded by headache which lasted about half-an-hour.

An EEG was reported to show random spiking from the right anterior temporal region. Thereafter air encephalography was carried out, and this seemed to precipitate a severe attack:

At the onset an epigastric sensation and angor animi occurred, and on two occasions at this stage the pulse was regular and of normal volume. It is probable, though not certain, that there was slight clouding of consciousness at this time. In some attacks, the pulse then ceased abruptly, and the heart became silent. Within a second or so the patient became pale and restless; if cardiac arrest continued for five seconds or more consciousness was lost, all muscular tone was reduced and slight twitching of hands and lips occurred. The longest period of observed asystole was eight seconds. An E.C.G. recording was made continuously for about one hour, and this shewed complete sino-auricular block during the periods that

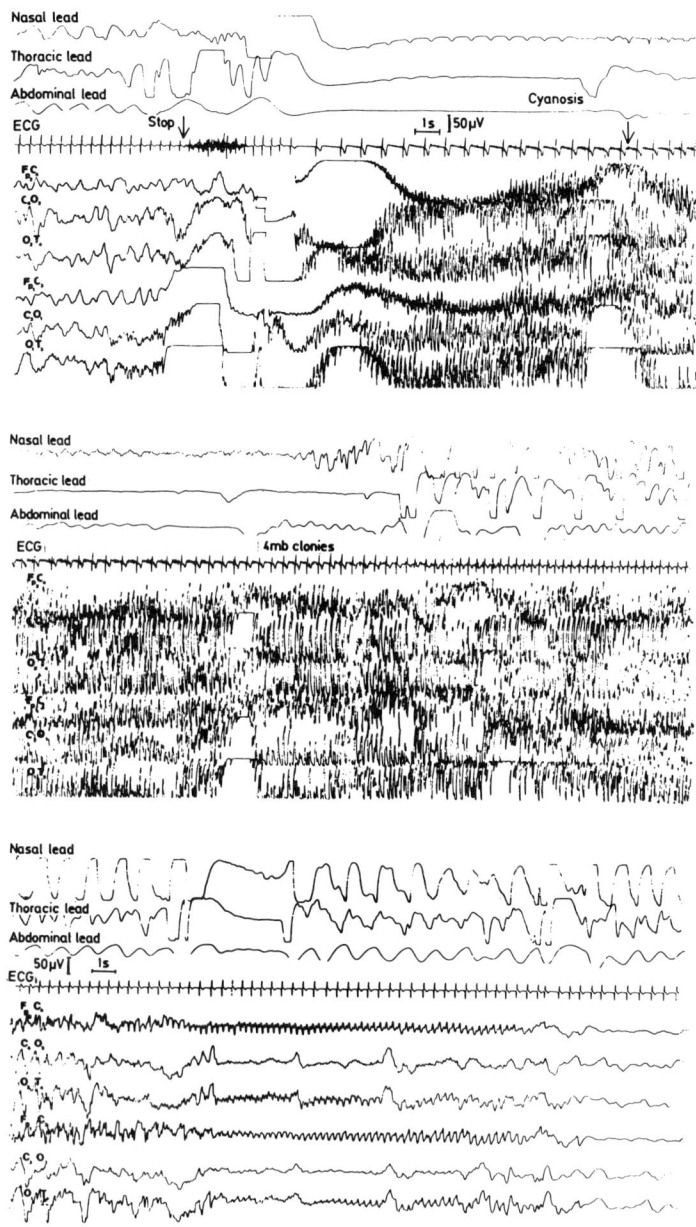

Fig. 12.1. Seizure triggered in infant boy by milk feed. (*a*) Feeding was stopped at the first arrow. Oxygen was given by mask after the second arrow. Respiratory obstruction is recorded on the three respiratory leads (nasal, thoracic, abdominal). EEG discharge starts at the left occipital area with secondary generalization. Short bradycardia is seen on the ECG trace. (*b*) The whole period of respiratory obstruction lasted 37 seconds. The term '4mb clonies' = clonic jerks of the four limbs. (*c*) There was a short (5 secs.) central respiratory pause without bradycardia or clinical symptoms. (Reproduced by permission from Navelet *et al.* 1989.)

130

the pulse could not be felt. Unfortunately concomitant E.E.G. recordings were not possible. Flushing of the face and opening of the eyes marked the end of an attack . . . These episodes were extremely distressing to the patient, and on the view that a vagal discharge was part of their mechanism, intravenous atropine was given. The attacks ceased at once, and the patient was subsequently maintained on tincture of belladonna by mouth. During a four month period of observation she had no further attacks of loss of consciousness, though she reported further episodes with epigastric sensations and angor animi. She was later given additional dilantin.

(The effect of this treatment was not stated by the authors.) It is absolutely certain that this woman had anoxic seizures from asystolic syncope, and almost certain that these were a sequel to a simple partial temporal lobe epileptic seizure (the alternative explanation would be that the epigastric sensation and 'angor animi' represented the symptoms of a vagal discharge of other mechanism). The findings of Devinsky *et al.* (1989), showing how small a proportion of simple partial seizures were detected by standard scalp EEG electrodes, make for difficulties even now in solving this sort of problem, more so in 1954.

Sinus arrest of up to eight seconds was reported in a generalized convulsive epileptic seizure by Varadi *et al.* (1983), and of eight and 10 seconds in two patients with right temporal epileptic seizures by Katz *et al.* (1983). Further asystoles have been reported as part of temporal or complex partial epileptic seizures by Gilchrist (1985), Kiok *et al.* (1986), Smaje *et al.* (1987), Howell and Blumhardt (1989) and Constantin *et al.* (1990); other examples have recently been published in abstract (DiLuzio and Rutecki 1989, Fincham *et al.* 1989, Radtke 1989); see also Case 12.3.

Bullard (1987) and Giroud *et al.* (1988) reported 'diencephalic seizures', in which bradycardia was a feature. A patient of Bullard seemed to respond to bromocriptine and morphine.

Most interesting of all from the point of view of mechanism is the patient of Ossentjuk *et al.* (1966), mentioned earlier (Chapter 11, pp. 112–114). One interpretation of the findings described would be that this young man had prolonged asystole as part of an epileptic seizure, but reasons for an opposing view, that this was an early example of an *anoxic-epileptic* seizure, have been elaborated in that chapter. It is even possible that this was the first recorded example of the triplet 'epileptic-anoxic-epileptic' seizure!

Summary
Epileptic seizures may include discharges which cause respiratory arrest, vagal-mediated bradycardia, or both. The *combination* is most likely to lead to clinical and EEG evidence of cerebral anoxia in the young, but in older patients prolonged isolated asystole—with convulsive syncope—may overshadow the triggering partial epileptic seizure.

Case histories
CASE 12.1
A boy began to have 'tonic' seizures before the age of 6 months. They were described as grunting with going blue and stiff. The first episodes observed in hospital were witnessed

when he was attached to an ECG and an apnoea monitor. A typical description was as follows.

Whilst in dreaming (REM) sleep, both the apnoea and heart monitors began sounding their alarms. He was very grey around the lips, hands and feet, his limbs were trembling, he was salivating, his mouth was tight, and his arms and legs were rigid. There was no shaking. His eyes were staring at first and then rolled into the back of the head. The episode appeared to last for five minutes. Oxygen and suction was given. He was very pale and listless thereafter for about 20 minutes. The ECG trace showed a heart rate of 40 per minute with no P waves (Fig. 12.2a).

Later, combined EEG/ECG monitoring was conducted with cassette recording. First two channels of EEG were employed (Figs. 12.2c,d) and later seven channels (Figs. 12.2e,f). Inspection of the tapes revealed non-focal generalized incremental fast spiking with simultaneous loss of sinus rhythm on the ECG, an asystole of up to three seconds and a nodal escape rhythm with absent P waves, the ECG abnormalities beginning synchronously with the EEG spiking.

Ocular compression induced the same degree of bradycardia with nodal escape on ECG as was present in his spontaneous epileptic seizure (Fig. 12.2b).

The degree of bradycardia with seizures became less with time. Complete seizure control required phenytoin and carbamazepine. At follow-up four years later the boy had mild mental impairment.

Comment. These epileptic seizures were initially mistaken for anoxic seizures because insufficient information was monitored simultaneously. Although non-convulsive syncope has been reported with a heart rate of 40 per minute (as in swallowing syncope—Woody and Kiel 1986), such a degree of bradycardia could not have resulted in a motor anoxic seizure. Furthermore, the duration was far too long. From an EEG point of view these seizures were of immature tonic-clonic type (presumably secondarily generalized).

CASE 12.2
A 3-month-old boy of supposedly normal development began to have frequent severe tonic seizures daily. In these episodes he was rigid with his arms out or bent, sometimes above his head or drawn towards his face. He was either blue, indeed often very cyanosed, or else predominantly pale, and afterwards he was extremely pale and lifeless. 30 or more episodes were captured during a 24-hour EEG/ECG cassette recording and samples are shown in Figure 12.3. The striking findings were marked vagal bradycardia at the onset of the fast EEG spiking and severe postictal depression of the EEG. High phenytoin levels inhibited the seizures, but mental impairment is now considerable.

Comment. The pronounced vagal component to these epileptic seizures added to their frightening aspect. From the EEG point of view they may have been immature tonic-clonic seizures, with the tonic phase predominating (as in Case 12.1).

CASE 12.3
This 7-month-old boy had Sturge–Weber syndrome with cerebral calcification on the right. Of his earlier history his family doctor wrote: 'The previous colour changes that I observed last approximately 10 to 15 seconds. The child becomes initially flushed, particularly around the port wine stain, and then a dusky mild cyanosis appears. During this time the child tends to lie with the head and eyes deviated to the left, and seems limp and totally unresponsive to external stimuli. Following this colour change there is a brief period as he looks around, and then he seems to return to normal fairly suddenly.'

Admission to Intensive Care was precipitated by the following incident. 'When I arrived to examine the child the mother was changing him, and he was lying limply across the mother's knee. She said that he felt cold and looked unwell, and indeed I was quite horrified

132

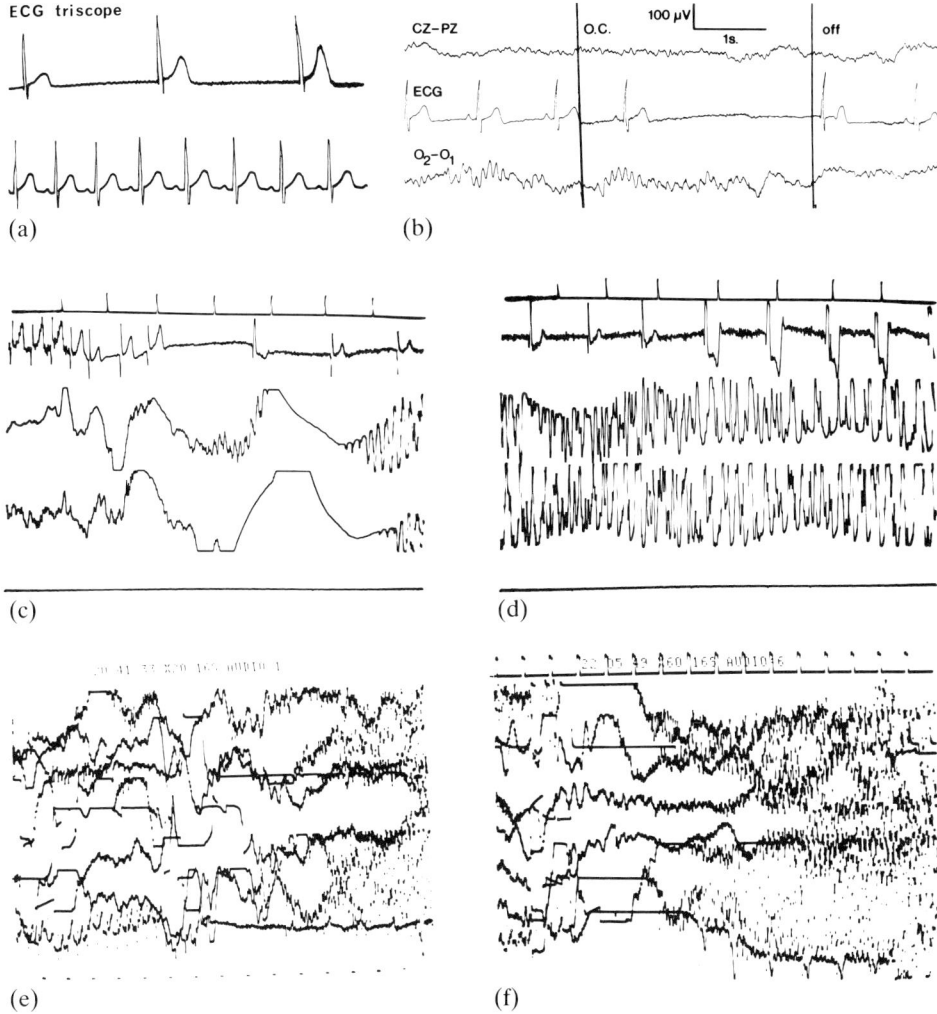

Fig. 12.2. Investigation of an infant with frequent 'tonic' seizures (Case 12.1).

(*a*) Appearance of bedside ECG monitor screen at time of attack. Upper trace is 'frozen', showing heart rate of 42 per minute with absent P waves. In lower trace ongoing heart rate is 120 to 140 per minute, with sinus rhythm (screen width = 3.6 secs.).

(*b*) Brief ocular compression induces asystole of 2.8 secs. with loss of P wave from succeeding QRS.

(*c*) ECG plus two-channel EEG cassette recording. Time markers in seconds. Minor slowing of heart rate in first second, then asystole for 1.8 secs. EEG: bilateral 10-per-second activity slowing to eight-per-second, and movement artefacts.

(*d*) Later in the same seizure. Continuing bradycardia with escape rhythm on ECG channels; fast spikes about seven per second on EEG channel.

(*e*) Seven-channel EEG/ECG cassette recording. Time markers in seconds. Much movement artefact, but asystole of 3.2 seconds at onset of epileptic seizure with incremental generalized fast spike at eight per second.

(*f*) Same recording system and time markers as in (*e*), but showing onset of a different seizure. Artefact hides precise onset of severe bradycardia with escape rhythm, but onset very close to start of generalized incremental fast spiking.

133

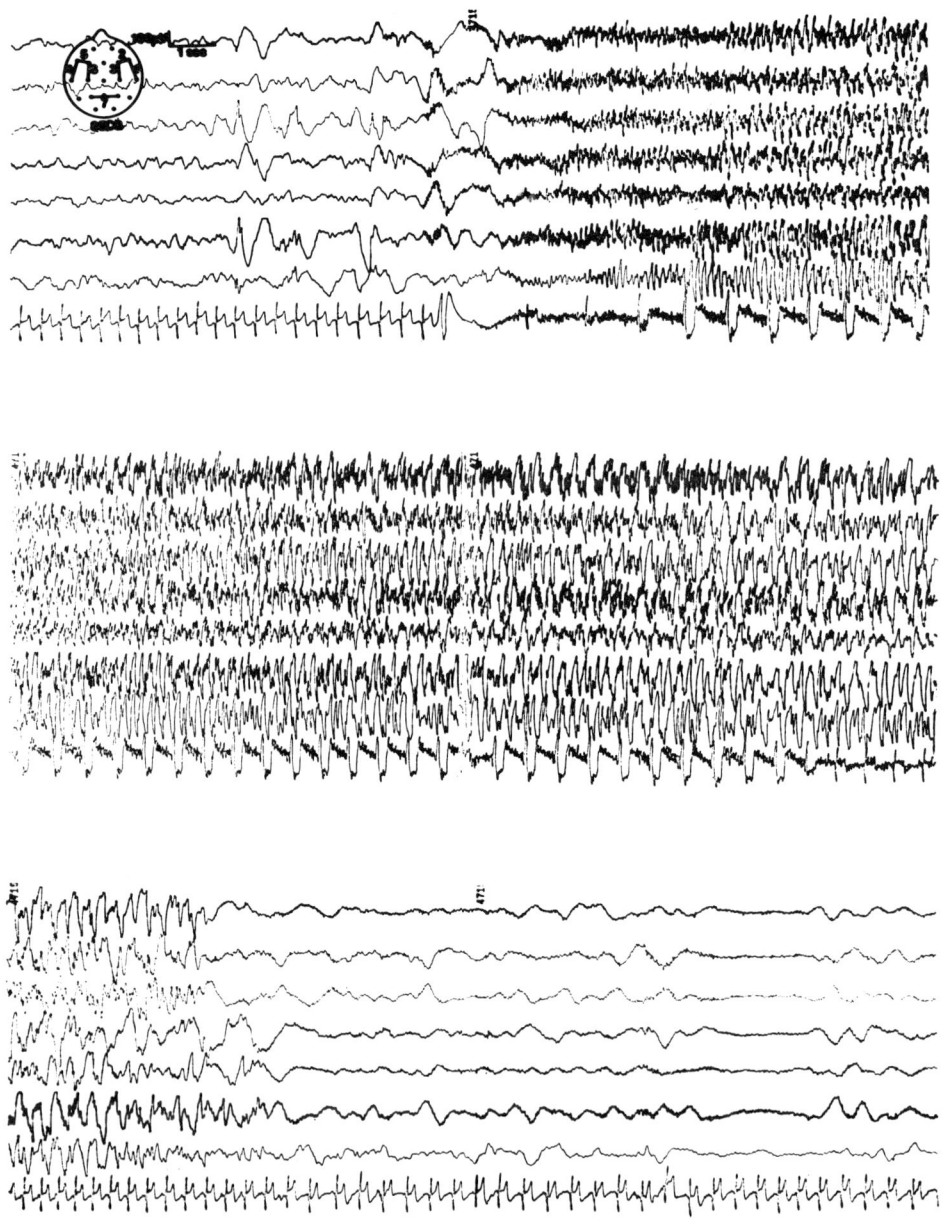

Fig. 12.3. Sections of cassette EEG/ECG recording of beginning and end of tonic seizure in 3-month-old boy (Case 12.2). Severe bradycardia occurs at onset of appearance of generalized epileptic discharge. A preceding focal origin could not be detected with the scalp electrodes. Duration of fast spiking was about 90 seconds, concluding marginally later on the left than on the right. Note generalized EEG flattening about 10 seconds after the conclusion of the epileptic seizure.

by his appearance. He felt very cold to the touch, had the grey appearance of a shocked child, and had a pulse rate of 210. While listening to the heart beat to accurately assess the rate, I noticed the left arm being brought upwards in a stiff manner, the head rolling backwards to the left, and the heart rate slowing dramatically to complete asystole over the course of 5 seconds or so. This was followed by total absence of heart sounds for some 15–20 seconds associated with very deep cyanosis of the child, not just on the port wine stain but around the lips and neck as well. I started cardiac massage by squeezing the chest between thumb and fingers, and after possibly five to ten squeezes was able to hear an irregular heart beat at a rate of approximately 30 per minute. This gradually picked up, and as it did the child took one very deep breath, which improved the colour enormously. Within five minutes he seemed considerably better but still quite pale and cold to the touch and quite drowsy, but alert to external stimuli. The pupils were normal size and reacting at that stage.'

Comment. The family doctor's observations were confirmed on polygraphic recording. Partial epileptic seizures led to apnoea and profound bradycardia with asystole. Carbamazepine was effective without the need for additional cardiac pacing.

13
PSYCHIC AND PSYCHOGENIC SEIZURES

This chapter gives a brief account of psychic events which can be classed as seizures, albeit neither epileptic nor anoxic; psychiatric disorders or derangements which lead to the invention or induction of epileptic and non-epileptic seizures; and the question of psychogenic epileptic and anoxic seizures. Overlaps will inevitably occur.

Hysteria

Hysterical conversion reactions (Bangash *et al.* 1988) may be difficult to distinguish from malingering or feigning, or from true Munchausen syndrome (see below). What is being referred to here is the main type of what Gastaut (*e.g.* 1974) calls 'psychic seizures'. This is a better term than 'non-epileptic seizures' (Trimble 1986), which of course ignores the large population of anoxic seizures. It is also to be preferred to the term 'psychogenic seizures' because, as indicated below, epileptic and anoxic seizures may be psychogenic. The term 'hysterical seizures' has a pejorative tone, and implies accuracy of the psychiatric diagnosis. At any rate, I am calling these episodes *psychic seizures*, and the summary of their distinction from epileptic and anoxic seizures has been given in Tables 5.IV and 5.XI. These distinctions have been elaborated by Gulick *et al.* (1982). As those authors pointed out, psychic seizures can be stereotyped, but the jerking episodes do not have appropriate EEG accompaniment (Aicardi 1986). The use of video–EEG monitoring increases the examiner's ability to recognize the character of the episodes (Duchovny *et al.* 1988) and, at any rate in older subjects, the use of suggestion and intravenous saline has been used to provoke hysterical psychic seizures during the EEG (Cohen and Suter 1982). The close resemblance between this sort of psychic seizure (Ramani 1987) and complex partial epileptic seizures of frontal lobe origin (Williamson 1986) may require very careful assessment and the use of biochemical studies (Trimble 1986).

In children, incest or other sexual abuse has been reported as a provocation (Goodwin *et al.* 1979, Gross 1979). Epileptic seizures may coexist.

Aggression, rage and dyscontrol

These are commonly just what they seem (*i.e.* rage is rage, not epilepsy). The patients may also have epileptic seizures, but such needs diagnosis on other grounds (Ramani 1987).

Panic

Blackouts may be a feature of panic disorder, a diagnosis made on the basis of at least four of the following features: (i) dyspnoea; (ii) palpitations; (iii) chest pain and other discomfort; (iv) choking or smothering sensations; (v) dizziness, vertigo or unsteadiness; (vi) sense of unreality; (vii) paraesthesiae; (viii) hot and cold flushes, (ix) sweating; (x) faintness; (xi) trembling or shaking; (xii) fear of dying, going crazy or doing something uncontrolled during an attack (Herskowitz 1986). These children have anxiety or depression.

Hyperventilation

The hyperventilation syndrome, well-known in adults (Perkin and Joseph 1986), also occurs in children, and clearly it may be a part of panic disorder as above. The symptoms can be reproduced by getting the child to hyperventilate, and indeed hyperventilation often leads to secondary hyperventilation at the stage shortly afterwards when the normal child has a low desire to breathe.

A particular type of hyperventilation occurs in certain mental disorders, particularly Rett syndrome (Hagberg *et al*. 1983, Southall *et al*. 1988*a*), and it may also be responsible for a succeeding apnoea which leads to a true respiratory syncope (Tassinari *et al*. 1976). A controversial view of how hyperventilation affects the brain has been given by Patel and Maulsby (1987).

Munchausen syndrome

Munchausen syndrome may present as prominent seizures both in the adult (Savard *et al*. 1988) and in the child (Croft and Jervis 1989). Status epilepticus may be mimicked (Savard *et al*. 1988).

Meadow syndrome

Meadow syndrome (Munchausen syndrome by proxy—see Chapter 8) may have various manifestations related to seizures. The mother may teach the child that he or she has epilepsy, so that the child then invents the episode (Croft and Jervis 1989); she may invent the story of seizures as in Meadow's original description (1984) (Case 13.2); or she may actively induce anoxic seizures by suffocation (Cases 8.5–8.7, 16.2, 16.3).

Psychogenic epileptic seizures

Whether 'stress convulsions' (Friis and Lund 1974) have some such mechanism is debatable, but there is no doubt that the self-induction of epileptic seizures, particularly by flickering light, is common (Andermann *et al*. 1962, Gastaut and Tassinari 1966, Aicardi and Gastaut 1985). A particularly subtle method of psychogenic epileptic seizure induction involves slow active eye closure (Darby *et al*. 1980), a feature which can be detected by careful observation of the eye closure 'artefact' on EEG. In so far as certain partial epileptic seizures may be inhibited by conditioning therapy (Forster 1972), it is likely that the opposite effect may also be possible.

Psychogenic anoxic seizures

The effects of hyperventilation and (voluntary) apnoea have been alluded to. Anoxic seizures associated with bradyarrhythmias (Stevens 1987) or ventricular tachyarrhythmias (Brodsky *et al*. 1987) may be related to psychological stress.

More directly, the rare patient may compulsively induce cerebral ischaemia directly (Case 13.3). In the case of Lai and Ziegler (1983) a girl pressed her carotid until she slumped and jerked, sometimes with a Valsalva manoeuvre superimposed, and later developed epileptic seizures of possible temporal lobe origin.

Murphy *et al.* (1981) described a 12-year-old boy who died after the voluntary combination of a 'mess trick' and a 'fainting lark' (Howard *et al.* 1951). In detail, he had had breath-holding spells in infancy but thereafter was well. In the weeks before his death he had been observed to hyperventilate, perform a Valsalva manoeuvre and subsequently to become transiently unconscious (the 'fainting lark'). Four days before his hospital admission he was seen to fall limp after neck (presumably carotid) massage. Finally, in the playground at school, he simultaneously hyperventilated and massaged his neck. He then did a Valsalva manoeuvre which was enhanced by a friend giving him a bear hug from behind (the 'mess trick'). He took several steps and then fell backwards with shallow respirations and bradycardia; death occurred three days later. Post-mortem revealed only a small subdural haematoma, but extensive ischaemic-hypoxic cerebral damage was evident.

Case histories
CASE 13.1

A 10½-year-old girl had a five-year history of unusual episodes every morning. The description was that every day she started squealing at about 8am as if frightened. She would try to fight people and run about the living room squealing with a look of terror and her face chalk white, and on occasion she tried to eat a beetle or a spider. Two of her four siblings were said to have epilepsy. Episodes of blankness had been observed during an inpatient stay in the referring hospital but 24-hour EEG cassette recording was normal.

It transpired that her father had been molesting her. After the incest had been stopped, the episodes ceased.

Comment. Although it is helpful to know that the EEG is normal during a supposed 'psychic' seizure (Aminoff *et al.* 1988*a*), partial epileptic seizures cannot be excluded in this way and additional information is necessary as in this case.

CASE 13.2

A 4-year-old girl was said to have up to 10 seizures daily. Three hypopigmented macules on the skin of her trunk hinted at the possible diagnosis of tuberous sclerosis. No seizures were observed by the staff of the children's hospital when she was admitted with her mother. Soon afterwards, the mother began daily visits to the adult psychiatric hospital elsewhere in the city while the child remained at the children's hospital. The mother assured the adult psychiatrist that the seizure frequency continued to be 10 daily whereas, as before, none were observed by the children's hospital staff.

Comment. A case of 'passive' Meadow syndrome in which seizures were invented but not induced.

CASE 13.3

The mother of a 12-year-old boy convinced the trainee neurologist that her son had generalized tonic-clonic epileptic seizures. Supposedly facial flushing was followed by rigidity and jerking of all the limbs, and then pallor and somnolence. Closer questioning indicated that minor injuries preceded these attacks. For example, his father said: 'I was in the living room and he was in the kitchenette. I heard a thump and went ben [in there]. He was lying on the floor. When I lifted him up he went rigid like a board. His eyes went to the top of his head. I thought he was not breathing and I started blowing into his mouth. He started to come out of it. He said the last thing he remembered was banging his shoulder blade. He was a bit white about the nostrils but *compos mentis*.' However, a further episode at school added an additional dimension. The teacher turned round from the blackboard to discover the boy on the floor. She went to him and pulled his scarf from his neck and went for help. He had a red face but she cannot remember if his eyes were open or closed. He recovered quickly. The girls in the class then told the teacher that the boy had done this to himself by pulling his scarf tightly around his own neck.

Comment. This boy had a tendency to vagocardiac convulsive syncope, but it is not clear whether self-strangulation or carotid sinus sensitivity was responsible for his classroom collapse.

14
FUNNY TURNS AND FUNNY ATTACKS

This chapter deals with episodes whose mechanisms are not clearly epileptic or anoxic, nor sufficiently peculiar to find a place in the chapter on psychic seizures.

Of these disorders of miscellaneous mechanism, some are very common, others rare, many trivial but of concern to the individual or the parents or the teachers, others of serious import. The list of entities is by no means complete and, given an open mind, 'new' funny turns keep turning up. The order of presentation follows that employed in the introductory chapter on differential diagnosis (Chapter 5) and does not reflect the seriousness or importance of the episodes.

Daydreams
These are universal but do come to medical attention (Case 4.10). When longer, they may be classified as 'gratification' phenomena (Cases 14.1, 14.2). Arguably one could classify these episodes in the 'psychic' section (as in Chapter 5).

Tics
The extensive subject of tics is well discussed by Lees (1985). The basis of tics, which is neurophysiologically different from that of willed imitated tics, might give clues about the much more complex motor phenomena discussed in the previous chapter. Lees classified childhood tics into *acute transient tics* which are usually simple, *i.e.* involving a single muscle group, and remit spontaneously within a year; *persistent simple or multiple tics*, being one or more tics which persist for several years before disappearing in or around adolescence; and *chronic simple or multiple tics*, where usually one tic persists into adult life. A large number of motor acts may be included, and if one imagines any short movement that one could effect then it is likely that it may be present as a tic. Movements involving cephalad musculature are most commonly involved, that is, muscles about the eyes, face, neck and shoulders. In *Gilles de la Tourette syndrome*, multiple body and vocal tics begin in childhood and wax and wane, and they are often associated with more complex movements of a compulsive nature.

Benign neonatal sleep myoclonus
Myoclonus in slow (non-REM) sleep in the newborn (Cases 15.1, 15.2) may be sufficiently dramatic and rhythmic to provoke the neonatologist to prescribe anti-epileptic drugs in heavy dosages (see Case 15.1). In this rather common disorder the EEG does not change, epilepsy is not present and the outcome is normally good (Coulter and Allen 1982, Resnick *et al.* 1986).

Benign myoclonus of early infancy
Benign myoclonus of early infancy (Lombroso and Fejerman 1977) is probably

better called *benign non-epileptic infantile spasms* (Dravet *et al.* 1986). Runs of spasms occur without any EEG accompaniment. In fact, the onset of each spasm may be a myoclonic jerk, so either term is appropriate for this harmless condition, important in differential diagnosis. Non-epileptic myoclonus occurs in many serious neurological disorders.

Hyperekplexia
Hyperekplexia (incorrectly called hyperexplexia) is best known as a dominantly inherited startle disorder (Suhren *et al.* 1966, Morley *et al.* 1982). Older patients fall abruptly to the ground, commonly backwards, on startle which may be quite slight as, for instance, bumping someone on a crowded pavement. A fractured skull or other injury may result. The startle may be incapacitating, and older patients run the risk of being mismanaged in two distinct ways. On the one hand they may be misdiagnosed as having 'akinetic epilepsy'. Perhaps worse, they may be regarded as neurotic and denied the medication—commonly clonazepam—which allows normal symptom-free living.

The initial presentation of affected individuals is in the neonatal period. They are stiff babies, and the condition may be mistaken for spastic tetraplegia. The stiffness fluctuates, and myoclonic and particularly tonic seizures of non-epileptic type may occur on minimal startle or without obvious stimulus. These tonic seizures may impede respiration and lead to apnoea, bradycardia and fatal syncope. Vigevano *et al.* (1989) describe an original method of aborting these 'stiffness seizures', by holding the baby by the head and legs and forcibly flexing the neck and trunk. They point out that hyperekplexia is an important avoidable cause of sudden infant death.

Cataplexy
If cataplexy presents in a young child it is more likely to be on the basis of a neurological disorder (Case 14.4) than a symptom of narcolepsy, in particular ophthalmoplegic neurolipidosis (Kandt *et al.* 1982; see also Case 4.10 in Stephenson and King 1989). Cataplexy, which is atonia most commonly induced by the emotion provoking laughter, should not be confused with a gelastic epileptic seizure in which laughter is a component (Jacome and Risko 1984). True gelastic epileptic seizures warrant a search for a hamartoma of the tuber cinereum by CT or MR imaging (Curatolo *et al.* 1984).

'Oculomotor apraxia'
The peculiar head thrusts or fixed eye positions in very young children with impairment of saccadic eye movement may lead to diagnostic confusion. Cogan's oculomotor apraxia (Cogan 1966) and ataxia telangiectasia (see Case 9.3 in Stephenson and King 1989) are examples of such conditions.

Subacute sclerosing panencephalitis (SSPE)
Small spasms or droops which occur in runs several seconds apart at the presentation of post-measles SSPE are thought to be of brainstem origin. By the

time this feature is evident, teachers will have noted slowing or regression of school performance, and stereotyped complex waves resembling those seen in 'periodic spasms' will be present on the EEG. Whether this phenomenon should be regarded as an epileptic one is debatable (anti-epileptic medications may actually help).

Intussusception
Although it is much more common for infantile spasms to be regarded as colic, occasionally the converse misdiagnosis is made.

Tetany
This is most often secondary to the hyperventilation syndrome. Its induction while taking the blood pressure in a child with 'grand mal' and chronically sore eyes may point to hypoparathyroidism.

Benign infantile dystonia
Willemse (1986) described four infants who manifested dystonic postures up to several times a day. Episodes might last only a few seconds. The movement was often an endorotation of an upper limb with backward flexion of the hand. The children were normal in between and at follow-up.

Benign paroxysmal torticolis in infancy
In this disorder, reviewed by Deonna and Martin (1981), episodes of torticollis in otherwise normal infants lasted at least hours. The possible relationship of this to migraine has been discussed by Hockaday (1988). The head tilt is not as dramatic as in Sandifer syndrome (see below).

Sandifer syndrome
In Sandifer syndrome (Werlin *et al*. 1980), the contortions of the neck are more dramatic and the important gastro-oesophageal reflux or hiatus hernia is expected. This may develop in a neurologically intact child as well as in one with pre-existing cerebral palsy. Distinction has to be made with the acute dystonic reaction which may follow drugs used for the treatment of reflux, the latest report of which concerned bethanechol (Shafir *et al*. 1986).

Alternating hemiplegia
In the syndrome of alternating hemiplegia of infancy (Verret and Steele 1971, Krägeloh and Aicardi 1980) the episodes of one-sided weakness associated with autonomic phenomena and drooling normally dominate, but non-epileptic tonic seizures may be prominent at an early stage.

Shuddering (pre-essential tremor)
In familial essential tremor, episodes of stiffening, shivering or shuddering may begin in infancy, the episodes decreasing in frequency as the child gets older (Vanasse *et al*. 1976). Given the family history (and examination), the diagnosis

should be apparent. Shuddering without a family history may perhaps reflect sodium glutamate intolerance (Reif-Leher and Stemmermann 1975).

Chin trembling
Prominent chin trembling may be seen in the very young and has been described as associated with nocturnal jerking in more than one generation (Johnson *et al.* 1971).

Benign paroxysmal vertigo of childhood
This condition was originally described by Basser (1964), and has most recently been reviewed by Deonna (1988). The child stops, immobile, looking frightened and possibly pale. The onset and end are sudden. Vomiting may be provoked. Even a very young child may describe vertiginous symptoms. Although one might expect vestibular nystagmus in such a situation, parents do not generally describe this.

Paroxysmal kinesigenic choreoathetosis
This is the only paroxysmal choreoathetosis likely to be seen in the young. The diagnostic aspect of the history is that the episodes are precipitated by movement (Basser 1964), such as getting up to stand after having sat quietly for a while, or when starting to walk. The attacks last from several seconds up to half a minute, and may occur several times a day depending on the motor activity of the child. In the first years they may seem to get worse and then later on may become less troublesome. They are characterized by peculiar movements which are called choreoathetosis but are not particularly like the choreoathetosis seen in static neurological disorders. When at their worst the episodes are embarrassing and may be regarded as hysterical psychic seizures.

Paroxysmal choreoathetosis not induced by onset of movement is a rare disorder in childhood in which prolonged dystonic attacks occur infrequently; they may begin *during* exercise (see Chapter 15).

Acquired paroxysmal movement disorders are worth recognizing, although some of the patients described by Erickson and Chun (1987) appear to have had startle epilepsy as usually defined (Saenz-Lope *et al.* 1984).

Gratification
More dramatic than the daydreams of older people are the complex ritualistic trances of older infants and toddlers. Sometimes it looks as if the child has eidetic imagery and is watching a television in the sky. Mostly parents can 'switch off the programme' (as it were) by passing their hand in front of the child's face; when they cannot, diagnosis is more difficult. An extension of this is something which looks like masturbation particularly in infant girls, rocking with thighs adducted and staring eyes.

Miscellaneous phenomena
Many other paroxysmal events which do not seem to fit any category may be

described by parents of young infants. Sometimes the episodes are of serious import like the paroxysmal hyperventilation and hemifacial spasms of Joubert syndrome (King *et al.* 1984). Similar events may presage epileptic seizures in babies before mental impairment is obvious and before EEG accompaniments are apparent, but this is an ill-explored field.

Stereotypies in mental impairment

Many varieties of complex movement develop in certain mentally impaired children, particularly those with autistic features. Characteristic of these is that they invoke primary sensations such as smell, visual movement, sound, touch, erotic sensation and pain. Rhythmic movements may be particularly prominent. On the whole these phenomena coexist with a profound impairment of the understanding of meaning or symbolic thought.

Case histories

CASE 14.1

An 8-month-old boy was referred with a diagnosis of infantile spasms. For one month he had had up to 20 episodes a day, without apparent loss of consciousness, in which he would extend his arms, all four limbs would quiver and his face would grimace. He seemed vacant during these episodes but could be snapped out of it instantly by a cuddle and would recover immediately. There was no regression of his normal development.

Comment. Although non-epileptic infantile spasms or myoclonus have been well described, such a diagnosis may be difficult without home video-recording at the least. In this case there was not positive evidence of a well-known disorder and reassurance was given, so far justified.

CASE 14.2

A 5-year-old boy had been prescribed sodium valproate for suspected 'epilepsy' because of daily episodes occurring in front of the television. 'One minute he is watching the TV and the next he is into it. He is on cloud nine. You can shout his name. If you go right up to him and shout he will stop. He makes weird wee noises, wee screeching sounds and does odd things to his hands as if he is hallucinating. He puts his hands into his hair and breathes quite heavy, and he rocks.'

CASE 14.3

A 15-year-old boy with Prader–Willi syndrome under excellent weight control collapsed when laughing, and had been doing this for at least five years. He was completely atonic during these episodes but his mother determined that he could remember precisely what was spoken to him during the period of time that he was collapsed. He had no apparent disorder of sleep or other evidence of narcolepsy.

Comment. Cataplexy is not recognized as a feature of Prader–Willi syndrome, but there was no other convincing explanation for his 'funny' turns.

15
FITS AND FAINTS IN SPECIAL SETTINGS

Clues to the diagnosis of paroxysmal phenomena or 'attacks' often come from the setting in which they have occurred. This chapter brings together a number of situations in which certain types of event may be more or less probable. It includes mention of a variety of triggering factors, in particular some of those which can induce both epileptic and non-epileptic seizures. Some clinical situations, diseases and syndromes are referred to, but the list is incomplete, as otherwise the whole of medicine would be incorporated.

Sleep
Sleep is both a mechanism for seizures and suchlike and also a setting or trigger for others. Some aspects of this huge subject will be mentioned.

The common phenomena of sleep are well known, in particular the myoclonic jerk, the hypnagogic hallucination and the nightmare. *Pavor nocturnus* may occur nightly and cause much distress as the parents find their young child sitting up crying in apparent terror and showing no awareness of them. The violent repetitive jerks of *jactatio capitis nocturna*, in which the head is involved, or the rhythmic banging of an arm cause annoyance to the family but are not confused with other epileptic or non-epileptic disorders. Exaggerated myoclonus, however, may be (see, for example, Cases 15.1–15.4, 15.12), especially in the neonate (Coulter and Allen 1982, Blennow 1985, Resnick *et al*. 1986). The difficulty in distinguishing epileptic from non-epileptic seizures in the newborn has recently been well discussed (Volpe 1989).

Narcolepsy is seldom recognized before late childhood or early adult life, and associated cataplexy is easily recognized in so far as a stimulus such as strong laughter is inevitably involved. More important in relation to daytime sleepiness are microsleeps (Guilleminault *et al*. 1975), which may resemble absences in obstructive sleep apnoea. Obstructive sleep apnoea may be related to tonsillar hypertrophy (Case 15.5), and may be a complicating factor in various syndromes such as Down and Prader–Willi.

Nocturnal anoxic seizures are very uncommon, and when they do occur they indicate paroxysmal ventricular tachyarrhythmia such as in one of the QT disorders (see Chapter 8). Asystole with sinus arrest has been reported during REM sleep in young adults either with some sort of syncopal disturbance at night or without any nocturnal symptoms (Guilleminault *et al*. 1984). In theory, vagal-mediated asystole during an REM sleep associated nightmare might be sufficient to produce an anoxic seizure, but this has not been reported.

Tonic sleep-associated seizures of presumed non-epileptic mechanism (Lugaresi and Cirignotta 1981, Rajna *et al*. 1983; see also Case 5.2) and also sometimes presenting with daytime somnolence (Maccario and Lustman 1990) have been described.

145

Case histories
CASE 15.1
This girl was admitted to the neonatal intensive care unit after starting to twitch and jerk at the age of 2 days. The twitching was apparently right-sided at first and later left-sided, and seemed refractory to medication. Sedation was so great that for a time she required ventilation. After the first week or two the duration of the twitching was much less, lasting only a matter of seconds, and most often seen in the right upper limb. The parents thought that sometimes external noise started off the twitching, which was characterized by slow repetitive jerks. On intensive questioning the parents asserted most firmly that the jerking and twitching was always in her sleep or in the drifting phase between wakefulness and sleep, and that it had never occurred when she was fully alert. Phenytoin which she had been prescribed was discontinued and she remained well.

Comment. This baby suffered from the effects of excessive anti-epileptic medication because of failure to recognize that in the neonate, as at other ages, not all seizures are epileptic. Epidemiological studies are not available, but benign infantile sleep-associated myoclonus (Coulter and Allen 1982) seems to be sufficiently often misdiagnosed as epileptic myoclonus to warrant considerable emphasis.

CASE 15.2
A 4-month-old girl had had seizures since the first week of life and had been treated with phenobarbitone, pyridoxine and then phenytoin.

The detailed story was as follows. Twitching was first noticed at the age of a few days. At first the episodes were observed four or five times a day, lessening to less than once a day after the age of 7 weeks and less than once a week at the age of 3 months. The onset was always during sleep and never when she was wide awake. Just before the start of the twitching she had been breathing in a normal audible manner. Episodes began with a slow low-amplitude rotatory jerking, with one or both hands twitching at about two per second. With each movement the hand was thrown out with a combination of supination and external rotation. These repetitive movements might occur either continuously during the several minutes of the attack or stop and start again intermittently. Simultaneous repetitive movements of the lower limbs might also be present with small amplitude extensions of the knees.

On examination the baby was found to have spectacularly advanced development and no abnormalities.

Comment. As with Case 15.1, the diagnosis was benign sleep-associated myoclonus.

CASE 15.3.
The parents of this 20-month-old boy were concerned that he might have a form of epilepsy because his father was said to be so affected. From the age of 5 months the child had had episodes for no apparent reason in which his eyes would start turning in then drift up. His mother would pick him up and he would then go to sleep for a couple of hours. This might happen to him once or twice a day for three or four days at a time. The father's 'epilepsy' had ceased four years previously and the description was that attacks always occurred sitting or standing. He had a warning of dizziness, a buzzing sound in his head and a feeling of being sick, then 'he conked out [collapsed] and twisted and fell asleep for hours, pure white in colour'.

Comment. This infant had a variant of normal drowsy behaviour on falling asleep. This was only brought to the physician's attention because of a false supposition that if epilepsy was hereditary it was likely to show itself first in infancy. As it turned out, the father had vasovagal syncope.

CASE 15.4
An 8½-month-old boy had nodding episodes from the age of 3 months, which the parents described as seizures. They only occurred when he was having a bottle feed or when he was very sleepy. His head would jerk backwards and forwards. His mother mimed this one-per-second nod, which was sometimes so slight that it was only felt rather than seen. In some of the episodes his left arm seemed to tremble. His mother mimed a pronation quiver. She said the whole episode never lasted more than a minute, and if the bottle was taken out of his mouth his eyes would open and he would stop. 20 episodes had been noted but the frequency was declining.

Comment. Another example of a hypnagogic phenomenon of no sinister significance.

CASE 15.5
A 4-year-old boy was said to have seizures in sleep, with twitching of the limbs and stiffness. In fact the 'twitching' was a vibration which occurred during obstructed inspiration, and the 'stiffness', apnoeic pauses.

Comment. The 'tonic-clonic' seizures were the motor association of obstructive apnoeas, related to the boy's tonsil and adenoid hypertrophy. Had his nocturnal sleep disturbance been sufficient to make him have daytime microsleeps simulating epileptic absences, the superficial misdiagnosis would have been even more convincing!

Reflux
Gastro-oesophageal reflux
Gastro-oesophageal reflux is so common in infants that evidence relating it to seizures has to be examined most carefully (Walsh *et al.* 1981, McFadyen *et al.* 1983). Furthermore, the tendency of reflux to improve with age means that double-blind crossover studies with placebo are necessary to demonstrate the effectiveness of specific therapies (Euler 1980).

Epileptic seizures may be associated with reflux at onset (Navelet *et al.* 1989) but the cause and effect relationship is not clear (Jeffery *et al.* 1983). The difficulty in interpretation may be that the same neurological disorder predisposes both to the reflux and to the seizure or apnoea (Walsh *et al.* 1981, Mahony *et al.* 1988; see also Chapter 12).

An important and striking non-epileptic seizure was described by Spitzer *et al.* (1984) as the *awake apnoea syndrome*; the features were summarized by Orenstein and Orenstein (1988): 'An awake infant fed within the previous hour and then placed in a supine or seated position, frequently having a prior history of regurgitation, has sudden cessation of breathing associated with initial staring, rigid or opisthotonic posturing, and plethora, followed by hypotonia and cyanosis or pallor. No coughing, choking, or gagging occurs.' In the index case described by Spitzer *et al.* a gasp occurred at the conclusion of the episode, as also in Case 15.6.

Gastro-intestinal reflux may also be a basis of Sandifer syndrome (Werlin *et al.* 1980) with tonic lateral twisting of the neck.

Nasopharyngeal reflux
Nasopharyngeal reflux has been demonstrated as a cause of awake apnoea with cyanosis, bradycardia and junctional escape rhythm in preterm infants (Plaxico and Loughlin 1981), episodes occurring during feeds.

Case history
CASE 15.6

A 6-month-old girl presented with a history of severe 'startle reaction' since the age of 10 weeks. She had runs of these every one or two weeks. All episodes occurred when she was awake, usually at least an hour after her feeds. Typically she would be lying down playing quietly when there would be an abrupt indrawing of air or gasp and her limbs would stretch out abruptly and her body become rigid. The upper limbs would be extended and abducted and the fists clenched. There would be a noise as if she was trying to breathe, and her arms would shake, vibrating. She would go a terrible colour, pale and grey. Within a minute she would give another gasp and a loud scream and look extremely startled. The poor colour would last for 30 minutes after the episode and she would then be back to normal. She had never vomited.

Lower-oesophageal pH study showed significant gastro-oesophageal reflux with the pH being below 4 for 17 per cent of the study. With treatment to thicken her feeds together with cimetidine and cisapride there was marked improvement.

Comment.   This is a typical example of the awake apnoea syndrome as described by Spitzer *et al.* (1984). What happens to the EEG in these reflux-induced episodes is not known, but any changes would be anoxic, not epileptic.

Bathing and water immersion

There is considerable literature on fits and faints after water immersion, but not all of it addresses the differential diagnosis critically.

Definite and probable true epileptic seizures have been described from Japan. In the case of Morimoto *et al.* (1985) the epilepsy included tonic, tonic-clonic and hemiclonic epileptic seizures with developmental stagnation after the age of 1 year. The child also had myoclonus and clearly had polymorphous epilepsy similar to 'severe myoclonic epilepsy in infants' (see Roger *et al.* 1985). Epileptic seizures were evidently induced by several triggers, of which hot water immersion was one. When, at the age of 21 months, she was immersed in water at 40°C, the frequency of EEG spikes progressively increased over the next 10 minutes until a tonic epileptic convulsion occurred. In another Japanese report (Onuma *et al.* 1972) probable complex partial epileptic seizures were *almost always* precipitated by hot water immersion from the age of 2 years.

In the remaining cases, all with an onset between the ages of 3 and 7 months, diagnosis is not so clear. In three reports the authors recognized the syncopal nature of the infants' attacks. Sheldon's (1952) Case 2 did not collapse on being immersed in a bath but rather on being removed from it, white and limp. The same applied to Jeavons' (1983) Case 1. Bower (1974*a,b*) described an infant whose father was a general practitioner with recent paediatric experience. This girl had four episodes from the age of 3 months, all within 30 to 60 seconds of being put in her bath. She went quiet and pale, vomited and became completely limp and unconscious, recovering after about a minute.

The infants in four other reports are described as having *epilepsy* after bathing or water immersion (Mofenson *et al.* 1965, Keipert 1969, Stensman and Ursing 1971, Shaw *et al.* 1988.) The first of these referred to a 7-month-old boy who had 'eyes rolling, followed by twitching of the upper limbs, and a generalized convulsion with cyanosis and unconsciousness.' Apnoea was noted at the conclusion. No EEG was obtained during an episode, and interictal EEGs were normal. Keipert's patient was a 5-month-old boy whose mother 'said that as soon as his body was immersed in water he became quiet, his arms flopped to his sides, his head became slack and rolled around, he was very pale and looked very tired and exhausted. Although he became limp and quiet, the mother felt that he still knew her.' In an attack in a bath in hospital 'he became quiet, developed a far away look in his eyes and appeared out of touch with his surroundings. He was temporarily apnoeic and the lips became blue. The pulse rate and volume were normal. The limbs showed increased tone. When lifted from the bath he lay quiet and relaxed without signs of recognition. He then became irritable with a gradual return to consciousness over the next 10 minutes.' Again, no EEG was obtained during an attack and, as with all these four infants, interictal EEGs were normal. The boy described by Stensman and Ursing became blue and stiff when immersed in a bath at the age of 7 months. Further episodes began when he was 5½ years of age, after the family had moved to a new house. 'About thirty seconds after he was put in hot water, he became unconscious. His face turned cyanotic and the whole body became stiff. He made automatic movements with his tongue and jaw but no sphincter relaxation occurred. The attack lasted one to two minutes.' Later an attack was precipitated in hospital under EEG control: 'A short while after the patient had been placed in hot water, he reported a feeling of well-being; a few seconds later, he became unconscious and his face turned cyanotic. He bent his head forward, and a general increase in muscle tone was observed. He made automatic movements with his tongue and jaw as well as with the right arm. About one minute later, the patient had paroxysms of coughing. No sphincter relaxation occurred. During the last part of the attack, his face turned deep red. The whole attack lasted two minutes.' The EEG is reported as showing initially focal delta activity on the left, but inspection of the figure does not suggest marked asymmetry. During the seizure proper, the EEG did not contain spikes but diffuse generalized slowing which continued 'for some minutes while the patient was still in the bath'. In the most recent report by Shaw et al., a 5-month-old boy was reported to have become cyanosed 'approximately one minute after being immersed in a bath of warm water at home. He also became limp, rolled his eyes upwards and developed noisy, shallow breathing.' It was not possible to induce episodes in hospital, but the child was visited at home and an attack was induced in his bath while a two-channel EEG was recorded on cassette tape. 'After 30 seconds he began to stare and became cyanosed, pale and hypotonic. The attack lasted for two minutes, after which he was sleepy for 10 minutes.' Inspection of the published EEG reveals muscle potentials at onset followed by diffuse slowing during the seizure. The authors suggest that slowing is more prominent on the left, but this asymmetry is not convincing. In summary, these four infants with 'epilepsy' on immersion in warm water had (i) consistent precipitation by a stimulus known to induce syncope, (ii) when recorded, no EEG evidence of a specific epileptic mechanism, (iii) when recorded, an EEG appearance consistent with cerebral hypoxia/ischaemia, and (iv) normal interictal EEG and normal development. My impression is that all these episodes were infantile syncopes, convulsive or otherwise, although the mechanism or mechanisms of the anoxic seizures must remain speculative. (See also Cases 9.2, 9.37.)

Venepuncture, injections and immunizations
Reflex asystole has now been well documented after venepuncture (Duvernoy *et al.* 1980, Hand and Schröder 1980, Roddy *et al.* 1983) and after injections (Braham *et al.* 1981), with a latency of as little as six seconds (Braham, *personal communication—see* Fig. 7.4, p. 48). Many other episodes have been inferred (*e.g.* Poles and Boycott 1942, Tizes 1976, Nash and Horton 1978), although not always recognized as such (Lloyd-Smith and Tatlow 1958*a,b*; Ziegler *et al.* 1978; Lin *et al.* 1982, Gautier-Smith 1983).

Much more controversial has been the question of the nature of the seizures following immunization containing pertussis antigen. The present author's studies have suggested that children who have such seizures may have a lower threshold to both anoxic and epileptic seizures (Stephenson and Ounsted 1982, Stephenson 1983*a*). Whatever the mechanism, the fine analysis of the National Childhood Encephalopathy Study (Bellman 1983, Stephenson 1988) indicates that such events are not harmful. Other studies confirm the safety of pertussis vaccine (Shields *et al.* 1988, Walker *et al.* 1988), which is now generally accepted (Nicoll and Rudd 1989). (See also Cases 9.1, 9.16, 9.27, 9.33.)

Case histories
CASE 15.7
A 7-year-old boy had absences and convulsions. The absences were typical three-per-second spike-wave absences which were hyperventilation activated, were abolished by sodium valproate and relapsed when he was not on this drug. The convulsions, which began at the age of 3 years, were usually brought on by fright or by seeing blood. Several occurred after venepuncture or attempted venepuncture, and the heart rate thereafter was noted to be about 20 per minute. The seizures were tonic in type and were prevented by atropine. He therefore had a maintenance therapy of combined sodium valproate and atropine sulphate.

Comment. Knowing that this boy had typical epileptic absences, it was easy for the attending doctors to assume that his venepuncture-induced reflex anoxic seizures were epileptic also. Interestingly, anoxic-epileptic seizures (see Chapter 11) did not occur.

CASE 15.8
A 1-year-old boy was referred with a history of 'epileptiform' seizures. Most of the episodes actually occurred after bumping his head and were characterized by rigidity and arching of the back, and variable colour between blue and white. He had a strong family history of epilepsy. The father said that he had not seen the first of his wife's 'epileptic fits' but he did see the most recent one. He said that she was lying flat and then became very pale, pure white and rigid. Her back seemed to arch, her legs and arms bent and she froze. The doctors and nurses who were with her asked him to go away so he did not see her coming out of it, but when he spoke to her later she did not remember anything about it. In fact, the episode had occurred just as the needle was being taken out of her arm after donating a pint of blood.

Comment. Reflex anoxic seizures (vagocardiac convulsive syncope) are so common that they are likely to be witnessed by those in any branch of medicine, not only in the blood transfusion service. It is surprising that the father was given the impression that he had witnessed a 'true epileptic seizure'.

CASE 15.9

Gautier-Smith (1983), in 'Problem cases of epilepsy in driving', wrote: 'The distinction between fits and faints can be extremely difficult and a fit can be provoked by a faint. On the one hand, lack of awareness of a syndrome such as micturition syncope may lead to an erroneous diagnosis of epilepsy, and on the other, a condition which on the history alone may sound like syncope can turn out to be epilepsy. A woman complained of having fainted on several occasions over the years, each episode having occurred when blood was being taken from her. It was decided to check her haemoglobin and the specimen was taken with the patient lying down and using the sphygmomanometer cuff as a tourniquet. The patient had a major tonic/clonic convulsion within seconds of the introduction of the needle, she did not exhibit pallor and her blood pressure, taken within seconds of the onset of the fit, was mildly elevated.'

Comment. This is the best available published example of how difficult it may be to distinguish an anoxic from an epileptic seizure. The distinguished neurologist interpreted what he saw as a 'major tonic/clonic convulsion' (and of course one cannot say in retrospect that this was not an anoxic-epileptic seizure), and in support of it not being syncopal he stressed the supine posture, the lack of pallor and the mild elevation of the blood pressure taken immediately. In fact the mechanism of venepuncture fits is cardio-inhibitory rather than vasodepressor so that, as shown in Chapter 9, the observations were entirely compatible with this syncopal mechanism. The onset and often also the conclusion of the period of asystole precede the motor components of the seizure and so it is not surprising to find rebound arterial hypertension as soon as it is manually possible to measure the blood pressure.

CASE 15.10

Elective tonsillectomy was postponed after this 5-year-old girl had a 'grand mal seizure' after her premedication. Evidently atropine was given intramuscularly into the left lateral thigh while she was lying down and then an analgesic cream was rubbed into the back of her left hand. Within a minute she complained of a headache and immediately went into a state of tonic flexion with her head turning to the left, followed by tonic extension and limpness, then went a very white yellow colour. In the past she had had about six other simple faints with fevers and with tonsillitis, and, at age 3½ years, a similar episode with fainting and stiffness preceded by a headache when she was kneeling after getting out of bed in the morning.

Comment. Vagally-mediated cardiac standstill after atropine injection is not truly paradoxical in that the latency is far too short to allow a vagal-blocking effect. Surgeons and anaesthetists commonly misinterpret these convulsive syncopes (see also Case 9.33).

CASE 15.11

A 5-year-old girl had repeated drop attacks following minor trauma, annoyance, and on one occasion following immunization.

A normal EEG was recorded but when she got off the EEG table she fell over, the colour drained from her face, and having been laid on the trolley she became stiff with a couple of twitches. She was incontinent of urine and vomited, and then was very pale and sleepy.

Comment. This girl demonstrated one of the mechanisms of immunization seizures. With her story an EEG was not indicated (Stephenson and King 1989), but having had the test it was a pity that the ECG channel was disconnected before her (presumed) cardiac asystole.

CASE 15.12

There was great concern in this family that the 7-month-old boy had whooping cough vaccine damage. Following immunization at the age of 4 months he was slightly jittery and when seen in the next 24 to 36 hours was irritable and minimally fevered. About 36 hours after the immunization, that is on the second night, he began to have something like a small fit as he was dropping off to sleep. This happened when he appeared to be asleep but was still sucking on his comforter. It was characterized by repeated slow jerks of the arms, with or without the legs, lasting for 15 to 30 seconds, following which he was apparently in a complete sleep. Since then the parents had noticed this brief repetitive slow bilateral jerking, frequently at the onset of sleep, on average about every 36 hours. Otherwise he had been progressing well, but he had not had any further immunizations—as his father said, 'He certainly won't get another against the whooping cough.' Both his parents often had single body jerks on falling off to sleep, and the father had had seizures with fever between the ages of 2 and 6 years.

Comment. This boy's benign and non-epileptic myoclonus was attributed to pertussis immunization. Although this procedure is no longer thought to have brain-damaging consequences (Stephenson 1988), public and professional attribution is likely to persist.

Blood and gore
Collapse or motor seizure on the sight of blood or the perception of injury is almost certainly vasovagal or vagal (Chapter 9) in mechanism (Greenfield 1951, Connolly *et al.* 1976, Engel 1978, Hand and Schröder 1980, Yule and Fernando 1980). Fears relating to the dentist are prominent. Some examples follow, but see also Cases 9.7–9.9, 9.14, 9.17–9.19, 9.22, 9.25, 9.37 and 9.38. It should be emphasized that from the histories given, *none* of the patients referred to in Cases 15.18 and 15.19 had epilepsy. The details illustrate how eminent neurologists may be misled by the 'malignant vasovagal syndrome'.

Case histories
CASE 15.13
An 8-year-old boy had had fainting fits since the age of 2½, mostly associated with cuts or infections or seeing blood, but once at breakfast with no apparent trigger. Recent stimuli included seeing the family doctor taking blood from his father, talking about the word blood, gutting fish, scratching or cutting himself, getting bruised, falling in the playground, and watching an illusionist on the television putting a knife through someone's arm. The episodes often occurred when sitting, with no warning. His eyes would roll, his colour would go slightly, he would go completely limp like a piece of rubber, then completely rigid with his eyes up. After one minute his eyes would still be rolling and the colour still out of him, then gradually he would start to come round, rather frightened, and would be able to get up in about 15 minutes. Sometimes there was a warning of a few seconds before these episodes.

A previous ocular compression at the age of 5 years had led to gross bradycardia with a series of asystoles of seven, four, four, five and three seconds, followed by 22 seconds of gross EEG slowing down to one per second, accompanied by closing of the eyes, moaning, upward deviation of the eyes, flexion of the upper limbs and then crying with pallor.

Comment. This boy's story suggested vagal-mediated cardio-inhibitory syncopes with blood as a predominant provoking feature, and he was perhaps graduating to blood-illness-injury phobia. Note the non-epileptic television seizure (Stephenson 1978c).

CASE 15.14
A 3-year-old girl was said to have had some sort of spasms or jumps from the second day of life for about a week. She was referred with a comment that her mother gave a very clear

account of a 'grand mal epileptic seizure'. In fact, it was a hot day and she had been running; she came into the kitchen and saw her young friend cut a finger on glass and draw blood. She said: 'I don't feel well' and then went a horrible grey colour. Her mother caught her before she hit the kitchen floor and lifted her up flat. 'She started jumping, first the legs, then the whole body, very hard to hold, and her eyes open, and she wasn't aware, and her hands were flying.' Her mother nearly dropped her because of the strong 'jumps'. The upper limbs were flexed and made about four large jerks or spasms. Then there was a snort which the mother thought was choking and then she was flat out again. The lips were discoloured a shade of blue and the rest of her was white. Then after a few minutes she woke and said she was very sleepy. She was covered with beads of sweat and lay and kept closing her eyes, and then was all right.

Comment. Another example of the dramatic nature of motor seizures after reflex asystole. The sight of blood may have this effect at a surprisingly young age. (The 'jumps' in the newborn period have no evident significance.)

CASE 15.15

A 12-year-old boy had been on carbamazepine for epilepsy for some years. He had microcephaly and a mild learning disability which he had inherited from his mother. The seizures began at the age of 7 and his mother insisted that he was 'allergic to blood'. She knew this because all his fits had occurred after seeing blood or other people injured. Taking blood for carbamazepine level (which was in fact zero) did not induce an episode, but his mother said that they should have shown him someone 'with his face bashed and the blood gushing and spurting', as that is what precipitated his first fit.

Comment. There are no data on whether a person with intellectual impairment or other neurodevelopmental disorder is more likely to receive a diagnosis of epilepsy after recurrent seizures. In this case it took substantial time and effort to elicit the story of 'allergy to blood'.

CASE 15.16

A 10-year-old girl was referred with a diagnosis of 'epileptic seizures'. The family members had not witnessed any of these, but her class teacher described an episode. The girl was in the biology class dissecting ox eyeballs. After a momentary warning of her stomach and eyes 'feeling funny' the next thing she knew she was lying on the ground talking to the teacher, who was saying, 'Don't get up quickly.' The teacher said that she turned round and suddenly the child was on the floor. Her eyes were rolling and her limbs were in awkward postures, with her arms slightly splayed and her elbows bent, and she made flailing movements which from the description sounded like repeated extensions. The total number of jerks was no more than half a dozen. She had the colour out of her face during the episode, but flushed up quickly on recovery. She came to looking disorientated.

Comment. Bearing in mind the stimulus, this case history might be entitled 'ocular compression *au naturel*'!

CASE 15.17

A 4½-year-old boy was said to have had a grand mal seizure in the receiving bay of the operating theatre before induction for an orchidopexy. He had had trimeprazine (Vallergan, 70mg) as premedication. The attending nurse said that when he came into reception he was flushed and crying, fearing the operation ahead, and when cuddled sitting on the nurse's knee he said, 'I'm not feeling well', went pale and immediately into a seizure. His limbs went rigid, extended inwards (she mimed the posture) and when he was put onto the recovery trolley 'he twitched for 10 seconds'. In fact, only the arms and the legs were involved and it was more a shake or quiver than a twitch. The whole episode lasted no more than 20 seconds and he was then very pale and once again said he was not feeling well. His pulse was then about 50 per minute.

Comment. Avoiding premedication by injection does not prevent vagal attacks. The exact history here was typical of an anoxic seizure.

CASE 15.18
Sir Charles Symonds (1950) gave two histories and an additional comment.

A. The first was 'a young man who was liable to faint at the sight or thought of illness or even when examined by a doctor.' A diagnosis of epilepsy had been made by an Army medical officer who had seen an attack. When another medical officer began to examine him he noticed that the pulse rate was one in every three seconds, and then 'I had only time to take three more beats when it stopped completely, confirmed by auscultation, for 45 seconds, during which he had a fit, rolling eyes, rigidity, and a few convulsive movements. The pulse stopped before the fit by about 10 seconds.'

B. The second patient was 'a man of 61, whom I saw for an entirely different complaint, and the details which follow were obtained from his past history. He had as he said "fainted" on many occasions. The first was in his teens when he was taken to the doctor with influenza, the second at 19 after a cycle accident. He was not injured, but very much upset, and lost his senses suddenly fifteen minutes later. The next occasion was a year afterwards when he went to have a tooth out, and, feeling, as he said, in a blue funk, lost his senses and fell before getting into the dentist's chair. In this attack he passed urine. There was a similar episode at the dentist's a year later. Again he passed water. There were no more attacks precipitated by emotion, but on about a dozen occasions he had fainted at the onset of a febrile illness, influenza or bronchitis. The sequence was always the same. He would begin to yawn and continue yawning for ten to twenty minutes. If he could keep walking about this might end without further incident, but if he gave way and sat down his vision would suddenly become grey and he would lose his senses for a minute. In almost all these attacks he passed urine.

'These attacks, I believe, were epileptic for two reasons. The first is the occurrence of involuntary micturition in nearly all the attacks . . . The second reason is the prodromal yawning . .'

Symonds then made a further comment: 'There is next to be considered a rare but important group of patients who begin by having attacks in childhood or adolescence which we diagnose confidently as faints, but who go on to have attacks which we are sure are epileptic. The earlier attacks have the usual causes for a faint, but the liability appears excessive, the attacks are more frequent than usual and continue to a later age and when they have continued long enough we are not altogether surprised when we are confronted with the story of an attack this time without cause and characteristic of epilepsy.'

Comment. The first anecdote is a nice example of how long cardiac standstill lasts when vagal attacks occur 'in the field'. Another example of blood-illness-injury phobia is to be found in the report by Hand and Schröder 1980 (see also Table 9.I, p. 84).

With regard to the second patient, we now know (Chapter 9) that urinary incontinence occurs in about 10 per cent of anoxic seizures, at any rate in the experimental situation of asystole induced by ocular compression. Yawning as a prodrome to vasovagal syncope is also now well known. Of particular interest is the mention of attacks at the onset of febrile illnesses.

The comment in the final paragraph is a disturbing one and a justification for the emphasis put in this book on vagally mediated anoxic seizures. I would hope that neurologists now would, unlike Sir Charles Symonds, indeed be surprised and sceptical at the attack 'characteristic of epilepsy'.

CASE 15.19
Dr Denis Williams (1950) described two patients.

'*Case 1.*—An army officer aged 42 was undergoing dental treatment. 1% novocain had been injected, there was no pain and no apprehension. The dental surgeon said the patient suddenly went rigid, his pupils dilated, his eyes were open and he went into a tonic-clonic convulsion, with deviation of the head and body to the left. The convulsions lasted for 5 seconds, then he seemed normal. The patient said he suddenly felt ill, giddy, sweated profusely and then remembered no more until he found himself with his head in a basin. He was confused at that time. Afterwards he was cold and clammy, and the surgeon said that his pulse was thready. Important points are that the subject experienced no apprehension, or pain, that he was half lying throughout, and that the experience of the symptoms of fainting was momentary.

'His past history showed that he had had the following kinds of attacks:

'(1) In bed just before sleeping, about once a week he had a feeling of apprehension, thumping in the head, pounding of the heart, a hot clammy sensation and a feeling of pins and needles throughout the body. This disturbance seemed to last five minutes. It was never associated with loss of consciousness, incontinence or movement.

'(2) In the daytime on sudden bending and rising he had typical postural hypotension with loss of consciousness.

'(3) He had had repeated attacks of loss of consciousness in response to the sight of blood, accidents, or bomb casualties.

'(4) On hot days, once or twice each summer, he had had attacks of unconsciousness which from the description were syncopal. The symptoms were similar to those of his attacks of orthostatic syncope, but the course of events was more rapid.

'His only brother, a leader of a heavy rescue squad in the Civil Defence Services in London during the war, had never been upset by all kinds of horrible sights. Traumatic amputation of a finger did not greatly disturb him. He had lupus of the face and had to make frequent visits to hospital. He always had to be accompanied for treatment, because when he smelt the "smell of a hospital" he would fall to the ground unconscious with only the briefest warning. He might have time to say "I feel funny" then would fall, often hurting himself. He would have a tonic-clonic fit and be confused for a few minutes afterwards. He had never lost consciousness or even felt faint in response to any other stimulus.

'The patient was normal on full examination. The E.C.G. and the E.E.G. were both normal. Mechanical stimulation of the carotid sinus failed to produce any symptoms.

'Here then is an example of a man having orthostatic and reflex syncope, hypnagogic disturbances and epileptic attacks in response to special circumstances, with a family history of epilepsy in response to a highly specific situation.'

'*Case 2.*—A young man of 19 hurt his hand slightly in machinery. He was having it dressed by a nurse when he suddenly fell off the chair in a tonic-clonic fit, which the nurse witnessed in detail. He was confused afterwards. He was not pale before the attack and said he felt no great pain or apprehension while the wound was being dressed.

'His past history showed that he was a high-grade defective, three years behind his age, whose physical development was normal. He had had no convulsions in infancy. When 8 he had a tonic-clonic attack after he had cut his finger, and after that he had six attacks at irregular intervals, each precipitated by sight of blood or injury to himself. In each he went pale then blue, fell to the ground and had convulsive movements. In one he was incontinent. He had no attacks of any sort in any other circumstances.

'His mother, who was unstable emotionally, had periods of lack of emotional control when frustrated. At the height of her histrionic anger she would suddenly fall down, become cyanosed and have a tonic-clonic fit of short duration. She was usually incontinent in these attacks. The father, a brother and a sister were normal.

'On examination, both the patient and his mother were normal. Their E.E.G.s were normal. In this case there was a maternal history of epilepsy in response to emotion, in a boy who had syncopal and epileptic attacks after physical injury.'

Comment. These are further beautiful descriptions written by a neurologist at the height of his profession but, as with Case 15.18, before Gastaut (1956a) published on the distinction between anoxic and epileptic seizures.

In Case 1 our interpretation now would be that cardiac standstill occurred in response to the dental experience. This man had had various other syncopes and also what may have been panic attacks. His brother evidently had convulsive syncopes of similar vagal mechanism in response to a very specific provoking stimulus.

In Case 2 the vagal mechanism is clearly the same, though in a patient with mental impairment, and once again the attacks persist into adult life. The mechanism of the mother's attacks is speculative. Although psychogenic, the incontinence means that they were not purely psychic. They are likely to have been anoxic rather than epileptic but through what mechanism cannot be established now.

CASE 15.20

Gordon (1982) described a 12-year-old girl whose EEG and ECG were being monitored by four-channel cassette recording. 'While the child was wearing this apparatus she fell to the floor with the arms outstretched and stiff and with the legs adducted. When examined the eyes were glazed, and rolled upwards, and the limbs twitched. The whole attack lasted 45 seconds and appeared to be a typical epileptic seizure.' After recovery, the girl 'said that she had been suddenly frightened by seeing a baby brought into the ward with a tube coming out of the head (a scalp drip).' The tracing, which Dr Gordon has kindly allowed me to examine, shows an asystole of 14 seconds with eight seconds of EEG flattening and no spikes.

Comment. The nurse who witnessed this seizure thought it was typical 'grand mal'. As elegantly demonstrated, however, the girl's heart stopped when she thought she saw a baby's brains leaking out through a tube!

CASE 15.21

A 7-year-old girl had a history of six blackouts in two years, always preceded by stimuli such as a fright, the sight of blood, getting her nails cut, or a bump on the head. The most recent attack had occurred when she was lying in bed about 15 minutes after pulling out her first tooth. On this occasion her eyes rolled and she had marked twitching of limbs and seemed unconscious for 10 minutes, and was then pale and limp afterwards, but recovered quickly.

Comment. In the absence of heart disease, convulsive syncope in the supine position tends to provoke surprise or disbelief in the mind of the doctor. Another example of the 'vicious vagus' (de Bono, *personal communication*).

CASE 15.22

An 8-year-old girl had two seizures with an apparent aura of a peculiar taste in her mouth, and also some pale attacks without loss of consciousness or convulsions—again preceded by the peculiar taste. One of the episodes occurred after having her ears and throat examined by a doctor, but the most dramatic occurred after her brother's knee struck a loose tooth in her mouth. Her eyes rolled, her arms flexed and she shook all over for a few seconds and then came to, white, and feeling sick and sleepy. Further episodes with unconsciousness and twitching occurred after she had bumped her head and when she saw her brother cut his finger and draw blood.

Comment. The aura of a peculiar taste erroneously suggested complex partial epileptic seizures, but blood-injury provocation was typical of vagal attacks.

Head injury

Aside from psychological phenomena, the adverse outcome after blows to the head can be put into four groups. The best-known consequence is *concussion*, with or without additional pathology. Related in part to this is the so-called 'early epilepsy', that is to say, presumed true epileptic seizures occurring soon after, but not within the first minutes after, the injury. Easily mistaken for these epileptic seizures are the *reflex anoxic seizures* precipitated by bumps to the head, as discussed in Chapter 9. More perplexing for the child and the doctor (and these are not confined to children) are *confusional episodes* which, while in certain respects they resemble concussion, are almost certainly migraine (Haas and Sovner 1969, Haas and Lourie 1988).

Case history
CASE 15.23
This 2-year-old boy had had so many reflex anoxic seizures that the parents had lost count. Most of them occurred when he banged any part of his head. They did not hear any noise from him or hear the bang, but would find him stiff and yellow with his head going back and his eyes going up. He would give three or four jerks and stare, then when he came round he would be dazed.

After ocular compression there was an asystole of 10 seconds with no more than one second of EEG flattening. Synchronous video EEG/ECG recording confirmed that the anoxic tonic upper-limb flexion began at the time of the first QRS complex after the asystolic period; the extension and snorting occurred at the second systole after the period of cardiac standstill. His mother insisted that the natural attacks were distinctly worse than the one which we recorded.

Comment. The most typical reflex anoxic seizure. Such children are commonly regarded as having head injuries. (See also Cases, 4.8, 9.10, 9.21, 9.29, 9.32.)

Startle, surprise or fright

Once again it is helpful to separate the mechanisms involved in events triggered by startle. It may be sufficient to list these.
(1) *Epileptic.* Startle epilepsy (Gastaut and Tassinari 1966, Fariello *et al.* 1979, Saenz-Lope *et al.* 1984).
(2) *Anoxic.*
   i) (Vaso)vagal.
   ii) Ventricular fibrillation with or without QT disorder (see Chapter 8, pp. 66–67).
   iii) Hyperventilation, apnoea and Valsalva manoeuvre, including in Rett syndrome (Southall *et al.* 1988*a*).
(3) *Psychic.* Panic disorder (Herskowitz 1986).
(4) *Miscellaneous.*
   i) Hyperekplexia or startle disease (Vigevano *et al.* 1989).
   ii) Pathological startle in progressive neurological disorders, *e.g.* Tay–Sachs disease.

iii) Paroxysmal movement disorder in static neurological disease (Erickson and Chun 1987), though it may be difficult to distinguish some of these latter movement disorders from startle epilepsy proper.

Case histories

CASE 15.24

An 8-year-old boy with moderate mental impairment and relative microcephaly had been very troubled by falls for the past two-and-a-half years, apparently for no reason. 'Down he goes,' his parents said, 'with his toes knotted and his feet bent' for up to half a minute several times a day. A 24-hour eight-channel ambulatory cassette EEG recording was carried out but the EEG changes around the time of his reported falls were not obvious.

When the history was reviewed his parents were not aware of any clear trigger. However, his father said that if he was looking at something out of the window a little noise would make him 'hit the deck' (collapse), the noise being a sudden whisper or a small sound behind his back. During the consultation when his attention was distracted, tapping a tuning fork briskly on the desk instantly induced a brief tonic seizure with fall, recovery occurring within 10 seconds.

Comment. Startle epilepsy, as in this case, is an important diagnosis in that carbamazepine is often effective (Saenz-Lope *et al.* 1984).

CASE 15.25

This 3-month-old girl's mother had noted 'startles' since the age of 6 weeks. The mother, a nurse, thought they resembled a Moro response as if she had had a fright. She was pink in colour and she cried, but calmed down when cuddled. The baby had advanced development and was normal at follow-up.

Comment. The pathological startle of Tay–Sachs disease and other serious neurological disorders is associated with an abnormal neurodevelopmental state. Easy availability of medical services allows benign if poorly understood startles to come to attention.

CASE 15.26

A newborn baby girl was stiff and jittery. This was at first attributed to withdrawal from the benzodiazepines that the mother had been taking during the pregnancy. The hypertonicity became severe and the infant was frequently cyanosed. Improvement gradually occurred over months, but at the same time it became apparent that she would fall backwards if startled. Clonazepam in small dosage led to marked improvement.

Genealogical investigation revealed in this widely scattered family a dominant pattern of inheritance in which affected members were stiff, many having cerebral palsy, and had startle disease as adults. The affected adults were often regarded as neurotic and had difficulty in obtaining the benzodiazepine (commonly clonazepam) which abolished their pathological startle response.

Comment. Hyperekplexia is important to neonatologists, in that it is an important if unusual basis for preventable sudden infant death (Vigevano *et al.* 1989), and to family practitioners, who may need support in prescribing benzodiazepines lifelong.

Exercise

Exercise-induced epileptic seizures are rare but have been described (Ogunyemi *et al.* 1988). Most exercise-induced seizures are syncopes of cardiac mechanism. Aside from obstructive cardiac disease and pulmonary hypertension, ventricular tachyarrhythmias may be induced, particularly in those with QT disorders (pp. 66–67). Profound bradycardia and asystole of presumed vagal mechanism has been described in heavily trained athletes (*e.g.* Ector *et al.* 1984) and also during exercise (Milstein *et al.* 1989). Of the psychic phenomena, hyperventilation syndrome (Perkin and Joseph 1986) may be induced. Paroxysmal kinesigenic choreoathetosis does not occur during exercise but at the moment movement is initiated (Harel *et al.* 1987), commonly many times a day. By contrast, longer episodes in familial paroxysmal dystonic choreoathetosis occur rather occasionally during exercise itself (Plant *et al.* 1984, Kurland *et al.* 1987). Adolescents may have syncope (with or without anoxic seizure) during exercise on stretching with extended neck (Pelekanos *et al.* 1990).

Schools, places of worship and hairdressers
There must be some emotional content to these situations aside from the prolonged upright posture which seems to stimulate a high proportion of vagal anoxic seizures in children and adolescents. Because the threshold of asystole necessary for an anoxic seizure is lower in the upright position, it may be that anoxic seizures develop more easily, and in places of worship it is often physically difficult to fall down with a syncope, which may then become dramatically violent.

Whether there is an additional different mechanism in those many children who have convulsive syncope in hairdressers, or when having their hair cut or blow-dried at home, is not clear. They may be sitting or kneeling upright and may be having their neck flexed or extended, and they are having some sort of stimulus in the area of the highest cervical nerve roots and to some extent the ophthalmic portion of the trigeminal nerve. Whether this is in any way analogous to the reflex anoxic seizures induced by head bumps in toddlers (see below) is not clear.

At any rate, the important message is that predominantly tonic seizures in these settings are likely to be vagal-mediated anoxic seizures not requiring further investigations or special management. (See also Cases 9.6, 9.26 and 9.27.)

Case histories
CASE 15.27
The mother of a 9-year-old girl was called to the school because her daughter was said to have had a fit, not an ordinary faint. The teacher said it looked much like those of her own daughter, who also had fits. The girl was said to have become rigid from the waist up, with bent knees, eyes rolling, and a slight trickle of saliva coming from the side of her mouth. When she came round she did not lose her colour.

The child said that she was at assembly and had had no breakfast. She felt hot, and she told the girl next to her that she felt sick, her eyes had 'gone wrong', she 'could only see squares moving about, circles and triangles, kind of bluish grey', and she 'couldn't hear the teacher talking, only a buzzing sound.' When she came to she felt confused and tired, and for the next few days she slept a lot.

Comment. Often the teacher's first-hand description clarifies the true nature of a convulsive syncope in the classroom but in this case it was, one supposes, biased by her own child having 'fits'. In the event the history from the young patient made the syncopal diagnosis clear.

CASE 15.28

A 10-year-old boy had three fits all in chapel at mass. From his point of view, he would get pains in his stomach, then feel briefly dizzy. He would know what was going to happen as everything went black, he couldn't hear, his head was dizzy and painful, and he would feel sick. When he came to he wouldn't know what had happened except that he might have wet himself. From the point of view of observers, his mouth would go funny and his eyes roll, he would become completely stiff and it would be ages before he came round and then he would want to sleep. He would go bright red before the stiffness and then 'sheet white'.

Ocular compression induced an asystole of 22 seconds accompanied by a typical anoxic seizure. He became flushed before the main extension jerks of the anoxic seizure which occurred after the return of the ECG, and then he became pale and was incontinent of urine. Afterwards he said that he had had dizziness, stomach and head pains and the feeling of sickness, all precisely identical to the natural episode.

Comment. A good example of a typical case of vagal-mediated anoxic seizure reproduced in detail by ocular compression. With the church setting and this seizure history, further investigation would not normally be necessary.

CASE 15.29

While a 9-year-old girl was having her hair dried she became limp and slumped to the side. She had pallor and blue lips, and her hands were twisted in tonic fashion. The duration was only a few seconds before recovery. She later said that she had seen yellow spots.

CASE 15.30

An 8-year-old girl, with a previous history of febrile convulsions at the age of 9 months characterized by eyes rolling and being stiff, collapsed while having her hair cut. She fell back and stared and was stiff, in a decerebrate posture, with her eyes still open, ashen white, and then she cried not knowing what had happened. Later she had another faint in the road, being frightened of traffic.

CASE 15.31

An 8-year-old girl with a previous history of juvenile rheumatoid arthritis passed out while her mother was brushing her hair. She twitched all over for about half a minute, and then came round unaware of what had happened, very pale. Later, when walking along a road in Spain on a hot day, she said she had a pain in her stomach, bent forward as if going to be sick and fell down, 'ricocheting off the pavement with limbs thrashing, and then came round and didn't know anything about it except her pain.' She was very pale afterwards.

CASE 15.32

A 9-year-old boy had fainted every time his hair was cut for the past year. He would kneel down and have his hair sprayed and then cut damp. Family concern arose because the last episode was a 'wee fit', with spasm and brief twitching. The boy said that beforehand he felt funny, his lips had pins and needles, and his head was all drowsy and dizzy, and then he woke up as his mother was putting him on the couch. His father used to faint when he was at school.

CASE 15.33

An 11-year-old girl had a single generalized tonic-clonic convulsion lasting for several minutes while having her hair cut by her father, being drowsy afterwards. She was said to have had a probable faint two weeks previously, not preceded by emotional events.

In more detail, the first episode occurred in a shop. She was very warm and just fell over unconscious, limp and very white; afterwards she was thirsty. The story of the convulsion was that she was kneeling on the carpet having her hair cut, the colour drained from her face, she fell over and banged her head on the side of the fire, and as her parents were trying to get her up her arms and legs started twitching, with general jerks. There was a total of less than five jerks, then she came to a couple of seconds afterwards, not remembering anything and looking very pale, and then went to sleep for three or four hours.

CASE 15.34

A 15-year-old boy was said to have an EEG suggesting 'centrencephalic epilepsy'. He had been treated with phenobarbitone, which he said gave him headaches. In fact his first seizure occurred when he was recovering from an operation. His father found him on the carpet. The next episode occurred when he was about to sit. He keeled over and went stiff with his arms bent, his mouth clenched and the whites of his eyes staring. He came round slowly, not knowing where he was. The last episode occurred when he was sitting having his hair cut, with an identical sequence.

The operation referred to was an orchidopexy, and review of sections of the EEG showed no abnormalities.

Comment. This boy and the children described in Cases 15.29–15.33 provide examples of an apparently very common situation, in which some kind of hairdressing procedure is associated with a fainting fit, presumably from vagal-mediated cardiac inhibition. Often the subjects are kneeling (but not necessarily so), with various procedures involved including brushing, combing, cutting, damping and blow-drying. Dr Ian McKinlay *(personal communication)*, after one of his patients had cardiac standstill and convulsive syncope as EEG electrodes were being applied, suggested a local mechanism. At any rate, the setting is such that the diagnosis can be made without further investigation.

Television

Because in modern days so much time is spent in front of the television, any sort of episode may occur while watching it without being in any way 'causally' related. However, certain episodes may be specifically triggered. Best known is the situation in photosensitive or television epilepsy in which epileptic seizures of various forms may be induced by a slow flicker. The EEG response to stroboscopic activation appropriately carried out may help in clarifying the details of the diagnosis, bearing in mind that EEG photosensitivity is much more common than photosensitive epilepsy. The principles of management are now fairly well established, with advice to watch either a large screen from a considerable distance or to use only a small screen, to ensure the set is stable and well functioning, to keep the intensity of the television picture on the dim side, and if necessary to use methods that ensure that the television picture is seen by only one eye. The latter may be enabled by the use of polarized television glasses or more simply by the use of frosted glass in one frame and clear glass in the other, the glasses being used only while watching television. Some patients need sodium valproate.

The other television-associated disorder which it is important not to forget is reflex vagal-mediated convulsive syncope, which is usually associated with particular types of programme content (Hall 1978). Programmes about medical matters or animal biology, or even magicians pretending to pass instruments through the bodies or limbs of their victims may lead to such a sequel. Because EEG photosensitivity is common, it is important to clarify the diagnosis in one's own mind before ordering an EEG. Otherwise one may have a patient with television-induced anoxic seizures who is by chance found to have a photoparoxysmal response on EEG and who becomes mislabelled as having photosensitive epilepsy (Stephenson 1978c).

Case histories
CASE 15.35
A 4-year-old girl had had several fainting fits including two in which she had gone stiff. One episode had occurred when she was lying in the horizontal position. The stimuli had included a bump on the forehead, and banging her knee. The most dramatic episode occurred when she was watching an acupuncture on television while she was kneeling. On this occasion she said, 'Daddy, oh daddy!' and passed out white and stiff, banging her head on the concrete floor so that she was taken to hospital for X-ray.

Comment. Another example of the effect of gory television, with assumed cardiac standstill (see also Case 15.13).

CASE 15.36
A 14-year-old mentally impaired boy, supposedly epileptic, had his worst-ever episode while watching television (a habit which was rare for him). He had some sort of warning, fell, his eyes went up with the whites showing, he was blue, stiff, and rigid, and then there was some jerking and he was briefly dazed. The EEG with photic stimulation was normal, but ocular compression induced an asystole of 14 seconds followed by jerking of his lower limbs, cyanosis, and diffuse slowing of the EEG to one-and-a-half per second for 11 seconds. He responded to questions eight seconds later.

Comment. Mental impairment is no bar to reflex syncopes, but this lad was not able to state clearly what aspect of the television programme was alarming.

Alcohol
It is a popular conception that alcohol, or at any rate fluctuations in alcohol level from higher to lower levels, may increase the risk of epileptic seizures in those who already have epilepsy as defined. More commonly alcohol withdrawal is followed by epileptic or non-epileptic seizures in those who do not have epilepsy.

The seizures which follow alcohol withdrawal are often classed within the category of 'stress convulsions' (Friis and Lund 1974). It is often difficult to know from a description whether they are in fact epileptic or anoxic, or even a combination of the two. In some individuals I have come across because they were fathers of my patients, the description of post-binge seizures strongly suggested that these were anoxic (*e.g.* Case 15.37). Five cases of alcohol-related syncopes were reported by Fisher (1979).

In children, alcohol ingestion is of course well known to induce profound hypoglycaemia and coma thereby, but this should not lead to any diagnostic problems.

Case history
CASE 15.37
The 26-year-old father of a boy with febrile convulsions was on phenobarbitone for 'epilepsy'. He had had only two attacks, both in the morning after an evening with alcohol ingestion. In the first he jumped out of bed, blacked out, and fell back rigid with his cheeks sucked in and his legs shaking. Then he came to and vomited. In the second episode he had

just come out of the bath and was nearing the wash basin when he became rigid, blacked out, began shaking and bit his tongue. Then he came to, pure white. On ocular compression he had asystole for 12 seconds with a minor anoxic seizure which resembled the episodes described (although not so severe).

Comment. The stertorous inspiration with indrawing of cheeks and flapping of lips which occurred at the end of the ocular compression induced asystole resembled the description given of one of his natural attacks. It seems likely that this man's alcohol-related seizures were syncopal rather than epileptic, but as with so many of the individuals described in this book the epileptic label had been firmly applied. It is of interest that the adults with 'stress convulsions' described by Friis and Lund (1974) had a high incidence of febrile seizures in their children, as in this case.

Migraine, headache and vomiting

All aspects of migraine in childhood (Hockaday 1988) and the relationship between migraine and epilepsy (Andermann and Lugaresi 1987) have recently been reviewed in detail.

It is evident that migraine may be triggered by and may itself be a trigger for another event. The trigger of head trauma has been mentioned earlier (p. 157), and a headache similar to migraine may follow epileptic seizures or syncopes.

It is apparent that true epileptic seizures secondary to migraine attacks are distinctly rare and tend to be focal (partial). Uncommonly, this combination, with transient ischaemic attacks, is symptomatic of a mitochondrial disorder, so-called MELAS* (Montagna *et al.* 1988). More commonly, loss of consciousness or convulsion with migraine is syncopal: an anoxic seizure, probably with a vagal mechanism. Certainly a vagal mechanism was responsible for the syncopes which accompanied vomiting only during migraine in the case reported by Lewis *et al.* (1988) and Lewis and Henderson (1989). Such also was the mechanism in the patient in Case 15.41, in whom a clear migraine story evolved from previous intermittent abdominal pains (syncope through a vagovagal mechanism may also occur with vomiting not associated with migraine—Mehta *et al.* 1988*a,b*).

Case histories
CASE 15.38
This 8-year-old girl had a long history of headaches, often accompanied by vomiting and pallor. On one occasion when she bent over to wash her hair in the bath she went as if to faint and lost her colour completely, at the same time complaining of a sore head and feeling as if she would flop, improving when her head was put between her knees.

A dramatic episode occurred when she complained of headache after being taken out of her bath, and then had what was described as a generalized tonic-clonic epileptic seizure with many jerks and postictal stupor. The history is clarified in the following conversation with the mother, in which her videotaped mime corresponded well with the appearance of an anoxic seizure. Coincidentally or otherwise, the episodes of headache and abdominal pain markedly reduced after withdrawing chocolate, cheese and citrus fruits from her diet (see Egger *et al.* 1989).

Doctor: Tell me what your daughter did when she was having her hair dried . . ?
Mother: Well, she was just standing up and she had no sooner said she had a headache

*Mitochondrial encephalopathy with lactic acidosis and stroke-like episodes.

	than she just keeled over right on top of me, and then she seemed to go unconscious, and her hands went completely like that [arms out] rigid and then she started . . .
Doctor:	Go on.
Mother:	Well, she was shaking—I can't really do it very well, but it was like that [arms out]. Her whole body started shaking.
Doctor:	Can you do a bit more of it?
Mother:	Just her whole body started—like a convulsion.
Doctor:	OK, I just want you to do it till it's finished so that I can see. Her body is stiff . . .
Mother:	She is completely rigid, her legs and her arms seem to go out just like that [arms and legs out] and then her whole body starts shaking.
Doctor:	Her legs and arms are out like this [arms and legs out] . . .
Mother:	And completely rigid.
Doctor:	Head back?
Mother:	Head back and just shaking.
Doctor:	Right, well, I want to see how it finishes as well as the beginning . . .
Mother:	Well, she was out like that [arms and legs out] completely shaking and that, and her legs too, and it seemed to go on for a long time—I just can't really tell exactly how long it went on for. And then I just kind of grabbed her, put her head up and tried to feel for a pulse to see whether she was breathing or not. To me she wasn't breathing, she seemed to stop breathing.
Doctor:	How did she finish the thing?
Mother:	She went limp, she suddenly went . . . you know, after I got to her, her mouth opened and her tongue was back and I pulled her tongue forward, she started coughing, and when she started coughing her body went limp.
Doctor:	And then what?
Mother:	And she seemed to be like in a sleepy daze, very very sleepy and tired, absolutely no colour in her face—her face was whitish-grey. I pulled her forward and just cuddled her and she didn't know what had happened to her.
Doctor:	Did she make any responses at all?
Mother:	She spoke—'Yes.'
Doctor:	When?
Mother:	I just said, 'Are you all right?'—'Yes.'
Doctor:	How long after that . . ?
Mother:	I would say roughly 10 minutes—I wouldn't say that was completely accurate, but I'd say no more than 10 minutes.
Doctor:	It was 10 minutes before she said she was okay—what was she doing for that 10 minutes?
Mother:	Well, the shaking and then . . .
Doctor:	No, no—the end of the shaking, from then on, how long till she says . . ?
Mother:	Probably just about 10 minutes till she actually responded.
Doctor:	And what was happening during the 10 minutes?
Mother:	Well my other daughter, she phoned up the ambulance and they said it was on the way so in that time I just sat and cuddled her, and made sure she was all right.
Doctor:	And what was she doing while she was being cuddled?
Mother:	No response, just sitting there completely limp, at the time she was very sleepy.
Doctor:	What do you mean sleepy?
Mother:	Well she seemed to want to go to sleep at that . . .
Doctor:	Can you explain that more?
Mother:	Erm . . . very very tired.
Doctor:	And what do you mean, wanted to go to sleep?

164

Mother: She just seemed to want to close her eyes again and . . .
Doctor: She wanted to go to sleep since immediately she stopped this . . ?
Mother: Yes, she seemed to want to go back to sleep—I spoke to her all the time and asked her if she was all right, and, say another 10 minutes later, she seemed to be responding quite well and she was fine.
Doctor: But can you explain slightly more what it means by wanting to go to sleep?
Mother: Wanted to close her eyes.
Doctor: She opened them and closed them?
Mother: [Nodding] Yes.
Doctor: So she was opening and closing them . . .
Mother: I think she said, 'I want to go to sleep.' I can't be 100 per cent certain on that because I was so uptight. She just wanted to cuddle in and go back to sleep.
Doctor: That was immediately at the end of the fit, that's what you'd say?
Mother: No, I wouldn't say I was completely accurate because at the time I was very very upset.
Doctor: In a panic was it?
Mother: In a panic—complete panic. I have never experienced anything like it.

Comment.   This is an example of rather prolonged history-taking. The outcome of the story is that the child probably had an anoxic seizure, but considerable interrogation was necessary to disperse the original conception of a grand mal epileptic seizure. The 'mal' of an anoxic seizure may be quite 'grand'.

CASE 15.39
A 9-year-old girl from the South of England was referred with the following story.
  In the first place she had a total of about 25 febrile convulsions between the ages of 12 months and 7 years. These, which were associated with earache or sore throat and feeling hot, consisted of eye rolling and gagging noises, usually at about 3am, with shaking all over, twitching and shivering.
  Next came a total of five episodes brought on by external pain, the first at 3 years and the last 18 months before referral. They would happen if she bumped her head or squeezed her finger in a door. She would not scream or cry but just drop 'like a sack of coal'. Her jaw would be completely firm and stiff; her eyes would roll; she would shake really violently as if very cold, like a coarse shiver; and she would choke and make a gagging noise. The whole thing would last several seconds, and then she would wake looking white and then go to sleep or be sick. Afterwards she would not remember everything, and would even forget that, for example, she had squeezed her finger in the door.
  She began to have headaches 12 months before the referral, and subsequently had a total of five attacks associated with headaches. She would come up to her parents and say that she had a bad headache and they would see in her eyes a glazed look. If she was able to swallow a soluble analgesic at the time and lie down then she would not have a fit. But if she was unable to have an analgesic and the headache became very bad she would then just drop on the ground and lie and twitch. She would give two large jerks, her eyes would stare and she would be really white with blue lips. Then she would come to as quickly as she used to do after the episodes induced by external pain.
  Her mother disclosed that when she was between three and six months pregnant she had a total of four blackouts with no warning except that she felt hot seconds before. The first of these was just after she had gone to the toilet. The next thing she knew, her work mates were leaning over her saying that she had been jerking around and moaning.

Comment.   This was a complex case. The febrile seizures seemed likely to have an epileptic basis although the child did not have unprovoked epilepsy. Clear-cut anoxic seizures were precipitated by painful stimuli of the kind which are well known to induce vagocardiac syncope. It seemed likely that the episodes associated with headache were of the same mechanism. The child's mother seemed to have syncopes of similar origin.

CASE 15.40
A 10-year-old boy had had many episodes since the age of 9 or 10 months. All these were precipitated by some sort of injury like a bump or a knock, or a hurt to the knee. With a latency of a few minutes he would feel his tummy sore; this would continue for half an hour and he would become pale. On one occasion this occurred on a rugby pitch: he was going about in a dazed condition and had to be sent off. His mother was concerned that he might have drowned if he had gone to the bath or the shower. These episodes were not helped if he lay down, or even if he was held upside down by his feet.

Comment. It is speculative as to whether this child's episodes were similar to the confusional migraine described after head bumps.

CASE 15.41
A 9-year-old girl had had episodes of abdominal pain, vomiting and loss of consciousness since the age of 3½. Her mother had classical migraine, on one occasion having had numbness on one side during an attack in pregnancy.

The first episode occurred when she was in a car and vomited and passed out for a second. Then for two years there were no episodes but no sickness either. At the age of 5½ she had three episodes in the same day with vomiting and loss of consciousness. Since then, episodes had occurred every two or three weeks. They would happen particularly under conditions of excitement such as going a long journey, to a pantomime, or far out into the hills, or at a karate class.

The parent's description was that she would complain of a sore tummy and would want to lie down. She would feel hot and the colour would drain from her face; she would become very white and vomit slightly. Then despite lying on the ground she would lose consciousness and become limp and her eyes would roll. Sometimes she would become stiff when coming round and slightly jerky. She would open her eyes and then vomit—'like a fountain, out it comes'— and she would faint again. The most recent episode was when she was away in the hills and the snow. She had an abdominal pain, felt sick, tried to be sick and passed out three times, being jerky when she did so. Evidently she could have abdominal pain without losing consciousness, but if she actually vomited she always felt faint and usually lost consciousness.

The child herself said that it wasn't really a sore tummy pain, but 'my chest gets all blocked up, I feel all funny, I can hardly breathe and then my sickness comes out. When I wake up the voices are all funny, sort of like a radio in the background with the reception not very good.' Before the faint her vision goes 'like an atmosphere when it's dark with wee tiny dots going round and round'; then, 'when I'm fainting my arms and legs go all tingling.' She said that the episodes were brought on by travelling and sometimes in the car when her father was driving.

She was given ipecacuanha, and her EEG and ECG were monitored under videotape control while she lay supine. With each vomit, and beginning before the vomit was expelled, there was gross bradycardia with sinus arrest and asystolic pauses of up to eight seconds (Fig.15.1a).

Later, after she was found unconscious with her face in a pool of vomit, it was decided to insert a transvenous ventricular demand pacemaker. Since then she has had no further trouble (Fig.15.1b).

Comment. Negative feedback ought to make the vagovagal reflex self-terminating, but the frequency of anoxic seizures associated with migraine-associated vomiting or even vomiting

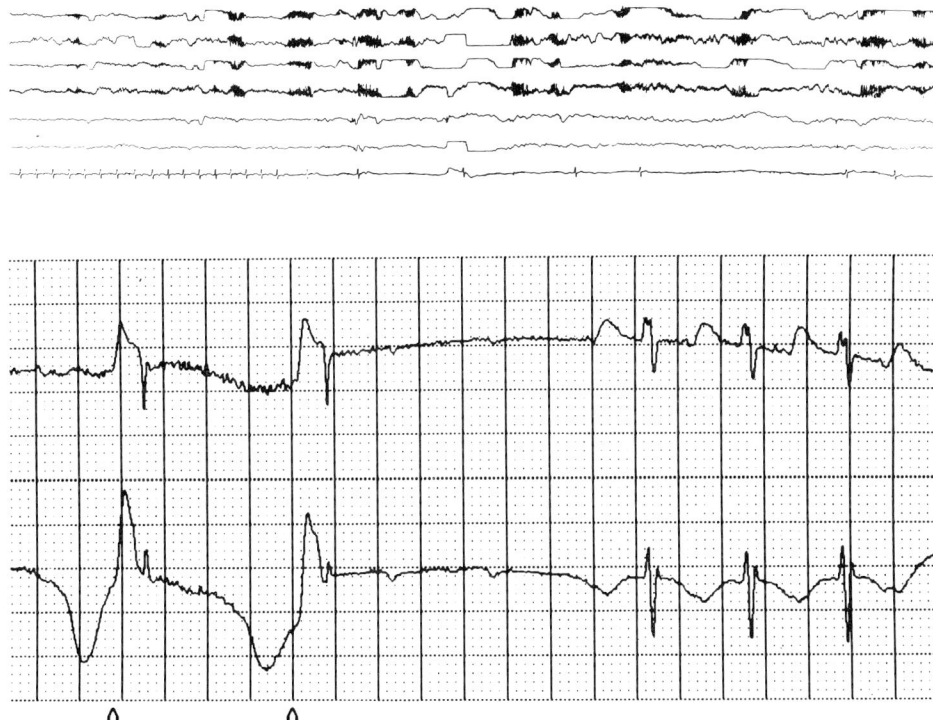

Fig. 15.1. *(a)* EEG/ECG recording after ipecacuanha in a 9-year-old girl with emerging migraine who had simple or convulsive syncope when she vomited (Case 15.41). EEG montage is not important, but shows clusters of muscle potentials related to retching. Note sinus arrest with gross bradycardia and asystolic intervals up to seven seconds. *(b)* Vomiting was again induced by ipecacuanha one month after pacemaker insertion. Frequent episodes of sinus arrest and complete atrioventricular block were promptly aborted by paced ventricular complexes, indicated by the markers in this two-channel ECG sample.

of uncertain cause suggested that transvenous pacemaker therapy was the treatment of choice.

Abdominal pain

Like headache, abdominal pain or discomfort may be both a manifestation of a seizure and also a trigger. The rising epigastric discomfort preceding complex partial epileptic seizures of temporal lobe origin is well known, but brief premonitory abdominal discomfort may also be the initial symptom of a vagal convulsive syncope *e.g.* Cases 15.28, 15.42). Pre-ictal abdominal pain occurred in our patient with paroxysmal pulmonary hypertension (Case 8.8), and has been described in QT disorders (see Chapter 8).

Epileptic seizures induced by abdominal discomfort are said to be exceptionally rare. One such case was described by Gastaut and Tassinari (1966). This

167

concerned a child aged 9 years with encephalopathy following measles, in whom myoclonic jerks with multiple spike and wave discharges could be provoked by an enema or the injection of prostigmine. Clinically, severe colicky pain preceded the clouding of consciousness and jerking in his natural seizures. Comments made to me by parents of severely disabled children suggest that this phenomenon may not actually be as rare as has been supposed. Vasovagal syncopes are of course easily induced by sudden severe abdominal pain of organic origin, but in practice it is often difficult to tell whether the abdominal pain is the trigger or represents the onset of a vasovagal syncope.

Case history
CASE 15.42
This 10-year-old girl was kneeling while her mother changed her earrings. She started to complain of a sore tummy (later she said that she also felt some round-and-round dizziness very briefly, but nothing else); within seconds, despite her mother having stopped touching her ears, she fell over onto her left side, moaning, and with her right arm and leg 'twitching'. The twitching was in fact a series of repeated extension jerks in an extended posture, the total number of jerks being no more than three. She was only down for a few seconds, with her eyes open, then she came to and jumped back onto her knees and burst out crying looking chalk white.

Comment. A typical example of the common phenomenon of abdominal pain as an aura of a vagal attack.

Asthma and coughing
Patients who are prone to paroxysmal cough may have syncopes or seizures which lead to diagnostic confusion. Asthma is a well-known example (Haslam and Freigang 1985). Some evidence has been offered to suggest that cerebral concussion is a mechanism (Keer and Eich 1961), but the evidence is overwhelming that in most cases the seizures are anoxic, repeated Valsalva manoeuvres being the mechanism, leading to abrupt loss of cerebral perfusion (Sharpey-Schafer 1953a,b). In the latter paper, Sharpey-Schafer wrote: 'The occurrence of fits during syncope after coughing is likely to be more misleading to neurological than to circulatory workers, who are probably aware that a fit can occur in any normal subject if the blood flow to the brain is sufficiently reduced. If the subject is a known epileptic the full seizure is more easily induced by methods of lowering the blood pressure. Two of the present cases had a history of epilepsy and grand mal after violent coughing.' However, only rarely in old people are actual epileptic seizures induced by coughing (Morgan-Hughes 1966). EEGs during the convulsion induced by coughing have clearly shown pure and typical anoxic changes (DeMaria *et al.* 1984). In the series of Haslam and Freigang (1985), five of the 12 asthmatic children had been inappropriately treated with anti-epileptic drugs because of convulsive movements and urinary incontinence during attacks.

Rarely, cough syncope may be a manifestation of hindbrain malformation (Larson *et al.* 1974). The mechanism probably involves acute changes in the pressure relationships of the cerebrospinal fluid above and below the foramen magnum (Williams 1976).

Diabetes mellitus

By far the most common episodic cerebral events in diabetes relate to insulin-induced hypoglycaemia. Episodes resembling generalized convulsive epileptic seizures and also transient focal neurological deficits may be seen. Hypoglycaemia is a potent stimulus to vagal mechanisms, so that vagal syncopes, convulsive or otherwise, may occur. In older patients autonomic neuropathy may allow postural hypotension. Further, at least in adult life, cerebral blood flow may be unstable (Dandona *et al.* 1979). A common concern is whether the patient has epilepsy proper, either secondary to previous hypoglycaemia-induced cerebral damage, or coincidentally present. I am not aware of population data which help with this question, but EEG abnormalities are evidently more frequent in those with previous severe hypoglycaemic episodes (Soltész and Acsádi 1989).

Tonic attacks with decline in consciousness in diabetic coma indicate impaired cerebral perfusion and the need for urgent intracranial pressure monitoring (Balakrishnan *et al.* 1989).

Case history

CASE 15.43

This 7-year-old boy had a history of seizures since infancy in three different situations. First, from the age of 10 months he had jerking convulsions with low blood glucose thought to be a manifestation of ketotic hypoglycaemia. Many finger-prick tests for blood glucose were done at this time. Second, he had jerking fits with fevers from 2 to 3 years of age. Third, since the age of 4½ he had faints or brief convulsions if he pricked his finger. In a recent episode he had a sore throat and was given glucose supplements. He was lethargic and went upstairs; the parents heard a thud at the top and rushed up to find him into a convulsion. He was rigid and white and colourless, with his hands jerking back five or six times, his head back, his tongue back and his teeth clamped down. Then he relaxed and he promptly sat up and could answer questions, but was drowsy, feeling very weak, and had no feeling in his arms. He was taken to the Accident and Emergency department. His finger was pricked for a blood glucose estimation and he had a mild convulsion sitting on his father's knee. The glucose level was not low.

Comment. Irrespective of the metabolic disorder, actual or imagined, seizures with blood sampling are likely to be vagal-mediated syncopes.

Fever and febrile illness

The problem of febrile seizures is well known to all who care for ill children and to those who deal with adults who have epilepsy. This subject has recently been reviewed in depth, and in this section I will restrict the bibliography to publications not included in the list of more than 400 references in Wallace's monograph *The Child with Febrile Seizures* (1988). My approach to the definition is the same as that of Wallace when she said, 'A febrile seizure is best defined as any seizure of cerebral origin which occurs in association with any feverish illness', provided that one does not use Wallace's definition of a seizure as 'an episode of alteration in motor, sensory or behavioural function with or without loss of consciousness but always accompanied by a sudden excessive discharge of cerebral neurones.' The matter is arguably more complex, as recently summarized by Stephenson and King (1989), the alternatives being as follows.

(1) The convulsion is not a seizure in either of the accepted senses of an epileptic or anoxic seizure, being a rigor or, for example, an hallucination.
(2) The seizure is a febrile syncope similar to a syncope suffered by adults with influenza and fever.
(3) The seizure reflects the presence of a gene for one or other type of epilepsy, and may predict to a certain extent the occurrence of that type of epilepsy in later childhood. For example, the febrile seizure may predict absence epilepsy or epilepsy with generalized tonic-clonic seizures or benign focal epilepsy of childhood with Rolandic spikes or epilepsy with complex partial seizures.
(4) The febrile seizure may be the beginning of polymorphous epilepsy, otherwise called severe myoclonic epilepsy of infancy.
(5) The seizures may reflect static focal pathology. This may be overt with obvious neurological signs in a baby, or covert. The latter is thought to be the basis of many cases of lateralized febrile seizures with later epilepsy and complex partial seizures.
(6) The febrile seizures when they are focal may represent the onset of a chronic progressive pathology, such as progressive neuronal degeneration of childhood (PNDC) or the chronic focal encephalitis of Rasmussen. An important situation is the coincidental tonic febrile seizure as the presenting symptom of a posterior fossa tumour.
(7) The febrile seizures may be a manifestation of an acute encephalopathy due to central nervous system infections. This may for example be due to virus invasion or pyogenic or tuberculous meningitis. If there is focal brain pathology the seizure accompanying the febrile illness will tend to be lateralized, whereas if there is generalized brain swelling, a tonic non-epileptic seizure with failure to localize pain may be the consequence.
(8) A febrile seizure may be a manifestation of a metabolic encephalopathy, the encephalopathy having been precipitated by the catabolism of the febrile illness. In this case the febrile seizure will often be a tonic non-epileptic one with loss of ability to localize, but lateralized seizures are also possible.

Epileptic seizures

Among those who use the term seizure as in this book, it is generally accepted that most febrile seizures have an epileptic mechanism (Gastaut 1973). Whether this is in fact so is less certain (McGreal 1956, Stephenson 1978*d*, Stephenson and Ounsted 1982). The only published example of a short febrile seizure was of epileptic mechanism and left temporal origin (Stephenson 1983*a*).

Early 'focal' febrile seizures were common antecedents to later complex partial epileptic seizures in the Minnesota population based case-control study (Rocca *et al.* 1987*a,b,c*). The conclusions of that study were summarized: 'Although our data are inadequate to draw conclusions, we would like to suggest that, in most cases, febrile seizures are linked to subsequent epilepsy through a preexisting liability of the brain to convulse, either genetically determined or induced by a lesion during brain development. A preexisting brain lesion is probably more common in febrile seizures followed by complex partial seizures, and manifests through focal febrile seizures. On the other hand, a genetically determined convulsive diathesis is probably more common in febrile seizures followed by generalized seizures, and manifests as nonfocal febrile seizures' (Rocca *et al.* 1987*b*). In this same study, febrile seizures were a predictor for later epileptic absences, and a prominent feature in these febrile convulsion histories was a tendency for multiple febrile seizures to occur within 24 hours (Rocca *et al.* 1987*a*).

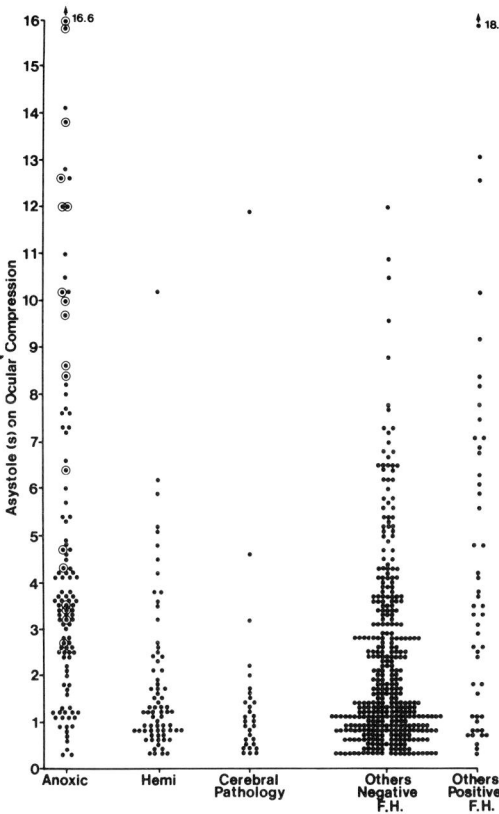

Fig. 15.2. Individual ocular compression asystole values in 630 children with febrile seizures. The circled dots denote 18 children who had reflex anoxic seizures from other stimuli (head bumps, etc.) as well as febrile convulsions. The 'others' are divided into those with or without a positive family history of febrile seizures in a first-degree relative. See text for further details. (Stephenson 1983a.)

Some additional support for an epileptic mechanism in a substantial proportion of children with febrile convulsions comes from a clinic-based study by Alvarez *et al.* (1983). These authors found 23 per cent of paroxysmal spike wave in drowsiness in the febrile seizure group compared with 2 per cent in normal controls.

Syncopes (anoxic seizures)
The idea that a proportion of febrile seizures are syncopal was proposed by McGreal (1956, 1957) and Gastaut and Gastaut (1957, 1958). More recent ocular compression studies added further weight to this proposal (Stephenson 1978*d*, Stephenson and Ounsted 1982) (Fig. 15.2). Some findings from Stephenson (1983*a*) are reproduced in Tables 15.I and 15.II. These data carry some weight, and as Aicardi (1986) wrote, 'There is no doubt, however, that at least some febrile

171

TABLE 15.I

Febrile convulsions and pain-induced seizures in the same child*

Number of children examined	28
Aged 3 years or over at test (range 10 months to 14 years)	20
Head bump a trigger	13
Asystole ⩾7 secs. on ocular compression	18 (64.3%)
EEG spikes	0
Fever/pain seizure type concordance	21 (75.0%)

*Adapted from Stephenson 1983*a*.

TABLE 15.II

Seizure description concordance: fever and pain triggers in the same child*

Fever	Pain or bump				
	Tonic	Jerks	Limp	Not known	Total
Tonic	11	1	—	—	12
Jerks	2	8	—	—	10
Limp	—	—	2	—	2
Not known	2	—	1	1	4
Total	15	9	3	1	28

*Adapted from Stephensen 1983*a*.

convulsions are anoxic rather than epileptic in mechanism' (see also Lennox-Buchtal 1973, Stephenson 1988*a*). In the light of further studies (Stephenson 1983*a*) there is no longer a clear indication for ocular compression in the context of febrile convulsion; to quote Aicardi again, 'At the moment, it would seem that the best and safest way of identifying febrile anoxic seizures is to obtain a precise description from parents or custodians.' Some such descriptions are given in Cases 9.2, 9.18, 9.25, 9.27 and 15.44.

As Jeavons (1983) pointed out, a past history of febrile convulsions is one of the five main reasons for the misdiagnosis of epilepsy (the other four being: an inadequate history; the occurrence of clonic movements, jactitations or incontinence; a family history of epilepsy; and an abnormal EEG). This error, in which the diagnosis of (vaso)vagal convulsive syncope in mid-childhood, adolescence or later is tilted toward that of 'grand mal' because of a previous history of febrile convulsions, applies even if the initial febrile convulsion was of epileptic mechanism. However, if the initial febrile seizure was a febrile syncope it is no surprise that later seizures have the same anoxic mechanism (Gastaut and Gastaut 1958).

Anoxic-epileptic

While it is clear that a febrile seizure characterized by tonic stiffening and immediate return to consciousness is compatible with an anoxic seizure or syncope, it does not follow that a febrile seizure which includes a definite repetitive clonic component is of pure epileptic mechanism (Stephenson and Ounsted 1982, Stephenson 1983a). The 'anoxic-epileptic' mechanism has been discussed in Chapter 11 and, as Case 15.45 illustrates, this can cause definite diagnostic confusion. It must be admitted, however, that technology is not yet available to allow population studies to test this point.

Miscellaneous mechanisms
The vibratory 'convulsion' or rigor is too well known to require description. Although there are no clear data on the relationship, it is worth bearing in mind that the same sort of causes of fever obtain when a fever is associated with seizures as when it is not, and occult bacteraemia has been found in about 5 per cent of simple febrile seizures (Chamberlain and Gorman 1988).

Movement disorders with other mechanisms may indicate acute cerebral pathology, as discussed below.

Meningitis and encephalitis
In overt encephalitis such as that due to herpes simplex virus 1, hemiclonic seizures followed by hemiparesis are likely to represent destructive cerebral pathology. In pyogenic meningitis, the range of events is greater:
(1) *Generalized* (in the sense of bilateral) short convulsions may have the same mechanism and significance as seizures with fever but without meningitis.
(2) Prolonged *hemiclonic* seizures may imply a secondary focal pathology.
(3) *Tonic* seizures with impaired ability to localize pain thereafter suggest a malignant anoxic mechanism, with brain swelling and compromised cerebral perfusion (Horowitz and Boxerbaum 1980). Case 15.46 is an unfortunate example.
(4) *Movement disorders* may imply secondary cerebral pathology (Burstein and Breningstall 1986).

The risk of later unprovoked epileptic seizures after encephalitis and meningitis has recently been studied in a population-based cohort (Annegers *et al.* 1988). The risk was markedly increased after virus encephalitis with or without early seizures, and after bacterial meningitis with early seizures, but not after aseptic meningitis nor after bacterial meningitis without early seizures. Not surprisingly, most of the later epileptic seizures were partial in type.

Long-term effects
From consideration of the various mechanisms and aetiologies, it is evident that various outcomes are possible, from the totally benign to the devastating. The extensive analyses of Nelson and Ellenburg referred to in Wallace (1988) have established that good prognosis of seizures with fever is associated with a lack of other pathology. There is strong evidence that long early convulsions are associated with adverse sequelae (Ounsted *et al.* 1987, Sagar and Oxbury 1987), but the explanation may lie in the aetiology more than in the seizure (Freeman 1989, Maytal *et al.* 1989).

Case histories
CASE 15.44

I first heard about this girl when she was 2 years of age. Her episodes had begun when she was 8 months old. By the age of 2 she had had about six major convulsions and about 20 smaller ones. They tended to occur when she was developing a fever (commonly they were the first sign of a fever) or when she was in a low state after an illness. They did not occur at the height of a fever. The immediate provocation was usually being thwarted or frustrated in not being able to come to her mother, or 'shock', the most severe attack occurring after she had fallen down stairs and bumped her head. Her mother's (written) description of these episodes is worth reporting in some detail:

'Usually, but not always, she screams and goes scarlet. Her mouth is wide open. If we anticipate matters at that stage we can abort the attack by breathing repeatedly into her mouth, but by the time her back arches and she goes still it is too late. Her teeth also clench and her eyes roll back, then limpness with convulsions occurs. In a severe attack there is a lot of limb movement during this convulsion. (I've not been able to persuade paediatricians that the limb movements while she is limp and unconscious are convulsions, but what are they if they aren't?) She goes waxy and ashen. Attempt to find her wrist pulse fails (I thought my icy panic was the culprit). Then she takes rasping heaves of breath that sound as if they are tearing her lungs apart. When the pulse returns it is uneven with long gaps. Normally she then becomes conscious but is clumsy and disorientated and ghostly pale. An example of the disorientation is after a bad attack in Paris when she didn't recognise her parents and started running around and falling about in a very distressed way and did not want to be pulled onto her mother's lap or cuddled by any member of the family. On one occasion she did not appear to become conscious at the conclusion. Her eyes opened and rolled around vacantly and she did not appear to see nor hear. She then became limp again and awoke 20 minutes later in an ambulance, in which, uncharacteristically, she went into the arms of the ambulanceman without complaint. She becomes very cold after the attacks and on several occasions we have been convinced that she had died.'

Comment. The 'febrile convulsions' in this case were clearly anoxic seizures, though whether they were vagocardiac or 'mixed' breath-holding episodes is uncertain.

CASE 15.45

This 17-month-old girl had episodes since the age of 11 months in which she went blue and then twitched. Before the first of these she had had more ordinary 'breath-holding attacks' since the age of 6 months. When restrained or annoyed she would hold her breath until she fell over, going slightly blue. The first twitching episode at 11 months led to an emergency admission to hospital with a discharge diagnosis of febrile convulsions. The story at the time was that at about 5pm, having been bathed in the kitchen sink, she cried and held her breath and fainted, then had shaking movements of the whole body with her eyes rolling. The blueness, twitching, salivation and staring eyes lasted seven minutes. She then became floppy with her eyes open and not responding. When she arrived at the Accident and Emergency department she was described as febrile, with a temperature of 38.5°C, and irritable, with a red, infected throat and inflamed tympanic membrane. Since then she had had about two episodes a week in which she would cry, hold her breath, start to turn blue, fall, and then be 'away', not breathing. Then there would begin clonic twitching of her flexed upper limbs with her eyes rolled up. The twitching would slow down at the end and she would go to sleep for a minute or two. The duration of twitching varied from one to 20 minutes. Most of the episodes had some cause, often seemingly for attention, but sometimes there was no apparent reason. She was a bright, intelligent, very active child who frequently bumped herself.

Ocular compression induced asystole of about 12 seconds, with a pure anoxic seizure without clonic twitching. An attempt was made to capture an episode by prolonged ambulatory cassette EEG/ECG recording. The episodes appeared to be completely inhibited during this period of several days recording, and thereafter the mother regarded the child as 'cured'.

Comment. Although episodes were not recorded by ambulatory monitoring, the history suggests anoxic-epileptic seizures which in the context of a febrile illness were *ipso facto* febrile convulsions.

CASE 15.46
A 4-year-old boy became ill at tea-time. The parents said that at 5pm he was tired and went to sleep. At 10pm he was delirious and had a 'convulsion'. Their description of this was that he was staring, with his pupils dilated, and he was tightening up. His arms were bent, rigid, and his fists clenched. He had wet himself. There was a slight shake—a tremble but not a twitch—and it did not affect his face. He did not come out of it. The family doctor arrived and gave diazepam and sent him to hospital.

The notes of the admitting hospital stated: 'Present complaint – febrile convulsion. Lethargic from five pm. Parents found him rigid and shaking. Temperature 39°. Pharynx: unable to visualise owing to teeth clenching. CNS: drowsy, postictal, no signs of meningism. Provisional diagnosis: febrile convulsion. Remains fitting intermittently – Paraldehyde four mls intramuscularly.' At 1am there was dramatic deterioration and he became apnoeic. He was ventilated from then on.

A third history was got directly from the doctor who admitted him to hospital. The boy was still tense and rigid on arrival and received a second dose (5mg) of rectal diazepam. He then became 'hypotonic' and 'postictal', but then had a further convulsion, a 'tonic-clonic seizure' in which his arms and then his legs became rigid. His arms extended and adducted (the doctor was wrestling to get intravenous access), the legs stiffened and he flushed, and then the arms flexed. The doctor reported that there was twitching at 180 per minute. In fact it wasn't actually a twitch, rather a low-voltage sine-wave movement more like a fast tremor. A further 10mg of diazepam was given, then another, and then he became more settled, although his temperature was still high. Then the tone in his arms began to increase again, and they were again extended and adducted so that the doctor gave 4ml of paraldehyde. By this time it was after midnight. He was then left asleep, but later on the nurse found him blue and mottled, and when the doctor came it was easy to intubate him with an endotracheal tube because he had no gag reflex.

Comment. This was a story of brain swelling due to *Haemophilus influenzae* meningitis with subsequent brain death. The trembling and stiffening were mistaken for tonic-clonic epileptic seizures. Diazepam or other anti-epileptic medications are absolutely contra-indicated when the mechanism of a seizure is likely to involve hypoxia, ischaemia or brain compression.

Hydrocephalus
'Hydrocephalus' covers a multitude of conditions and it is necessary to disentangle the effect of the disorder from its treatment. Again, as in most conditions in this book, by no means all the seizures suffered by these patients are epileptic.

In a series of 202 children with *shunted* hydrocephalus of congenital or acquired origin, reported by Stellman *et al.* (1986), 39 per cent had some kind of seizure, and 17 per cent recurrent (presumed) epileptic seizures and thus epilepsy. In a recent study of 190 patients with myelomeningocele (Chadduck and Adametz

175

1988) the frequency of (presumed) epileptic seizures in shunted patients was 22 per cent, whereas in those without shunts it was only 2 per cent despite a high incidence of ventriculomegaly. More than one shunt revision and shunt infections increased the likelihood of epileptic seizures. Similar findings have previously been found by Bartoshesky *et al.* (1985), who also pointed to the importance of associated cerebral malformation aside from Arnold–Chiari. In one patient in whom the malformation was a suprasellar arachnoid cyst, the epileptic seizures were of diencephalic type with symptoms of drowsiness, sweating, ocular revulsion, cyanosis and bradycardia (Giroud *et al.* 1988), and might have been mistaken for anoxic seizures.

Although it is evident that shunt blockage may be associated with epileptic seizures of various types, tonic seizures, whether or not asymmetrical or adversive, suggest brainstem herniation and must not be confused with epileptic seizures (Haines 1988). An example of such a case of a more chronic and intermittent nature was described in Case 10.2 and illustrated in Figures 10.1 and 10.2 (pp. 110, 111).

Anoxic seizures of a more conventional type may be a consequence of associated brainstem malformation as, for example, in infants with bilateral abductor vocal-cord paralysis (Holinger *et al.* 1978). Whether there is a true increase in the incidence of severe 'prolonged expiratory apnoea' (blue breath-holding) has not been established, but if there is, the mechanism may be analogous to that in exceptional cases of medullary neoplasm (Southall *et al.* 1987a) in which there is a potential anatomical basis for disruption of brainstem control mechanisms.

Down syndrome

Dr Mary King and I undertook a postal survey of 1000 families with one or more children with Down syndrome, the details of which have been presented at meetings but not yet published. Children with this chromosomal abnormality mostly do not have seizures, epileptic or non-epileptic, but the seizures they do have are to a certain extent distinctive. The infantile spasm appears to be the most characteristic epileptic seizure, occurring in about 2 per cent of our population sample. Because of the high prevalence of Down syndrome in the population, this disorder ought to account for a substantial proportion of the total of infantile spasms, but it seems that many go unreported (Stephenson 1983b). Other epileptic seizure types including myoclonic seizures are also noted in young children. In older individuals with Down syndrome 'grand mal' is reported but what this means is not clear. It has been suggested that the infantile spasms of Down syndrome are selectively responsive to pyridoxine, but this does not seem to be a feature specific to Down syndrome.

It is not clear whether the seizures with fever commonly called febrile convulsions are under-represented in Down syndrome. There is one intriguing report from Australia (Callaway 1978) of an association between severe febrile convulsions and D/G translocation. To my knowledge, one other example of this (a 14/21 translocation) has been noted (Ounsted, *personal communication*).

In our series, convulsive reflex anoxic seizures and non-convulsive syncopes appear to be over-represented. Many parents commented that 'everyone knows that Down syndrome children have this sort of reaction', one describing it as an 'active vagus nerve'. Autonomic oddities have been described in Down syndrome (Harris and Goodman 1968), but I am not aware of a reference to vagal syncopes in the literature. The small number of children with Down syndrome in whom I have performed ocular compression have all had anoxic seizures induced thereby, but these children were highly selected.

Other 'funny turns' in these patients relate to the various complicating disorders which they are heir to. Types of congenital heart disease may lead to anoxic seizures or indirectly, via ischaemic brain damage, to partial epileptic seizures.

Case history
CASE 15.47
A 3-year-old boy with Down syndrome had congenital heart disease and episodes of reflex syncope precipitated by temper or fright. At the time of the first episode his mother thought that he must have died because his heart stopped. She knew it had stopped because it was normally so easily seen and felt on account of his congenital heart disease.

Comment. Parents of Down syndrome children assert that this phenomenon is not rare (see also Case 9.36).

Rett syndrome
Rett syndrome (Hagberg *et al.* 1983) is now well known as a mentally handicapping disorder of girls, characterized by superficially normal development not proceeding beyond about the 10 month stage, followed by loss of purposeful use of the hands and then stereotypic repetitive hand movements. These girls have a multitude of fits and 'funny turns', the explanation of all of which is far from being known. In line with the increasing frequency of EEG spikes, particularly at night with advancing age, they do have epileptic seizures of one sort or another, but to add to the complexity the epileptic seizures may be induced by hypocapnia (Southall *et al.* 1988*a*). Hyperventilation in the awake state is a very striking component of this syndrome and it seems that this induces non-epileptic seizures of its own right secondary to the hypocapnia. Investigations are in order to see whether the use of acetazolamide or behaviour-altering management may prevent these episodes. Panic attacks, presenting as a form of psychic seizure, may also seem distressing. These girls also seem prone to syncopes or syncopal seizures from compulsive Valsalva manoeuvres (Gastaut *et al.* 1987).

Familial dysautonomia (Riley–Day syndrome)
Familial dysautonomia is a rare autosomal recessive disorder confined to Ashkenazi Jews. Afflicted children have frequent fevers and inappropriate temperature control: for example, fever may be higher after immunization and after serious infection such as pneumonia. It is not clear whether there is any increase in the frequency of epileptic seizures among these patients, but the incidence of their febrile convulsions and anoxic seizures of various sorts is remarkably high. In a large series of young Riley–Day children studied by Axelrod

et al. (1974), 40 per cent had a history of seizures. Of these, 60 per cent had seizures associated with hyperpyrexia, but I am not aware of published data on the mechanism of these febrile seizures. Of the remaining 40 per cent, half had seizures associated with severe breath-holding and half with hypoxia of other kinds. In this disorder there is a decreased sensitivity to hypercapnia and hypoxia: convulsions may occur during air flights, and deaths during underwater swimming. It is of interest that although a clinical appearance akin to a massive vasovagal reaction is common in this condition, there is no cardiac slowing on carotid massage (Axelrod, *personal communication*) nor on ocular compression (Stephenson, *unpublished observation*).

Tuberous sclerosis
Epileptic seizures occur in about one-half of those carrying the gene for this dominant disorder. If seizures have not presented by school age, mental development is normal. Patients with only simple partial epileptic seizures are likely to be intellectually unscathed, less so those with infantile spasms or complex partial myoclonic or tonic seizures.

Syncopes may accompany the paroxysmal supraventricular tachycardia which can result from cardiac rhabdomyomata. In autistic individuals (a likely sequel of infantile spasms of asymmetrical type), hyperventilation may lead to apnoea and syncope (Tassinari *et al.* 1976).

Self-injurious behaviour completes the unfortunate picture, particularly in those without symbolic thought.

16
FITS AND FAINTS: PROGNOSIS AND MANAGEMENT

Wisdom in treatment and general management derive from knowledge of prognosis. Barcroft's apocryphal remark that 25,000 individuals gave blood in the last great war without fatality is encouraging, but I am not aware of a 100 per cent follow-up of this cohort, even without case controls!

Between 1948 and 1954 Ounsted and his associates had the prescience to determine the National Health Service numbers of an unselected sample of 100 children with 'temporal lobe epilepsy'. The result (Ounsted *et al.* 1987) was a 100 per cent follow-up over more than 30 years. As Jean Aicardi wrote in the foreword to their book, 'Because the life of diseases, like life itself, is in permanent evolution, major fixed landmarks are necessary and the edifice of knowledge must be built on solid foundations.' This cannot be denied, but, notwithstanding the enormous achievement of determining prognosis from what has happened in the past, the march of time makes inevitable the difficulties in estimating prognosis now and thus determining what factors in treatment and management are of solid worth today. Following the dictum that truth comes more from error than from confusion, and inasmuch as the paroxysmal disorders described in this book are so many and so diverse, I propose to limit my comments to some particular aspects of the management of epileptic and anoxic seizures.

Epileptic and anoxic seizures have two things in common. One is that they may disappear with age. The other is that if they do not remit then they may become more obvious and powerful. The epileptic 'grand mal' of early childhood is mild compared with the full-blown tonic-clonic epileptic seizure of the full-grown adult. Likewise, the motor sequelae of a vagal syncope in early childhood are nothing to the dramatic extensions which signal transient asystole in an adult in peak physical condition.

More needs to be known about some aspects of the prognosis of both groups of conditions. In relation to the driving of motor vehicles (Spudis *et al.* 1986), although cardiac syncopes are obviously a hazard (Parsons 1986) it is not satisfactory for patients with vagal syncopes to be hindered from driving on dubious diagnostic or prognostic grounds (Case 16.1).

Epileptic seizures
Some neurologists have a remarkable zeal for the early treatment of epileptic seizures. I think this reflects a unitary view of epilepsy antipathetic to the notion that there can be a good epilepsy and a bad epilepsy. Certainly in paediatric practice parents are often mistrustful of drugs and may well accept that if no medication helps, then no medication may be helpful. While the results of trials of

chemicals which enhance inhibition or reduce excitation are awaited, more attention needs to be paid to the mechanism of action of corticosteroids and how such could be reproduced in other molecules. The remarkable effect of corticosteroids in removing spikes from the EEG, perhaps for months after the last dose, is a phenomenon by no means confined to early childhood and has yet no satisfactory explanation. Other approaches to neurotransmitter behaviour need to be explored. We have scarcely gone past acetylcholine (Hooshmand 1972, Wahlström 1978). The remarkable effects of pyridoxine (Krishnamoorthy 1983, Stephenson and Byrne 1983) cannot be total exceptions.

When Gregory Stores took a patient of mine with exceedingly severe epilepsy sand-sledging, canoeing and rock climbing, the boy was improved—how?

Anoxic seizures

The same enthusiasm for the active management and prevention of anoxic seizures arises from fear of their potential brain-harming effect (Simpson 1949). When I wrote to the *Lancet* (Stephenson 1985*b*) about prolonged expiratory apnoea or blue breath-holding, I was particularly concerned about the anxieties of thousands of parents whose management cornerstone is that *these attacks will not do harm*. I have the same concern in lesser degree about the insertion of pacemakers into the hearts of those who suffer reflex vagal syncopes. However, these episodes can be remarkably annoying, and if pacemakers are safe this is certainly an option for those who have ceased growing (see also Milstein *et al.* 1989).

Many other approaches have been proposed, for example atropine metho-nitrate (Stephenson 1979*a*), theophylline (Benditt *et al.* 1983), somatostatin (Greco *et al.* 1984, Hoeldtke *et al.* 1986), atropine sulphate (McWilliam and Stephenson 1984*a*), transdermal scopolamine (Palm and Blennow 1985, Abi-Samra *et al.* 1988) (although toxic psychosis has been reported after the latter drug in children—Sennhauser and Schwarz 1986), and disopyramide (Milstein *et al.* 1989). In addition to pacemaker implantation, surgical methods have included denervation of the sino-atrial node or thoracic vagectomy (Coryllos *et al.* 1981, 1984), and truncal vagotomy (Obel and Marchand 1971). Quite different methods of management are needed to prevent the type of tragic outcome seen in Cases 16.2 and 16.3: smother-proof pillows as strongly recommended to prevent death during adult *epileptic* seizures (Wilson 1989) are clearly not the answer!

Case histories
CASE 16.1
A senior clinical tutor was forbidden to drive because of 'epilepsy' diagnosed by two adult neurologists. The detailed story was as follows.

At age 18 years this woman fainted in a cinema when she had diarrhoea. Over the next seven years she had three or four bouts of becoming unconscious and incontinent on the first day of her period. On each occasion she felt faint first. From the age of 25 she had bouts at about four-year intervals. They were all associated with intense nausea, vomiting and diarrhoea. Loss of consciousness always occurred in the bathroom, without witnesses, except on one occasion when the bathroom was engaged. In that episode she passed out in the kitchen 'a bit stiff' according to a witness. On another occasion she was either on or beside

180

the lavatory pan, not being quite sure if she was going to be sick first. At the age of about 35, at a time when there was an epidemic of diarrhoea and vomiting, she passed out more than once. The first time was before being sick. She remembered going through to the bathroom, hanging on to the pan and taking deep breaths, then her left arm jerked a bit and she passed out again.

She indicated this story on her driving licence application form and was then referred to a neurologist who said that, on the history, 'this has to be epilepsy'. He ordered an EEG which showed a 'discharging focus from left temporal lobe'. He said that the epilepsy was so mild that he would not normally treat it, but if she needed to drive she would have to take phenytoin. Apparently the doctor then gave her phenobarbitone.

Five years later when she was doing clinical teaching, five of the class had diarrhoea and vomiting. While she herself was being sick she blacked out. Later that night she jumped out of bed, passed out again in the lavatory, came to incontinent of diarrhoea and then blacked out again. One year later while still on phenobarbitone she had another attack of diarrhoea and vomiting, felt sick, went to the lavatory and flaked out.

When she next applied for her driving licence she was referred to another neurologist who said, 'I have to say it's epilepsy', stopped her from driving and gave her phenytoin. She stopped this herself afterwards and has been fine on no therapy.

On appeal, in which I indicated that she would 'only be at some risk if driving a mobile portaloo during a cholera epidemic', her driving licence was restored, although it is still being reviewed every three years.

Comment. Neurologists who make diagnoses which affect an individual's right to drive have an awesome responsibility. It behoves them to recognize the difference between anoxic and epileptic seizures and to know which of the former may be hazardous to the driver of a motor vehicle.

CASE 16.2

A girl who was born by elective caesarean section because of breech presentation at 32 weeks gestation weighing 2.1kg was discharged home at the age of 4 weeks. She was subsequently admitted to hospital for investigation of apnoeic attacks. When these persisted without obvious cause she was transferred to a paediatric neurological unit at the age of 7 months. Several episodes of severe asphyxia accompanied by asystole occurred without explanation until one of the other parents on the ward noticed that the mother was intermittently suffocating the child. By this stage she had acquired a quadriplegia and developed infantile spasms which responded to steroids. At follow-up she had athetoid cerebral palsy with a degree of microcephaly but relative preservation of intellect.

Comment. On superficial observation apnoeic attacks developed into infantile spasms, but 'active' Meadow syndrome was the explanation for it all.

CASE 16.3

A 15-month-old boy was admitted as an emergency with a story of nocturnal tonic seizures for three weeks followed by status epilepticus and a clinical picture resembling encephalitis. He died after four weeks. The details of the story, as reconstructed later, were actually as follows.

He lived with his mother and his mother's parents. For about three weeks it was thought that he must be banging his face and getting bruises on it, particularly around the eyes. He still got bruises after his grandfather put padding on the cot, although no more once he was admitted to hospital. In fact, no-one ever saw him banging his face but the grandparents thought that he must have done so, otherwise how would he have got the bruises and the black eyes? Over the same period he had blue and stiff episodes. The mother said she saw all of these but the grandparents, although always trying to see them, never succeeded—by the time they got to him he was always out of it. On the night of his admission he was bouncing about at midnight and very lively, but at 3am the mother went to the grandfather and said that she could not wake him. His eyes were open and his face was white. On arrival he was pale with abnormal eye movements and pyramidal signs. He was afebrile and had a high blood-glucose level of 16mmol/l. At first he had no response to pain but later he flexed but had no visual response. The EEG showed slow stereotyped high-voltage complexes resembling those seen in herpes encephalitis. The white blood count showed severe neutrophil leukocytosis which persisted for five days, although with no evidence of infection. His neurological state gradually improved over the next four weeks and he was much improved on the evening of his death. He was then moved to a cubicle near the door at the far end of the ward away from the nurses' station, where he stayed with his mother. She got up later that night, she said, and found that he was looking at first a bit white, then turning a bit blue, at which point she told one of the nurses. The registrar who found him at 4am observed that he was pale, warm and pulseless, with no respirations and no pool of vomit. Cardiac massage was unsuccessful. General post-mortem revealed no abnormality but neuropathology showed, in summary, brainstem hypoxic damage, cerebral hypoxic damage, cerebellar hypoxic damage and watershed ischaemic damage. There was no evidence of encephalitis. His mother was charged with his murder.

Comment. Anoxic seizures from breath-holding or vagal-mediated asystole seem to be harmless, but when there is pressure from within, as in brain swelling or cerebrospinal fluid obstruction, or from without as in strangulation or suffocation, then irreversible brain damage may ensue. Epileptic seizures may then be generated, confusing the diagnostic picture. In this case the reader may be the judge, but the time for useful management had passed when this child arrived in hospital.

Conclusion
I would like to end this book by referring once more to Case 9.41 (pp. 106–107). This 5-year-old girl had 'white' and 'blue' seizures (see Fig. 9.7), most of which had no provocation that her parents could detect. Because these episodes were frequent and severe, not surprisingly intensive efforts were made to control them with anti-epileptic medications. Finally reflex anoxic seizures were diagnosed, she received atropine and she was better. Now she is at school, a fine girl with no seizures and no medication. She may feel like the mother in Case 9.21 who said, 'Oh, the vagus! Why don't the doctors know about this?' There is much to learn (DiMario *et al.* 1990)!

REFERENCES

Abi-Samra, F., Maloney, J.D., Fouad-Tarazi, F.M., Castle, L.W. (1988) 'The usefulness of head-up tilt testing and haemodynamic investigation in the workup of syncope of unknown origin.' *PACE*, **11**, 1202–1214.

Acker, D., Boehm, F.H., Askew, D.E., Rothman, H. (1973) 'Electrocardiogram changes with intrauterine contraceptive device insertion.' *American Journal of Obstetrics and Gynecology*, **115**, 458–461.

Adams, R. (1827) 'Cases of diseases of the heart accompanied with pathological observations.' *Dublin Hospital Reports*, **4**, 353–453.

Ahnve, S. (1985) 'Correction of the QT interval for heart rate: review of different formulas and the use of Bazett's formula in myocardial infarction.' *American Heart Journal*, **109**, 568–574.

Aicardi, J. (1986) *Epilepsy in Children.* New York: Raven Press.

—— (1987) 'The future of clinical child neurology.' *Journal of Child Neurology*, **2**, 152–159.

—— (1988) 'Epileptic syndromes in childhood.' *Epilepsia*, **29** (Suppl. 3), S1–S5.

—— Gastaut, H. (1985) 'Treatment of self-induced photosensitive epilepsy with fenfluramine.' *New England Journal of Medicine*, **313**, 1419.

—— —— Mises, J. (1988) 'Syncopal attacks compulsively self-induced by Valsalva's manoeuvre associated with typical absence seizures.' *Archives of Neurology*, **45**, 923–925.

Almquist, A., Goldenberg, I.F., Milstein, S., Chen, M-Y., Chen, X., Hansen, R., Gornick, C.C., Benditt, D.G. (1989) 'Provocation of bradycardia and hypotension by isoproterenol and upright posture in patients with unexplained syncope.' *New England Journal of Medicine*, **320**, 346–351.

Alvarez, N., Lombroso, C.T., Medina, C., Cantlon, B. (1983) 'Paroxysmal spike and wave activity in drowsiness in young children: its relationship to febrile convulsions.' *Electroencephalography and Clinical Neurophysiology*, **56**, 406–413.

Aminoff, M.J., Goodin, D.S., Berg, D.O., Compton, M.N. (1988a) 'Ambulatory EEG recordings in epileptic and nonepileptic children.' *Neurology*, **38**, 558–562.

—— Scheinman, M.M., Griffin, J.C., Herre, J.M. (1988b) 'Electrocerebral accompaniments of syncope associated with malignant ventricular arrhythmias.' *Annals of Internal Medicine*, **108**, 791–796.

Amyes, E.W., Mahony, D.V., Goodman, R.D. (1953) 'Adams–Stokes syndrome and cerebral anoxia. Occurrence in a pregnant woman without previous history of heart disease.' *Journal of Nervous and Mental Disease*, **117**, 334–340.

Andermann, F., Lugaresi, E. (Eds.) (1987) *Migraine and Epilepsy.* London: Butterworths.

Andermann, K., Berman, S., Cooke, P.M., Dickson, J., Gastaut, H., Kennedy, A., Margerison, A., Pond, D.A., Tizard, J.P.M., Walsh, E.G. (1962) 'Self-induced epilepsy: a collection of self-induced epilepsy cases compared with some other photoconvulsive cases.' *Archives of Neurology*, **6**, 49–65.

Anderson, D.P., Allen, W.J., Barcroft, H., Edholm, O.G., Manning, G.W. (1946) 'Circulatory changes during fainting and coma caused by oxygen lack.' *Journal of Physiology*, **104**, 426–434.

Annegers, J.F., Hauser, W.A., Beghi, E., Nicolosi, A., Kurland, L.T. (1988) 'The risk of unprovoked seizures after encephalitis and meningitis.' *Neurology*, **38**, 1407–1410.

Arnold, R.W., Hohberger, G.G., Gould, A.B., Jr. (1988) 'The oculocardiac reflux in identical twins.' *Archives of Ophthalmology*, **106**, 879.

Aschner, B. (1908) 'Ueber einen bisher noch nicht beschriebenen Reflex vom Auge auf Kreislauf und Atmung. Verschwinden des Radialpulsen bei Druck auf des Auge.' *Wiener Klinische Wochenschrift*, **21**, 1529–1530.

Auborg, P., Dulac, O., Plouin, P., Diebler, C. (1985) 'Infantile status epilepticus as a complication of 'near-miss' sudden infant death.' *Developmental Medicine and Child Neurology*, **27**, 40–48.

Axelrod, F.B., Nachtigal, R., Dancis, J. (1974) 'Familial dysautonomia: diagnosis pathogenesis and management.' *Advances in Pediatrics*, **21**, 75–96.

Balakrishnan, G., Skeoch, C.H., Stephenson, J.B.P., McWilliam, R.C., Hallworth, D., Sinclair, J.F. (1989) 'Intracranial pressure monitoring in a group of critically ill children.' *Archives of Disease in Childhood*, **64**, 427.

Ballardie, F.W., Murphy, R.P. (1983) 'Epilepsy: a presentation of the Romano–Ward syndrome.' *British Medical Journal*, **284**, 896–897.

Bangash, I.H., Worley, G., Kandt, R.S. (1988) 'Hysterical conversion reactions mimicking neurological disease.' *American Journal of Diseases in Childhood*, **142**, 1203–1206.

Barcroft, H., Edholm, O.G. (1945) 'On the vasodilation in human skeletal muscle during post-haemorrhagic fainting.' *Journal of Physiology*, **104**, 161–175.

—— —— McMichael, J., Sharpey-Schafer, E.P. (1944) 'Posthaemorrhagic fainting. Study by cardiac output and forearm flow.' *Lancet*, **1**, 489–490.

Baraff, L.J., Shields, W.D., Beckwith, L., Strome, G., Marcy, S.M., Cherry, J.D., Manclark, C.R. (1988) 'Infants and children with convulsions and hypotonic–hyporesponsive episodes following diphtheria–tetanus–pertussis immunization: follow-up evaluation.' *Pediatrics*, **81**, 789–794.

Bartoshesky, L.E., Haller, J., Scott, R.M., Wojick, C. (1985) 'Seizures in children with meningomyelo-cele.' *American Journal of Diseases of Children*, **139**, 400–402.

Basser, L.S. (1964) 'Benign paroxysmal vertigo of childhood (a variety of vestibular neuronitis).' *Brain*, **87**, 141–152.

Battaglia, A., Guerrini, R., Gastaut, H. (1989) 'Epileptic seizures induced by syncopal attacks.' *Journal of Epilepsy*, **2**, 137–146.

Bellman, M.H. (1983) *Serious Acute Neurological Diseases of Children.* Unpublished MD thesis, University of London.

Benditt, D.G., Benson, D.W., Kreitt, J., Dunnigan, A., Pritzker, M.R., Crouse, L., Scheinman, M.M. (1983) 'Electrophysiologic effects of theophylline in young patients with recurrent symptomatic bradyarrhythmias.' *American Journal of Cardiology*, **52**, 1223–1229.

Blanc, V.F., Hardy, J.F., Milot. J., Jacob, J.L. (1983) 'The oculocardiac reflex: a graphic and statistical analysis in infants and children.' *Canadian Anaesthetic Society Journal*, **30**, 360–369.

—— Jacob, J.L., Milot, J., Cyrenne, L. (1988) 'The oculorespiratory reflex revisited.' *Canadian Journal of Anaesthesia*, **35**, 468–472.

Blennow, G. (1985) 'Benign infantile nocturnal myoclonus.' *Acta Paediatrica Scandinavica*, **74**, 505-507.

Blumhardt, L. (1986) 'Ambulatory ECG and EEG monitoring in the differential diagnosis of cardiac and cerebral dysrhythmias.' *In:* Gumnit, R.J. (Ed.) *Intensive Neurodiagnostic Monitoring. Advances in Neurology, Vol. 46.* New York: Raven Press.

—— Smith, P.E.M., Owen, L. (1986) 'Electrocardiographic accompaniments of temporal lobe epileptic seizures.' *Lancet*, **1**, 1051–1056.

Bodensteiner, J.B., Brownsworth, R.D., Knapik, J.R., Kanter, M.C., Cowan, L.D., Leviton, A. (1988) 'Interobserver variability in the ILAE classification of seizures in childhood.' *Epilepsia*, **29**, 123–128.

Born, J.D., Albert, A., Hans, P., Bonnal, J. (1985) 'Relative prognostic value of best motor response and brain stem reflexes in patients with severe head injury.' *Neurosurgery*, **16**, 595–601.

Botez, M.I., Hausser, C.O. (1982) 'Falls.' *British Journal of Hospital Medicine*, **27**, 494–503.

Bower, B.D. (1974) 'Fits, faints and "funny turns" in young children.' *British Journal of Hospital Medicine*, **12**, 527–534.

—— (1984) 'Pallid syncope (reflex anoxic seizures).' *Archives of Disease in Childhood*, **59**, 1118–1119.

Braham, J., Hertzeanu, H., Yahini, J.H., Neufeld, H.N. (1981) 'Reflex cardiac arrest presenting as epilepsy.' *Annals of Neurology*, **10**, 277–278.

Bridge, E.M. (1949) *Epilepsy and Convulsive Disorders in Children.* New York: McGraw–Hill.

—— Livingston, S., Tietze, C. (1943) 'Breath-holding spells: their relationship to syncope, convulsions, and other phenomena.' *Journal of Pediatrics*, **23**, 539–561.

Brodsky, M.A., Sato, D.A., Iseri, L.T., Wolff, L.J., Allen, B.J. (1987) 'Ventricular tachyarrhythmia associated with psychological stress.' *Journal of the American Medical Association*, **257**, 2064–2067.

Brorson, L.O., Wranne, L. (1987) 'Long-term prognosis in childhood epilepsy: survival and seizure prognosis.' *Epilepsia*, **28**, 324–330.

Buja, G., Folino, A.F., Bittante. M., Canciani, B., Martini, B., Miorelli, M., Tognin, D., Corrado, D., Nava, A. (1989) 'Asystole with syncope secondary to hyperventilation in three young adults.' *PACE*, **12**, 406-412.

Bullard, D.E. (1987) 'Diencephalic seizures: responsiveness to bromocriptine and morphine.' *Annals of Neurology*, **21**, 609–611.

Burstein, L., Breningstall, G.N. (1986) 'Movement disorders in bacterial meningitis.' *Journal of Pediatrics*, **109**, 260–264.

Callaway, B.C. (1978) 'Febrile convulsions and DG translocation.' *Medical Journal of Australia*, **2**, 115.

Caralis, D.G., Varghese, P.J. (1976) 'Familial sinoatrial node dysfunction. Increased vagal tone a possible aetiology.' *British Heart Journal*, **38**, 951–956.

Chadduck, W., Adametz, J. (1988) 'Incidence of seizures in patients with myelomeningocele: a multifactorial analysis.' *Surgical Neurology*, **30**, 281–285.

Chamberlain, J.M., Gorman, R.L. (1988) 'Occult bacteremia in children with simple febrile seizures.' *American Journal of Diseases in Children*, **142**, 1073–1076.

184

Chen, H.I., Chai,C.Y. (1976) 'Integration of the cardiovagal mechanism in the medulla oblongata of the cat.' *American Journal of Physiology*, **231**, 454–461.

Choi, Y.S., Kim, J.J., Oh, B.H., Park, Y.B., Seo, J.D., Lee, Y.W. (1989) 'Cough syncope caused by sinus arrest in a patient with sick sinus syndrome.' *PACE*, **12**, 883-886.

Clancy, R.R. (1989) 'Interictal sharp EEG transients in neonatal seizures.' *Journal of Child Neurology*, **4**, 30–38.

—— Spitzer, A.R. (1985) 'Cerebral cortical function in infants at risk for sudden infant death syndrome.' *Annals of Neurology*, **18**, 41–47.

Clark, D.J., Chan, K.C., Gibbs, J.L. (1989) 'Propranolol induced bradycardia in tetralogy of Fallot.' *British Heart Journal*, **61**, 378–379.

Cogan, D.G. (1966) 'Congenital ocular motor apraxia.' *Canadian Journal of Ophthalmology*, **1**, 253–260.

Cohen, R.J., Suter, C. (1982) 'Hysterical seizures: suggestion as a provocative test.' *Annals of Neurology*, **11**, 391–395.

Connolly, J., Hallam, R.S., Marks, I.M. (1976) 'Selective association of fainting with blood–injury–illness fear.' *Behaviour Therapy*, **7**, 8–13.

Constantin, L., Martins, J.B., Fincham, R.W., Dagli, R.D. (1990) 'Bradycardia and syncope as manifestations of partial epilepsy.' *Journal of the American College of Cardiology*, **15**, 900–905.

Constantinou, J.E.C., Gillis, J., Ouvrier, R.A., Rahilly, P.M. (1989) 'Hypoxic–ischaemic encephalopathy after near miss sudden infant death syndrome.' *Archives of Disease in Childhood*, **64**, 703–708.

Cooper, A. (1836) 'Some experiments and observations on tying the carotid and vertebral arteries, and the pneumogastric, phrenic and sympathetic nerves.' *Guy's Hospital Reports*, **1**, 457–475.

Corbett, J., Butler, A., Kaufman, B. (1976) '"Sneeze syncope", basilar invagination and Arnold–Chiari type 1 malformation.' *Journal of Neurology, Neurosurgery and Psychiatry*, **39**, 381–384.

Coryllos, E.V., Mohtashemi, M., Delaney, T., Greensher, J. (1981) 'Thoracic vagectomy for vagal bradycardia in children.' *Lancet*, **2**, 526.

—— Delaney, T., Reitman, M., Mohtashemi, M., Kenisberg, K. (1984) 'Selective denervation of the S-A node in the treatment of progressive central vagal bradycardia.' *Journal of Pediatric Surgery*, **19**, 451–456.

Coulter, D.L. (1984) 'Partial seizures with apnea and bradycardia.' *Archives of Neurology*, **41**, 173–174.

—— Allen, R.J., (1982) 'Benign neonatal sleep myoclonus.' *Archives of Neurology*, **39**, 191–192.

Croft, R.D., Jervis, M. (1989) 'Munchausen's syndrome in a 4 year old.' *Archives of Disease in Childhood*, **64**, 740–741.

Culpeper, N. (1737) *A Directory for Midwives; or a Guide for Women in their Conception, Bearing (etc.).* London: Bettersworth & Hitch.

Curatolo, P., Cusmai, R., Finochi, G., Boscherini, B. (1984) 'Gelastic epilepsy and true precocious puberty due to hypothalamic hamartoma.' *Developmental Medicine and Child Neurology*, **26**, 509–514.

Dagnini, G. (1908) 'Interno ad un riflesso provocato in alcuni emiplegici collo stimolo della cornea e collo pressione sul bulbo oculare.' *Bollettino della Scienze Mediche*, **8**, 380.

Dandona, P., James, I.M., Woollard, M.L., Newbury, P., Beckett, A.G., (1979) 'Instability of cerebral blood-flow in insulin-dependent diabetics.' *Lancet*, **2**, 1203–1205.

Daniels, S.R., Bates, S.R., Kaplan, S. (1987) 'EEG monitoring during paroxysmal hyperpnea of Fallot: an epileptic or hypoxic phenomenon.' *Journal of Child Neurology*, **2**, 98–100.

Danner, R., Shewmon, A., Sherman, M.P. (1985) 'Seizures in an atelencephalic infant.' *Archives of Neurology*, **42**, 1014–1016.

Darby, C.E., de Korte, R.A., Binnie, C.D., Wilkins, A.J. (1980) 'The self-induction of epileptic seizures by eye closure.' *Epilepsia*, **21**, 31–41.

Davies, A.B., Stephens, M.R., Davies, A.G. (1979) 'Carotid sinus hypersensitivity in patients presenting with syncope.' *British Heart Journal*, **42**, 583–586.

Davis, J.M., Metrakos, K., Aranda, J.V. (1986) 'Apnoea and seizures.' *Archives of Disease in Childhood*, **61**, 791–793.

Dawkins, R. (1976) *The Selfish Gene.* Oxford: Oxford University Press.

Day, S.C., Cook, E.F., Funkenstein, H., Goldman, L. (1982) 'Evaluation and outcome of emergency room patients with transient loss of consciousness.' *American Journal of Medicine*, **73**, 15–23.

Dean, J.C.S. (1988) 'T waves in long Q-T syndromes.' *Lancet*, **2**, 171.

de Bono, D.P., Warlow, C.P., Hyman, N.M. (1982) 'Cardiac rhythm abnormalities in patients presenting with transient non-focal neurological symptoms: a diagnostic grey area?' *British Medical Journal*, **284**, 1437–1439.

DeMaria, A.A., Jr., Westmoreland, B.F., Sharbrough, F.W. (1984) 'EEG in cough syncope.' *Neurology*, **34**, 371–374.

deMay, C., Enterling, D. (1986) 'Variant responses to passive upright tilt.' *Lancet*, **2**, 221.

Deonna, T.W. (1988) 'Paroxysmal disorders which may be migraine or may be confused with it.' *In:* Hockaday, J.M. (Ed.) *Migraine in Childhood.* London: Butterworth.

—— Martin, D. (1981) 'Benign paroxysmal torticollis in infancy.' *Archives of Disease in Childhood*, **56**, 956–959.

Devinsky, O., Sato, S., Kufta, C.V., Ito, B., Rose, D.F., Theodore, W.H., Porter, R.J., (1989) 'Electroencephalographic studies of simple partial seizures with subdural electrode recordings.' *Neurology*, **39**, 527–533.

Dighton, D.H. (1974) 'Sinus bradycardia, autonomic influences and clinical assessment.' *British Heart Journal*, **36**, 791–797.

—— (1986) 'Vasovagal syncope.' *Lancet*, **1**, 982.

DiLuzio, T.A., Rutecki, P.A. (1989) 'Complex partial seizures associated with asystole.' *Epilepsia*, **30**, 705. (*Abstract.*)

DiMario, F.J., Chee, C.M., Berman, P.H. (1990) 'Pallid breath-holding spells. Evaluation of the autonomic nervous system.' *Clinical Pediatrics*, **29**, 17–24.

DiMicco, J.A., Gale, K., Hamilton, B., Gillis, R.A. (1979) 'GABA receptor control of parasympathetic outflow to heart: characterisation and brainstem localisation.' *Science*, **204**, 1106–1109.

Dobkin, B.H. (1978) 'Syncope in the adult Chiari anomaly.' *Neurology*, **28**, 718–720.

Donat, J.F., Wright, F.S. (1989) 'Sleep, epilepsy, and the EEG in infancy and childhood.' *Journal of Child Neurology*, **4**, 84-94.

Dravet, C., Bureau, M., Roger, J., (1985) 'Severe myoclonic epilepsy in infants.' *In:* Roger, J., Dravet, C., Bureau, M., Dreifuss, F.E., Wolf, P. (Eds). *Epilectic Syndromes in Infancy, Chilhood and Adolescence.* London: John Libbey.

—— Giraud, N., Bureau, M., Roger, J., Gobbi, G., Dalla Bernardina, B. (1986) 'Benign myoclonus of early infancy or benign non-epileptic infantile spasms.' *Neuropediatrics*, **17**, 33–38.

Driver, M.V., Selby, P.J. (1977) 'Apparent epilepsy due to the intermittent tachy-arrythmia (Romano–Ward) syndrome.' *Electroencephalography and Clinical Neurophysiology*, **43**, 289.

Duchowny, M.S., Resnick, T.J., Deray, M.J., Alvarez, L.A. (1988) 'Video EEG diagnosis of repetitive behavior in early childhood and its relationship to seizures.' *Pediatric Neurology*, **4**, 162–164.

Duvernoy, W.F.C., Nair, M.R.S., Zobl, E.G. (1980) 'Convulsive disorder mimicked by prolonged asystole and cured by permanent pacing.' *Heart and Lung*, **9**, 711–714.

Duvoisin, R.C. (1961) 'The Valsalva maneuver in the study of syncope.' *Electroencephalography and Clinical Neurophysiology*, **13**, 622–626.

—— (1962) 'Convulsive syncope induced by the Weber maneuver.' *Archives of Neurology*, **7**, 219–226.

Ector, H., Rolies, L., de Geest, T. (1983) 'Dynamic electrocardiography and ventricular pauses of 3 seconds or more: etiology and therapeutic indications.' *PACE*, **6**, 548–551.

—— Bourgois, J., Verlinden, M., Hermans, L., vanden Eynde, E., Fagard, R., de Geest. H. (1984) 'Bradycardia, ventricular pauses, syncope, and sports.' *Lancet*, **2**, 591–594.

Egger, J., Carter, C.M., Soothill, J.F., Wilson, J. (1989) 'Oligoantigenic diet treatment of children with epilepsy and migraine.' *Journal of Pediatrics*, **114**, 51–58.

Egli, M., Mothersill, I., O'Kane, M., O'Kane, F. (1985) 'The axial spasm—the predominant type of drop seizure in patients with secondary generalised epilepsy.' *Epilepsia*, **26**, 401–415.

Engel, G.L. (1962) *Fainting, 2nd Edn.* Springfield, IL: Charles C. Thomas.

—— (1978) 'Psychologic stress, vasodepressor (vasovagal) syncope, and sudden death.' *Annals of Internal Medicine*, **89**, 403–412.

Erickson, G.R., Chun, R.W.M. (1987) 'Acquired paroxysmal movement disorders.' *Pediatric Neurology*, **3**, 226–229.

Euler, A.R. (1980) 'Use of bethanechol for the treatment of gastroesophageal reflux.' *Journal of Pediatrics*, **96**, 321–324.

Faden, A., Spire, J-P., Faden, R. (1977) 'Fits, faints and the IUD.' *Annals of Neurology*, **1**, 305–306.

Fariello, R.G., Dorro, J.M., Forster, F.M. (1979) 'Generalized cortical electrodecremental event, clinical and neurophysiological observations in patients with dystonic seizures.' *Archives of Neurology*, **36**, 285–291.

Fejerman, N., Medina, C.S. (1986) *Convulsiones en la Infancia, 2nd Edn.* Buenos Aires: El Atenio.

Fenichael, G.M., Olson, B.J., Fitzpatrick, J. E., (1980) 'Heart rate changes in convulsive and nonconvulsive apnea' *Annals of Neurology*, **7**, 577–582.

Fildisevski, P. (1961) 'Diagnostic value of the oculocardiac reflex in differentiation of syncope and epileptic manifestations.' *In:* Gastaut, H., Meyer, J.S. (Eds.) *Cerebral Anoxia and the*

Electroencephalogram. Springfield, IL: Charles C. Thomas.

Fincham, R.W., Shivapour, E.T., Leis, A.A., Martins, J.B. (1989) 'Ictal bradycardia with syncope: a case report.' *Epilepsia*, **30**, 706. (*Abstract.*)

Fisher, C.M. (1967) 'A particular kind of syncope.' *Transactions of the American Neurological Association*, **92**, 230–231.

—— (1979) 'Syncope of obscure nature.' *Canadian Journal of Neurological Sciences*, **6**, 7–20.

Fitzpatrick, A., Sutton, R. (1989) 'Tilting towards a diagnosis in recurrent unexplained syncope.' *Lancet*, **1**, 658–660.

Forster, F.M., Roseman, E., Gibbs, F.A. (1942) 'Electroencephalogram accompanying hyperactive carotid sinus reflex and orthostatic syncope.' *Archives of Neurology and Psychiatry*, **48**, 957–967.

—— (1972) 'The classification and conditioning treatment of the reflex epilepsies.' *International Journal of Neurology*, **9**, 73–86.

Freeman, J.M. (1989) 'Status epilepticus: it's not what we've thought or taught.' *Pediatrics*, **83**, 444–445.

Friis, M.L., Lund, M. (1974) 'Stress convulsions.' *Archives of Neurology*, **31**, 155–159.

Gandevia, S.C., McCloskey, D.I., Potter, E.K. (1978) 'Reflex bradycardia occurring in response to diving, nasopharyngeal stimulation and ocular pressure, and its modification by respiration and swallowing.' *Journal of Physiology*, **276**, 383–394.

Gastaut, H. (1956a) 'La syncope nocturne des hypervagotoniques, sa differenciation d'avec l'epilepsie morpheique.' *Revue Neurologique*, **95**, 420–421.

—— (1956b) 'Etude electroencephalographique des syncopes.' *Revue Neurologique*, **95**, 541–549.

—— (1958) 'Syncope and seizure.' *Electroencephalography and Clinical Neurophysiology*, **10**, 571–572.

—— (1968) 'A physiopathogenic study of reflex anoxic cerebral seizures in children (syncopes, sobbing spasms and breath-holding spells).' *In:* Kellaway, P., Petersen, I. (Eds.) *Clinical Electroencephalography of Children.* Stockholm: Almquist & Wiksell.

—— (1973) *Dictionary of Epilepsy, Part 1. Definitions.* Geneva: World Health Organization.

—— (1974) 'Syncopes: generalized anoxic cerebral seizures.' *In:* Vinken, P.J., Bruyn, G.W. (Eds.) *Handbook of Clinical Neurology, Vol. 15: The Epilepsies.* Amsterdam: North–Holland.

—— (1980) 'Un syndrome névrotique méconnu de l'enfant oligophrene: les syncopes autoprovoquées de façon compulsive par manoevre de Valsalva.' *Bulletin de l'Academie Nationale de Médecine*, **164**, 713–717.

—— Broughton, R. (1972) *Epileptic Seizures.* Springfield, IL: Charles C. Thomas.

—— Fischer-Williams, M. (1957) 'Electro-encephalographic study of syncope: its differentiation from epilepsy.' *Lancet*, **2**, 1018–1025.

—— Gastaut, Y. (1957) 'Syncopes et convulsions. A propos de la nature syncopale de certains spasmes du sanglot et de certains convulsions essentielles hyperthermiques ou à froid.' *Revue Neurologique*, **96**, 158–163.

—— —— (1958) 'Electroencephalographic and clinical study of anoxic convulsions in children.' *Electroencephalography and Clinical Neurophysiology*, **10**, 607–620.

—— Tassinari, C.A. (1966) 'Triggering mechanisms in epilepsy: the electroclinical point of view.' *Epilepsia*, **7**, 85–138.

—— Bostem, F., Fernandez-Guardiola, A., Naquet, R., Gibson, W. (1961a) 'Hypoxic activation of the EEG by nitrogen inhalation.' *In:* Gastaut, H., Meyer, J.S. (Eds.) *Cerebral Anoxia and the Electroencephalogram.* Springfield, IL: Charles C. Thomas.

—— Fischer-Williams, M., Gibson, W., El Ouahchi, S. (1961b) 'Clinico-electroencephalographic study of reflex vaso-vagal syncope provoked by ocular compression.' *In:* Gastaut, H., Meyer, J.S. (Eds.) *Cerebral Anoxia and the Electroencephalogram.* Springfield, IL: Charles C. Thomas.

—— Regis, H., Infante, B. (1961c) 'Polygraphic study of carotid sinus hypersensitivity produced by intra-sinus stimulation (forced expiration): its application to the study of cough syncope.' *In:* Gastaut, H., Meyer, J.S. (Eds.) *Cerebral Anoxia and the Electroencephalogram.* Springfield, IL: Charles C. Thomas.

—— Vigoroux, R., Dell, M.B. (1961d) 'Polygraphic study of carotid sinus hypersensitivity produced by extra-sinus stimulation (compression of the carotid sinus).' *In:* Gastaut, H., Meyer, J.S. (Eds.) *Cerebral Anoxia and the Electroencephalogram.* Springfield, IL: Charles C. Thomas.

—— Fischgold, H., Meyer, J.S. (1961e) 'Conclusions of the international colloquium on anoxia and the EEG.' *In:* Gastaut, H., Meyer, J.S. (Eds.) *Cerebral Anoxia and the Electroencephalogram.* Springfield, IL: Charles C. Thomas.

—— Roger, J., Ouahchi, S., Timsit, M., Broughton, R. (1963) 'An electro-clinical study of generalised epileptic seizures of tonic expression.' *Epilepsia*, **4**, 15–44.

—— Broughton, R., De Leo, G. (1982) 'Syncopal attacks compulsively self-induced by the Valsalva manoeuvre in children with mental retardation.' *Electroencephalography and Clinical Neurophysiology*, **35** (Suppl.), 323–329.

—— Zifkin, B., Rufo, M. (1987) 'Compulsive respiratory stereotypies in children with autistic features: polygraphic recording and treatment with fenfluramine.' *Journal of Autism and Developmental Disorders*, **17**, 391–406.

Gauk, E.W., Kidd, L., Prichard, J.S. (1963) 'Mechanism of seizures associated with breath-holding spells.' *New England Journal of Medicine*, **268**, 1436–1441.

Gautier-Smith, P.C. (1983) 'Problem cases of epilepsy and driving.' *In:* Godwin-Austen, R.B., Espir, M.L.E. (Eds.) *Driving and Epilepsy - and Other Causes of Impaired Consciousness. Royal Society of Medicine Congress and Symposium Series No. 60.* London: Royal Society of Medicine with Academic Press.

Gesell, R., Mason, A., Brassfield, C.R. (1944) 'Acid humoral control of heart beat.' *American Journal of Physiology*, **141**, 312–321.

Gibbs, F.A., Davis, H., Lennox, W.G. (1935) 'Electroencephalogram in epilepsy and in conditions of impaired consciousness.' *Archives of Neurology and Psychiatry*, **34**, 1133–1148.

Gilchrist, J.M. (1985) 'Arrhythmogenic seizures: diagnosis by simultaneous EEG/ECG recording.' *Neurology*, **35**, 1503–1506.

Gilliatt, R.W., Roberts, R.C. (1986) 'Syncope and non-epileptic seizures.' *In:* Asbury, A.K., McKhann, G.M., McDonald, W.I. (Eds.) *Diseases of the Nervous System, Vol. 2.* London: Heinemann.

Giroud, M., Santreaux, J.L., Thierry, A., Dumas, R. (1988) 'Diencephalic epilepsy with congenital suprasellar arachnoid cyst in an infant.' *Child's Nervous System*, **4**, 252–254.

Gobbi, G., Bruna, L., Pina, A., Rossi, P.G., Tassinari, C.A. (1987) 'Periodic spasms: an unclassified type of epileptic seizure in childhood.' *Developmental Medicine and Child Neurology*, **29**, 766–775.

Golding, J., Butler, N. (1983) 'Convulsive disorders in the child health and education study.' *In:* Rose, F.C. (Ed.) *Research Progress in Epilepsy.* London: Pitman.

Goldstein, D.S., Spanarkel, M., Pitterman, A., Tolzis, R., Gratz, E., Epstein, S., Keiser, H.R. (1982) 'Circulatory control mechanisms in vasodepressor syncope.' *American Heart Journal*, **104**, 1071–1075.

Goodin, D.S., Aminoff, M.J. (1984) 'Does the interictal EEG have a role in the diagnosis of epilepsy?' *Lancet*, **1**, 837–839.

Goodridge, D.M.G., Shorvon, S.D. (1983) 'Epileptic seizures in a population of 6000.' *British Medical Journal*, **287**, 641–647.

Goodwin, J., Simms, M., Bergman, R. (1979) 'Hysterical seizures: a sequel to incest.' *American Journal of Orthopsychiatry*, **49**, 698–703.

Gordon, N. (1982) 'The differential diagnosis of epilepsy and the use of the ambulatory electroencephalogram.' *Journal of Electrophysiological Technology*, **8**, 15–18.

—— (1987) 'Breath-holding spells.' *Developmental Medicine and Child Neurology*, **29**, 810–814.

Gowers, W.R. (1907) *The Borderland of Epilepsy.* London: Churchill.

Greco, A.V., Ghirlanda, G., Barone, C., Bertoli, A., Caputo, S., Uccioli, L., Manna, R. (1984) 'Somatostatin in paroxysmal supraventricular and junctional tachycardia.' *British Medical Journal*, **288**, 28.

Greenfield, A.D.M. (1951) 'An emotional faint.' *Lancet*, **1**, 1302–1303.

Gross, M. (1979) 'Incestuous rape: a cause for hysterical seizures in four adolescent girls.' *American Journal of Orthopsychiatry*, **49**, 704–708.

Grossi, D., Nozzoli, C., Roca, M.E., Santostasi, R., Simone, F. (1987) 'Head-up tilt for triggering and diagnosing syncope.' *Functional Neurology*, **2**, 457–464.

Guilleminault, C., Billiard, M., Montplaisir, J., Dervent, W.C. (1975) 'Altered states of consciousness in disorders of daytime sleepiness.' *Journal of Neurological Sciences*, **26**, 377–393.

—— Pool, P., Motta, J., Gillis, A.M. (1984) 'Sinus arrest during REM sleep in young adults.' *New England Journal of Medicine*, **311**, 1006–1010.

Gulick, T.A., Spinks, I.P., King, D.W. (1982) 'Pseudoseizures: ictal phenomena.' *Neurology*, **32**, 24–30.

Gumnit, R.J. (1987) 'Terminology.' *In:* Gumnit, R.J. (Ed.) *Intensive Neurodiagnostic Monitoring. Advances in Neurology, Vol. 46.* New York: Raven Press.

Haas, D.C., Lourie, H. (1988) 'Trauma-triggered migraine: an explanation for common neurological attacks after mild head injury.' *Journal of Neurosurgery*, **68**, 181–188.

—— Sovner, R.D. (1969) 'Migraine attacks triggered by mild head trauma, and their relation to certain post-traumatic disorders of childhood.' *Journal of Neurology, Neurosurgery and Psychiatry*, **32**, 548–554.

Hagberg, B., Aicardi, J., Dias, K., Ramos, O. (1983) 'A progressive syndrome of autism, dementia, ataxia and loss of purposeful hand use in girls: Rett's syndrome.' *Annals of Neurology*, **14**, 471–479.

Haines, S.J. (1988) 'Decerebrate posturing misinterpreted as seizure activity.' *American Journal of Emergency Medicine*, **6**, 173–177.

Hainsworth, R. (1988) 'Fainting.' *In:* Bannister, R. (Ed.) *Autonomic Failure, 2nd. Edn.* Oxford: Oxford University Press.

Hall, D.M. (1978) 'Non-epileptic television syncope.' *British Medical Journal*, **2**, 205.

Hampton, F., Williams, B., Loizou, L.A. (1982) 'Syncope as a presenting feature of hindbrain herniation with syringomyelia.' *Journal of Neurology, Neurosurgery and Psychiatry*, **45**, 919–922.

Hand, I., Schröder, G. (1980) 'Die vago-vasale Ohnmacht bei der Blut-Verletzungs-Katastrophen-(BVK)-Phobie und ihre verhaltenstherapeutische Behandlung.' *Therapiewoche*, **30**, 923–932.

Harel, S., Yurgenson, U., Kutai, M. (1987) 'Paroxysmal kinesigenic choreoathetosis.' *Child's Nervous System*, **3**, 47–49.

Harris, W.S., Goodman, R.M. (1968) 'Hyper-reactivity to atropine in Down's syndrome.' *New England Journal of Medicine*, **279**, 407–410.

Haslam, R.H.A., Freigang, B. (1985) 'Cough syncope mimicking epilepsy in asthmatic children.' *Canadian Journal of Neurologic Sciences*, **12**, 45–47.

Henry, J.A., Woodruff, G.H.A. (1978) 'A diagnostic sign in states of apparent unconsciousness.' *Lancet*, **2**, 920–921.

Herskowitz, J., (1986) 'Neurologic presentations of panic disorder in childhood and adolescence.' *Developmental Medicine and Child Neurology*, **28**, 617–623.

Hockaday, J.M. (Ed.) (1988) *Migraine in Childhood.* London: Butterworths.

Hoeldtke, R.D., O'Doriso, T.M., Boden, G. (1986) 'Treatment of autonomic neuropathy with a somatostatin analogue SMS-201-995.' *Lancet*, **2**, 602–605.

Holinger, P.C., Holinger, L.D., Reichert, T.J., Holinger, P.H. (1978) 'Respiratory obstruction and apnoea in infants with bilateral abductor vocal cord paralysis, meningomyelocele, hydrocephalus and Arnold–Chiari malformation.' *Journal of Pediatrics*, **92**, 368–373.

Holmes, G.L., Sackellares, J.C., McKiernan, J., Regland, M., Dreifuss, F.E. (1980) 'Evaluation of childhood pseudoseizures using EEG telemetry and video tape monitoring.' *Journal of Pediatrics*, **97**, 554–558.

Hooshmand, H. (1972) 'Apneic seizures treated with atropine—report of a case.' *Neurology*, **22**, 1217–1221.

Horowitz, S.J., Boxerbaum, B., O'Bell, J. (1980) 'Cerebral herniation in bacterial meningitis in childhood.' *Annals of Neurology*, **7**, 524–528.

Howard, P., Leathart, G., Dornhorst, A.C., Sharpey-Schafer, E.P. (1951) 'The "mess trick" and the "fainting lark".' *British Medical Journal*, **2**, 382–384.

Howell, S.J.L., Blumhardt, L.D. (1989) 'Cardiac asystole associated with epileptic seizures: a case report with simultaneous EEG and ECG.' *Journal of Neurology, Neurosurgery and Psychiatry*, **52**, 795-798.

Ikeno, T., Shigematsu, H., Miyakoshi, M., Ohba, A., Yagi, K., Seino, M. (1985) 'An analytic study of epileptic falls.' *Epilepsia*, **26**, 612–621.

Jackson, J.H. (1899) 'On asphyxia in slight epileptic paroxysms—on the symptomatology of slight epileptic fits supposed to depend on discharge-lesions of the uncinate gyrus.' *Lancet*, **1**, 79–80.

Jacome, D.E., FitzGerald, R. (1982) 'Ictus emeticus.' *Neurology*, **32**, 209–212.

—— Risko, M. (1984) 'Pseudocataplexy: gelastic-atonic seizures.' *Neurology*, **34**, 1381–1383.

—— Suarez, M. (1987) 'Ictus emeticus induced by photic stimulation.' *Journal of Clinical Neurophysiology*, **4**, 293.

Jaeger, F.J., Maloney, J.D., Fouad-Tarazi, F.M. (1990) 'Newer aspects in the diagnosis and management of syncope.' *In:* Rapaport, E. (Ed.) *Cardiology Update.* New York: Elsevier.

Jeavons, P.M. (1983) 'Non-epileptic attacks in childhood.' *In:* Rose, F.C. (Ed.) *Research Progress in Epilepsy.* London: Pitman.

Jeffery, H.E., Rahilly, P., Read, D.J.C. (1983) 'Multiple causes of asphyxia in infants at high risk for sudden infant death.' *Archives of Disease in Childhood*, **58**, 92–100.

Jervell, A., Lange-Nielsen, F. (1957) 'Congenital deaf-mutism, functional heart disease with prolongation of the Q-T interval and sudden death.' *American Heart Journal*, **54**, 59–67.

Johnson, L.F., Kinsbourne, M., Renuart, A.W. (1971) 'Hereditary chin-trembling with nocturnal myoclonus and tongue-biting in dizygous twins.' *Developmental Medicine and Child Neurology*, **13**, 726–729.

Johnson, P. (1985) 'Prolonged expiratory apnoea and implications for control of breathing.' *Lancet*, **2**, 877–880.

189

Johnson, R.H., Lambie, D.G., Spalding, J.N.K. (1984) *Neurocardiology*. London: W.B. Saunders.

Kaada, B.R., Jasper, H. (1952) 'Respiratory responses to stimulation of temporal lobe, insula and hippocampal and limbic gyri in man.' *Archives of Neurology and Psychiatry*, **68**, 609–619.

Kahn, A., Riazi, J., Blum, D. (1983) 'Oculocardiac reflex in near miss for sudden infant death infants.' *Pediatrics*, **71**, 49–52.

Kandt, R.S., Emerson, R.G., Singer, H.S., Valle, D.L., Moser, H.W. (1982) 'Cataplexy in variant forms of Niemann–Pick disease.' *Annals of Neurology*, **12**, 284–288.

Kapoor, W.N., Karpf, M., Wieand, S., Peterson, J.R., Levey, G.S. (1983) 'A prospective evaluation and follow-up of patients with syncope.' *New England Journal of Medicine*, **309**, 197–204.

—— Peterson, J., Wieand, H.S., Karpf, M. (1987) 'Diagnostic and prognostic implications of recurrences in patients with syncope.' *American Journal of Medicine*, **83**, 700–708.

Karp, H.R., Weissler, A.M., Heyman, A. (1961) 'Vasodepressor syncope: EEG and circulatory changes.' *Archives of Neurology*, **5**, 94–101.

Katona, P.G., McLean, M., Dighton, D.H., Guz, A. (1982) 'Sympathetic and parasympathetic cardiac control in athletes and non-athletes at rest.' *Journal of Applied Physiology*, **52**, 1652–1657.

Katz, R.I., Tiger, M., Harner, R.N. (1983) 'Epileptic cardiac arrythmia: sino-atrial arrest in two patients. A potential cause of sudden death in epilepsy?' *Epilepsia*, **24**, 248. (*Abstract.*)

Keer, A., Eich, R.H. (1961) 'Cerebral concussion as a cause of cough syncope.' *Archives of Internal Medicine*, **108**, 248–252.

Keipert, J.A. (1969) 'Epilepsy precipitated by bathing: water-immersion epilepsy.' *Australian Paediatric Journal*, **5**, 244–247.

Kellaway, P. (1987) 'Intensive monitoring in children.' *In:* Gumnit, R.J. (Ed.) *Intensive Neurodiagnostic Monitoring. Advances in Neurology, Vol. 46.* New York: Raven Press.

Kelly, D.H., Krishnamoorthy, K.S., Shannon, D.C. (1980) 'Astrocytoma in an infant with prolonged apnoea.' *Pediatrics*, **66**, 429–431.

Kempster, P.A., Balla, J.I. (1986) 'A clinical study of convulsive syncope.' *Clinical and Experimental Neurology*, **22**, 53–55.

Kenny, R.A. (1986) *Unexplained Syncope*. Unpublished MD thesis, University College Galway.

—— Ingram, A., Bayliss, J., Sutton, R. (1986a) 'Head-up tilt: a useful test for investigating unexplained syncope.' *Lancet*, **1**, 1352–1355.

—— —— (1986b) 'Head-up tilt for unexplained syncope.' *Lancet*, **2**, 169–170.

—— Lyon, C.C., Ingram, A.M., Bayliss, J., Lightman, S.L., Sutton, R. (1987) 'Enhanced vagal activity and normal arginine vasopressin response in carotid sinus syndrome: implications for a central abnormality in carotid sinus hypersensitivity.' *Cardiovascular Research*, **21**, 545–550.

Keränen, T. (1987) 'The frequency of erroneous diagnosis of epilepsy.' *In:* Dam, D., Johannessen, S.I., Nilsson, B., Sillanpää, M. (Eds.) *Epilepsy: Progress in Treatment.* London: Wiley.

—— Sillanpää, M., Riekkinen, P.J. (1988) 'Distribution of seizure types in an epileptic population.' *Epilepsia*, **29**, 1–7.

King, M.D., Dudgeon, J., Stephenson, J.B.P. (1984) 'Joubert's syndrome with retinal dysplasia: neonatal tachypnoea as the clue to a genetic brain-eye malformation.' *Archives of Disease in Childhood*, **59**, 709–718.

Kiok, M.C., Terrence, C.F., Fromm, G.H., Lavine, S. (1986) 'Sinus arrest in epilepsy.' *Neurology*, **36**, 115–116.

Krageloh, I., Aicardi, J. (1980) 'Alternating hemiplegia in infants: report of five cases.' *Developmental Medicine and Child Neurology*, **22**, 784–791.

Kramer, R.E., Luaders, H., Goldstick, L.P., Dinner, D.S., Morris, H.H., Lesser, R.P., Wyllie, E. (1988) 'Ictus epilepticus: an electroclinical analysis.' *Neurology*, **38**, 1048–1052.

Krishnamoorthy, K.S. (1983) 'Pyridoxine-dependency seizure: report of a rare presentation.' *Annals of Neurology*, **13**, 103–104.

Kurland, R., Behr, J., Medved, L., Shoulson, I. (1987) 'Familial paroxysmal dystonic choreoathetosis: a family study.' *Movement Disorders*, **2**, 187–192.

Kussmaul, A., Tenner, A. (1859) *On the Nature and Origin of Epileptiform Convulsions Caused by Profuse Bleeding, and also of those of True Epilepsy.* (Translated by E. Bronner.) London: The New Sydenham Society.

Lagergren, H. (1988) '25 years of implanted intracardiac pacers.' *Lancet*, **1**, 636–638.

Lai, C.W., Ziegler, D.K. (1981) 'Syncope problem solved by continuous ambulatory simultaneous EEG/ECG recording.' *Neurology*, **31**, 1152–1154.

—— —— (1983) 'Repeated self-induced syncope and subsequent seizures.' *Archives of Neurology*, **40**, 820–823.

Landman, M.E., Ehrenfeld, L. (1952) 'Ventricular fibrillation following eyeball pressure in a case of paroxysmal supraventricular tachycardia.' *American Heart Journal*, **43**, 791–795.

Larson, S., Sances, A., Baker, J. (1974) 'Herniated cerebellar tonsils and cough syncope.' *Journal of Neurosurgery*, **40**, 524–528.

Laslett, E.E. (1909) 'Syncopal attacks associated with prolonged arrest of the whole heart.' *Quarterly Journal of Medicine*, **2**, 347–355.

Laxdal, T., Gomez, M.R., Reiher, J. (1969) 'Cyanotic and pallid syncopal attacks in children (breath-holding spells).' *Developmental Medicine and Child Neurology*, **11**, 755–763.

Lees, A.L. (1985) *Tics and Related Disorders*. Edinburgh: Churchill Livingstone.

Lehovský, M., Rostoková, R., Mertlíková, L. (1979) 'Poznámky k patofyziologii a léčbě afektivně respiračních křečí.' *Cskoslovenska Pediatrie*, **34**, 145–147.

Lennox, W.G., Lennox-Buchtal, M.A. (1960) *Epilepsy and Related Disorders, Vol. 1*. London: Churchill.

Lennox-Buchtal, M.A. (1976) 'A summing-up: clinical session.' *In:* Brazier, M.A.B., Coceani, F. (Eds.) *Brain Dysfunction in Infantile Febrile Convulsions*. New York: Raven Press.

Leviton, A., Cowan, L.D. (1981) 'Methodological issues in the epidemiology of seizure disorders in children.' *Epidemiological Reviews*, **3**, 67–89.

Lewis, N.P., Henderson, A. (1989) 'Stokes–Adams attacks with migraine.' *Lancet*, **1**, 165–166.

—— Fraser, A.G., Taylor, A. (1988) 'Syncope while vomiting during migraine attack.' *Lancet*, **2**, 400–401.

Lewis, T. (1932) 'A lecture on vasovagal syncope and the carotid sinus mechanism.' *British Medical Journal*, **1**, 873–876.

Li, W.W., Lombroso, C.T., Stephenson, J.B.P. (1989) 'Eradication of incapacitating self-induced ischaemic seizures by opioid receptor blockade.' *Epilepsia*, **30**, 679. (*Abstract.*)

Lin, J.T-Y., Ziegler, D.K., Lai, C-W., Bayer, W. (1982) 'Convulsive syncope in blood donors.' *Annals of Neurology*, **11**, 525–528.

Livingston, S. (1972) *Comprehensive Management of Epilepsy in Infancy, Childhood and Adolescence*. Springfield, IL: Charles C. Thomas.

Lloyd-Smith, D.L., Tatlow, W.F.T. (1958a) 'Syncope and seizure.' *Electroencephalography and Clinical Neurophysiology*, **10**, 153–157.

—— —— (1958b) 'Syncope and seizure.' *Electroencephalography and Clinical Neurophysiology*, **10**, 573–574.

Lombroso, C.T., Fejerman, N. (1977) 'Benign myoclonus of early infancy.' *Annals of Neurology*, **1**, 138–143.

—— Lerman, P. (1967) 'Breathholding spells (cyanotic and pallid infantile syncope).' *Pediatrics*, **39**, 578–581.

Lown, B., Temte, J.V., Reich, P., Gaughan, C., Regestein, Q., Hai, H. (1976) 'Basis for recurring ventricular fibrillation in the absence of coronary heart disease and its management.' *New England Journal of Medicine*, **294**, 623–629.

Lucet, V., Toumieux, M.C., Pajot, N., Monod, N. (1984) 'Hypertonie vagale paroxystique du nourrisson. A propos de 14 observations.' *Archives Françaises de Pédiatrie*, **41**, 527–531.

Lugaresi, E., Cirignotta, F. (1981) 'Hypogenic paroxysmal dystonia: epileptic seizure or a new syndrome?' *Sleep*, **4**, 129–138.

Luxon, L.M., Crowther, A., Harrison, M.J.G., Coltart, D.J. (1980) 'Controlled study of 24-hour ambulatory electrocardiographic monitoring in patients with transient neurological symptoms.' *Journal of Neurology, Neurosurgery and Psychiatry*, **43**, 37–41.

Maccario, M., Lustman, L.I. (1990) 'Paroxysmal nocturnal dystonia presenting as excessive daytime somnolence.' *Archives of Neurology*, **47**, 291–294.

MacFadyen, U.M., Hendry, G.M.A., Simpson, H. (1983) 'Gastro-oesophageal reflux in near-miss sudden infant death syndrome or suspected recurrent aspiration.' *Archives of Disease in Childhood*, **58**, 87–91.

McGreal, D.A. (1956) 'Observations on febrile convulsions.' American Journal of Diseases of Children, 92, 504–505.

—— (1957) *Convulsions in Childhood: a Clinical and Electroencephalographic Study of 500 Children Under the Age of Seven*. Unpublished MD thesis, University of St. Andrews.

McLaran, C.J., Gersh, B.J., Osborn, M.J., Wood, D.L., Sugrue, D.D., Holmes, D.R., Hammill, S.C. (1986) 'Increased vagal tone as an isolated finding in patients undergoing electrophysiological testing for recurrent syncope: response to long-term anticholinergic agents.' *British Heart Journal*, **55**, 53–57.

McNamara, B.A. (1984) 'Generalised seizure occurring with argon laser photocoagulation.' *Annals of Ophthalmology*, **16**, 548–550.

McRae, J.R., Wagner, G.S., Rogers, M.C., Canent, R.V. (1974) 'Paroxysmal familial ventricular fibrillation.' *Journal of Pediatrics*, **84**, 515–518.

McWilliam, R.C., Stephenson, J.B.P. (1984a) 'Atropine treatment of reflex anoxic seizures.' *Archives of Disease in Childhood*, **59**, 473–485.

—— —— (1984b) 'Rapid bedside technique for intracranial pressure monitoring.' *Lancet*, **2**, 73–75.

—— —— (1985a) 'Bedside intracranial monitoring.' *Lancet*, **2**, 341.

—— —— (1985b) 'Life-threatening intracranial hypertension in Reye's syndrome treated with intravenous thiopentone.' *European Journal of Pediatrics*, **144**, 383–384.

Mahony, M.J., Migliavacca, M., Spitz, L., Milla, P.J. (1988) 'Motor disorders of the oesophagus in gastro-oesophageal reflux.' *Archives of Disease in Childhood*, **63**, 1333–1338.

Mallinson, F.B., Coombes, S.K. (1960) 'A hazard of anaesthesia in ophthalmic surgery.' *Lancet*, **1**, 574–575.

Maloney, J.D., Jaeger, F.J., Fouad-Tarazi, F.M., Morris, H.H. (1988) 'Malignant vasovagal syncope: prolonged asystole provoked by head-up tilt.' *Cleveland Clinic Journal of Medicine*, **55**, 542–548.

Mameli, P., Mameli, O., Tolu, E., Padua, G., Giraudi, D., Caria, M.A., Melis, F. (1988) 'Neurogenic myocardial arrhythmias in experimental focal epilepsy.' *Epilepsia*, **29**, 74–82.

Mangin, P., Krieger, J., Kurtz, D. (1982) 'Apnea following hyperventilation in man.' *Journal of the Neurological Sciences*, **57**, 67–82.

Mathis, A., Bec, P., Arne, J-L., Camuzet, F., Lloveras, A-M. (1982) 'Rupture traumatique au cours d'une compression des globes oculaires par application thérapeutique du réflexe oculo-cardiaque.' *Bulletin de Sociétés d'Ophtalmologie de France*, **82**, 1437–1438.

Maulsby, R., Kellaway, P. (1964) 'Transient hypoxic crises in children.' *In:* Kellaway, P., Petersen, I. (Eds.) *Neurological and Electroencephalographic Correlative Studies in Infancy.* New York: Grune & Stratton.

Maytal, J., Shinnar, S., Moshec, S.L., Alvarez, L.A. (1989) 'Low morbidity and mortality of status epilepticus in children.' *Pediatrics*, **83**, 323–331.

Meadow, R. (1984) 'Fictitious epilepsy.' *Lancet*, **2**, 25–28.

Mehta, D., Farrell, T.G., Joy, M., Ward, D., Camm, A.J. (1988a) 'Syncope and vomiting.' *Lancet*, **2**, 790–791.

—— Saveymuttu, S.H., Camm, A.J. (1988b) 'Recurrent paroxysmal complete heart block induced by vomiting.' *Chest*, **94**, 433–435.

Meyer, J.S., Waltz, A.G. (1961) 'Relationship of cerebral anoxia to functional and electro-encephalographic abnormality.' *In:* Gastaut, H., Meyer, J.S. (Eds.) *Cerebral Anoxia and the Electro-encephalogram.* Springfield, IL: Charles C. Thomas.

Milam, S.B., Giovanitti, J.A., Israelson, H. (1986) 'Faint in the supine position.' *Journal of Periodontology*, **57**, 44–47.

Milstein, S., Buetikofer, J., Lesser, J., Goldenberg, I.F., Benditt, D.G., Gornick, C., Reyes, W.J. (1989) 'Cardiac asystole: a manifestation of neurally mediated hypotension-bradycardia.' *Journal of the American College of Cardiology*, **14**, 1626–1632.

Mizrahi, E.M., Kellaway, P. (1987) 'Characterization and classification of neonatal seizures.' *Neurology*, **37**, 1837–1844.

Mofenson, H.C., Weymuller, C.A., Greensher, J. (1965) 'Epilepsy due to water immersion. An unusual case of reflex sensory epilepsy.' *Journal of the American Medical Association*, **191**, 600–601.

Monod, N., Peirano, P., Plouin, P., Sternberg, B., Bouille, C. (1988) 'Seizure-induced apnea.' *Annals of the New York Academy of Sciences*, **533**, 411–420.

Montagna, P., Gallassi, R., Medori, R., Govoni, E., Zeviani, M., diMauro, S., Lugaresi, E., Andermann, F. (1988) 'MELAS syndrome: characteristic migrainous and epileptic features and maternal transmission.' *Neurology*, **38**, 751–754.

Morgan-Hughes, J.A. (1966) 'Cough seizures in patients with cerebral lesions.' *British Medical Journal*, **2**, 494–496.

Morimoto, T., Hayakawa, T., Sugie, H., Awaya, Y., Fukuyama, Y. (1985) 'Epileptic seizures precipitated by constant light, movements in daily life, and hot water immersion.' *Epilepsia*, **26**, 237–242.

Morley, D.J., Weaver, D.D., Garg, B.P., Markand, O. (1982) 'Hyperexplexia: an inherited disorder of the startle response.' *Clinical Genetics*, **21**, 388–396.

Morquio, L. (1901) 'Sur une maladie infantile et familiale caracterisée par des modifications permanentes du pouls, des attaques syncopales et epileptiformes et la mort subite.' *Archives de Médecine des Enfants*, **4**, 467–475.

Moss, A.J., Rockoff, M. (1981) 'EEG monitoring during cardiac arrest and resuscitation.' *Journal of the American Medical Association*, **246**, 2750–2751.

—— Schwartz, P.J. (1982) 'Delayed repolarization (QT or QTU prolongation) and malignant ventricular arrhythmias.' *Modern Concepts of Cardiovascular Disease*, **51**, 85–90.

—— —— Crampton, R.S., Locati, E., Carleen, M.A. (1985) 'The long QT syndrome: a prospective international study.' *Circulation*, **71**, 17–21.

Murphy, J.V., Wilkinson, I.A., Pollack, N.H. (1981) 'Death following breath holding in an adolescent.' *American Journal of Diseases of Children*, **135**, 180–181.

Mutani R., Bergamimi, R., Fariello, R. (1970) 'A case of status epilepticus of tonic expression (so-called "reticular epilepsy").' *Epilepsia*, **11**, 321–326.

—— Fariello, R., Accatino, G., Brocchi, G. (1971) 'Sincope anossica o crisi epilettica?' *Minerva Medica*, **62**, 2518–2523.

Nash, E.S., Horton, J.N, (1978) 'Cardiac standstill following venepuncture: a report of the subsequent management of the case.' *British Journal of Oral Surgery*, **16**, 70–72.

Natelson, B.H. (1985) 'Neurocardiology. An interdisciplinary area for the 80s.' *Archives of Neurology*, **42**, 178–184.

Navelet, Y., Wood, C., Robieux, C., Tardieu, M. (1989) 'Seizures presenting as apnoea.' *Archives of Disease in Childhood*, **64**, 357–359.

Nelson, D.A., Mahru, M.N. (1963) 'Death following digital carotid artery occlusion.' *Archives of Neurology*, **8**, 640–643.

—— Ray, C.D. (1968) 'Respiratory arrest from seizure discharges in the limbic system.' *Archives of Neurology*, **19**, 199–207.

Neri, G., Martini-Neri, M.E., Katz, B.E., Opitz, J.M. (1984) 'The Perlman syndrome: familial renal dysplasia with Wilms tumour, fetal gigantism and multiple congenital anomalies.' *American Journal of Medical Genetics*, **19**, 195–207.

Neville, B.G.R. (1972) 'The origin of infantile spasms: evidence from a case of hydranencephaly.' *Developmental Medicine and Child Neurology*, **14**, 644–656.

Nicoll, A., Rudd, P. (Eds.) (1989) *British Paediatric Association Manual of Infections and Immunizations in Children*. Oxford: Oxford University Press.

Obel, P., Marchand, L. (1971) 'Successful treatment by vagotomy of 2 patients with peptic ulcer and Stokes–Adams (vasovagal) syncope.' *American Journal of Cardiology*, **28**, 731–734.

O'Brien, I.A.D., O'Hare, P., Corrall, R.J.M. (1986) 'Heart rate variability in healthy subjects: effect of age and the derivation of normal ranges for tests of autonomic function.' *British Heart Journal*, **55**, 348–354.

O'Donohoe, N.V. (1985) *Epilepsies of Childhood, 2nd Edn*. London: Butterworths.

Ogunyemi, A.O., Gomez, M.R., Klass, D.W. (1988) 'Seizures induced by exercise.' *Neurology*, **38**, 633–634.

Oller-Daurella, L. (1985) 'Epilepsy with generalised convulsive seizures in childhood.' *In:* Roger, J., Dravet, C., Bureau, M., Dreifuss, F.E., Wolf, P. (Eds.) *Epileptic Syndromes in Infancy, Childhood and Adolescence*. London: John Libbey.

Onrot, J., Wiley, R.G., Fogo, A., Biaggioni, I., Robertson, D., Hollister, A.S. (1987) 'Neck tumour with syncope due to paroxysmal sympathetic withdrawal.' *Journal of Neurology, Neurosurgery and Psychiatry*, **50**, 1063–1066.

Onuma, T., Fukushima, Y., Takeda, T., Osawa, T., Sato, T. (1972) 'A case of epilepsy precipitated by hot water immersion.' *Clinical Neurology*, **12**, 386–393. *(Japanese.)*

Oren, J., Kelly, D., Shannon, D.C. (1986) 'Identification of a high-risk group for sudden infant death syndrome among infants who were resuscitated for sleep apnoea.' *Pediatrics*, **77**, 495–499.

Orenstein, S.R., Orenstein, D.M. (1988) 'Gastroesophageal reflux and respiratory disease in children.' *Journal of Pediatrics*, **112**, 847–858.

Ossentjuk, E., Elink Sterk, C.J.O., Storm van Leeuwen, W. (1966) 'Flicker-induced cardiac arrest in a patient with epilepsy.' *Electroencephalography and Clinical Neurophysiology*, **20**, 257–259.

Ounsted, C., Lindsay, J., Richards, P. (1987) *Temporal Lobe Epilepsy, 1948–1986: a Biographical Study*. Clinics in Developmental Medicine, No. 103. London: Mac Keith Press with Blackwell Scientific; Philadelphia: Lippincott.

Palm, L., Blennow, G. (1985) 'Transdermal anticholinergic treatment of reflex anoxic seizures.' *Acta Paediatrica Scandinavica*, **74**, 803–804.

Pampiglione, G., Waterston, D.J. (1961) 'EEG observations during changes in venous and arterial pressure.' *In:* Gastaut, H., Meyer, J.S. (Eds.) *Cerebral Anoxia and the Electro-encephalogram*. Springfield, IL: Charles C. Thomas.

Panayiotopoulos, C.P. (1989) 'Benign nocturnal childhood occipital epilepsy: a new syndrome with nocturnal seizures, tonic deviation of the eyes, and vomiting.' *Journal of Child Neurology*, **4**, 43–48.

—— Obeid, T., Waheed, G. (1989) 'Differentiation of typical absence seizures in epileptic syndromes.' *Brain*, **112**, 1039–1056.

Parsons, M. (1986) 'Fits and other causes of loss of consciousness while driving.' *Quarterly Journal of Medicine*, **58**, 295–303.

Patel, V.M., Maulsby, R.L. (1987) 'How hyperventilation alters the electroencephalogram: a review of controversial viewpoints emphasising neurophysiological mechanisms.' *Journal of Clinical Neurophysiology*, **4**, 101–120.

Paulson, G. (1963) 'Breath holding spells: a fatal case.' *Developmental Medicine and Child Neurology*, **5**, 246–251.

Pearson, R.S.B. (1945) 'Sinus bradycardia with cardiac asystole.' *British Heart Journal*, **7**, 85–90.

Peiper, A. (1939) 'Das "Wegbleiben".' *Monatschrift für Kinderheilkunde*, **79**, 236–240.

Pelekanos, J.T., Dooley, J.M., Camfield, P.R., Finley, J. (1990) 'Stretch syncope in adolescence.' *Neurology*, **40**, 705–707.

Perkin, G.D., Joseph, R. (1986) 'Neurological manifestations of the hyperventilation syndrome.' *Journal of the Royal Society of Medicine*, **79**, 448–450.

Phizackerley, P.J.R., Poole, E.W., Whitty, C.W.M. (1954) 'Sino-auricular heart block as an epileptic manifestation.' *Epilepsia*, **3**, 89–96.

Picornell-Darder, I., Carrasco, J.L., Rostain, J.C., Naquet, R.A. (1978) 'Study on the Valsalva manoeuvre in young healthy subjects.' *Electroencephalography and Clinical Neurophysiology*, **45**, 648–654.

Pignata, C., Farina, V., Andria, G., del Giudice, E., Striano, S., Adinolfi, L. (1983) 'Prolonged Q-T interval syndrome presenting as idiopathic epilepsy.' *Neuropediatrics*, **14**, 235–236.

Plant, G.T., Williams, A.C., Earl, C.J., Marsden, C.D. (1984) 'Familial paroxysmal dystonia induced by exercise.' *Journal of Neurology, Neurosurgery and Psychiatry*, **47**, 275–279.

Plaxico, D.T., Loughlin, G.M. (1981) 'Nasopharyngeal reflux and neonatal apnea.' *American Journal of Diseases of Children*, **135**, 793–794.

Poles, F.C., Boycott, M. (1942) 'Syncope in blood donors.' *Lancet*, **2**, 531–535.

Radtke, R.A. (1989) 'Cardiac asystole: an epileptic arrhythmia?' *Epilepsia*, **30**, 705-706. (*Abstract.*)

Rajna, P., Kundra, O., Halacsz, P. (1983) 'Vigilance level-dependent tonic seizures. Epilepsy or sleep disorder.' *Epilepsia*, **24**, 725–733.

Ramani, V. (1987) 'Intensive monitoring of psychogenic seizures, aggression and dyscontrol syndromes.' *Advances in Neurology*, **46**, 203-217.

Ramet, J., Praud, J.P., D'Allest, A.M., Carofilis, A., Dehan, M., Guilleminault, C., Gaultier, C. (1988) 'Effect of maturation on heart rate response to ocular compression test during rapid eye movement sleep in human infants.' *Pediatric Research*, **24**, 477–480.

Rasmussen, V., Hauns, S., Skagen, K. (1978) 'Cerebral attacks due to excessive vagal tone in heavily trained persons: a clinical and electrophysiological study.' *Acta Medica Scandinavica*, **204**, 401–405.

Rawles, J.M., Pai, G.R., Reid, S.R. (1989) 'A method of quantifying sinus arrhythmia: parallel effect of respiration on P-P and P-R intervals.' *Clinical Science*, **76**, 103–108.

Regis, H., Toga, M., Righini, C. (1961) 'Clinical, electroencephalographic and pathological study of a case of Adams–Stokes syndrome.' *In*: Gastaut, H., Meyer, J.S. (Eds.) *Cerebral Anoxia and the Electroencephalogram*. Springfield, IL: Charles C. Thomas.

Reif-Leher, L., Stemmermann, M.G. (1975) 'Monosodium glutamate intolerance in children.' *New England Journal of Medicine*, **4**, 1204-1205.

Rendle-Short, J. (1972) 'The physiopathology of breath-holding attacks: a hypothesis.' *Australian Paediatric Journal*, **8**, 92–94.

Rennie, J.M., Arnold, R. (1984) 'Asystole in the prolonged QT syndrome.' *Archives of Disease in Childhood*, **59**, 571–573.

Resnick, T.J., Moshe, S.L., Perotta, L., Chambers, H.J. (1986) 'Benign neonatal sleep myoclonus.' *Archives of Neurology*, **43**, 266-268.

Robinson, B.J., Johnson, R.H. (1988) 'Why does vasodilatation occur during syncope?' *Clinical Science*, **74**, 347–350.

Rocca, W.A., Sharbrough, F.W., Hauser, W.A., Annegers, J.F., Schoenberg, B.S. (1987*a*) 'Risk factors for absence seizures: a population-based case-control study in Rochester, Minnesota.' *Neurology*, **37**, 1309–1314.

—— —— —— —— —— (1987*b*) 'Risk factors for generalized tonic-clonic seizures: a population-based case-control study in Rochester, Minnesota.' *Neurology*, **37**, 1315–1322.

—— —— —— —— —— (1987*c*) 'Risk factors for complex partial seizures: a population-based case-control study.' *Annals of Neurology*, **21**, 22–31.

Roddy, S.M., Ashwal, S., Schneider, S. (1983) 'Venepuncture fits: a form of reflex anoxic seizure.' *Pediatrics*, **72**, 715–718.

Rodin, E. (1987) 'An assessment of current views on epilepsy.' *Epilepsia*, **28**, 267–271.

Roger, J., Dravet, C., Bureau, M., Dreifuss, F.E., Wolf, P. (1985) *Epileptic Syndromes in Infancy, Childhood and Adolescence.* London: John Libbey.

Romano, C., Gemme, G., Pongiglione, R. (1964) 'Aritmie cardiache rare dell'eta pediatrica.' *Clinica Pediatrica*, **45**, 656–683.

Rosen, C.L., Frost, J.D., Bricker, T., Tarnow, J.D., Gillette, P.C., Dunlavy, S. (1983) 'Two siblings with recurrent cardiorespiratory arrest: Munchausen syndrome by proxy or child abuse?' *Pediatrics*, **71**, 715–720.

Ross, E.M., Peckham, C.S. (1983) 'Seizure disorder in the National Child Development Study.' *In:* Rose, F.C. (Ed.) *Research Progress in Epilepsy.* London: Pitman.

—— West, P.B., Butler, N.R. (1980) 'Epilepsy in childhood: findings from the National Child Development Study.' *British Medical Journal*, **1**, 207–210.

Ross, R.T. (1989) *Syncope.* Philadelphia: W.B. Saunders.

Rossen, R., Kabat, H., Anderson, J.P. (1943) 'Acute arrest of the cerebral circulation in man.' *Archives of Neurology and Psychiatry*, **50**, 510–528.

Rossiter, E.J.R., Luckin, J., Vile, A., Ganly, N., Hallowes, R., Pearson, R.D. (1970) 'Convulsions in the first three years of life.' *Medical Journal of Australia*, **2**, 735–740.

Saenz-Lope, E., Herranz, F.J., Masdeu, J.C. (1984) 'Startle epilepsy: a clinical study.' *Annals of Neurology*, **16**, 78–81.

Sagar, H.J., Oxbury, J.M. (1987) 'Hippocampal neuron loss in temporal lobe epilepsy: correlation with early childhood convulsions.' *Annals of Neurology*, **22**, 334–340.

Sapire, D.W., Casta, A. (1985) 'Vagotonia in infants, children, adolescents and young adults.' *International Journal of Cardiology*, **9**, 211–222.

—— —— Safley, W., O'Riordan, A.C., Balsara, R.K. (1983) 'Vasovagal syncope in children requiring pacemaker implantation.' *American Heart Journal*, **106**, 1406–1411.

—— Shah, J.J., Black, I.F.S. (1979) 'Prolonged atrioventricular conduction in young children and adolescents. The role of increased vagal tone.' *South African Medical Journal*, **55**, 669–673.

Savard, G., Andermann, F., Teitelbaum, J., Lehmann, H. (1988) 'Epileptic Munchausen's syndrome: a form of pseudoseizures distinct from hysteria and malingering.' *Neurology*, **38**, 1628–1629.

Scherrer, U., Vissing, S., Morgan, B.J., Hanson, P., Victor, R.G. (1990) 'Vasovagal syncope after infusion of a vasodilator in a heart-transplant recipient.' *New England Journal of Medicine*, **322**, 602–604.

Schott, G.D., McLeod, A.A., Jewitt, D.E. (1977) 'Cardiac arrhythmias that masquerade as epilepsy.' *British Medical Journal*, **1**, 1454–1457.

Schwartz, P.J. (1985) 'Idiopathic long QT syndrome: progress and questions.' *American Heart Journal*, **109**, 339–411.

Scott, O., Macartney, F.J., Deverall, P.B. (1976) 'Sick sinus syndrome in children.' *Archives of Disease in Childhood*, **51**, 100–105.

Selleger, C., Adamec, R., Morabia, A., Zimmerman, M. (1988) 'Vasovagal syncope during recto-sigmoidoscopy: report of a case.' *PACE*, **11**, 346–348.

Sennhauser, F.H., Schwarz, H.P. (1986) 'Toxic psychosis from transdermal scopolamine in a child.' *Lancet*, **2**, 1033.

Shafir, Y., Levy, Y., Beharab, A., Nitzam, M., Steinherz, R. (1986) 'Acute dystonic reaction to bethanecol—a direct acetylcholine receptor agonist.' *Developmental Medicine and Child Neurology*, **28**, 646–648.

Sharpey-Schafer, E.P. (1953a) 'Effects of coughing on intrathoracic pressure, arterial pressure and peripheral blood flow.' *Journal of Physiology*, **122**, 351–357.

—— (1953b) 'The mechanism of syncope after coughing.' *British Medical Journal*, **2**, 860–863.

Shaw, N.J., Livingston, J.H., Minns, R.A., Clarke, M. (1988) 'Epilepsy precipitated by bathing.' *Developmental Medicine and Child Neurology*, **30**, 108–111.

Sheldon, W. (1952) 'Syncopal attacks in infancy.' *Great Ormond Street Journal*, **3**, 20–22.

Shields, W.D., Nielsen, C., Buch, D., Jacobsen, V., Christenson, P., Zachau-Christiansen, B., Cherry, J.D. (1988) 'Relationship of pertussis immunization to the onset of neurologic disorders: a retrospective epidemiologic study.' *Journal of Pediatrics*, **113**, 801–805.

Shinebourne, E.A., Anderson, R.H., Bowyer, J.J. (1975) 'Variations in clinical presentation of Fallot's tetralogy in infancy: angiographic and pathogenetic implications.' *British Heart Journal*, **37**, 946–955.

Simpson, K. (1949) 'Deaths from vagal inhibition.' *Lancet*, **1**, 558–560.

195

Smaje, J.C., Davidson, C., Teasdale, G.M. (1987) 'Sino-atrial arrest due to temporal lobe epilepsy.' *Journal of Neurology, Neurosurgery and Psychiatry*, **50**, 112-113.

Soltész, G., Acsádi, G. (1989) 'Association between diabetes, severe hypoglycaemia, and electro-encephalographic abnormalities.' *Archives of Disease in Childhood*, **64**, 992–996.

Southall, D.P. (1988) 'Role of apnea in the sudden infant death syndrome: a personal view.' *Pediatrics*, **81**, 73–84.

—— Talbert, D.G. (1987) 'Sudden atalectasis apnoea braking syndrome.' *In:* Hollinger, M.A. (Ed.) *Current Topics in Pulmonary Pharmacology and Toxicology, Vol. 2.* New York: Elsevier.

—— —— Johnson, P., Morley, C.J., Salmons, S., Miller, J., Helms, P.J. (1985) 'Prolonged expiratory apnoea: a disorder resulting in episodes of severe arterial hypoxaemia in infants and young children.' *Lancet*, **2**, 571–577.

—— Lewis, G.M., Buchanan, R., Weller, R.O. (1987*a*) 'Prolonged expiratory apnoea (cyanotic 'breath-holding') in association with a medullary tumour.' *Developmental Medicine and Child Neurology*, **29**, 789–793.

—— Stebbens, V., Abraham, N., Abraham, L. (1987*b*) 'Prolonged apnoea with severe arterial hypoxaemia resulting from complex partial seizures.' *Developmental Medicine and Child Neurology*, **29**, 784–789.

—— —— Rees, S.V., Lang, M.H., Warner, J.O., Shinebourne, E.A. (1987*c*) 'Apnoeic episodes induced by smothering: two cases identified by covert video surveillance.' *British Medical Journal*, **294**, 1637–1641.

—— —— Shinebourne, E.A. (1987*d*) 'Sudden and unexpected death between 1 and 5 years.' *Archives of Disease in Childhood*, **62**, 700–705.

—— Kerr, A.M., Tirosh, E., Amos, P., Lang, M.H., Stephenson, J.B.P. (1988*a*) 'Hyperventilation in the awake state: a potentially treatable component of Rett syndrome.' *Archives of Disease in Childhood*, **63**, 1039–1048.

—— Thomas, M.G., Lambert, H.P. (1988*b*) 'Severe hypoxaemia in infants with pertussis.' *Archives of Disease in Childhood*, **63**, 598–605.

—— Samuels, M.P., Talbert, D.G. (1990) 'Recurrent cyanotic episodes with severe arterial hypoxaemia and intrapulmonary shunting: a mechanism for sudden death.' *Archives of Disease in Childhood*, **65**, 953–961.

Spitzer, A.R., Boyle, J.T., Tuchman, D.N., Fox, W.W. (1984) 'Awake apnea associated with gastroesophageal reflux: a specific clinical syndrome.' *Journal of Pediatrics*, **104**, 200–205.

Spudis, E.V., Penry, J.K., Gibson, P. (1986) 'Driving impairment caused by episodic brain dysfunction. Restrictions for epilepsy and syncope.' *Archives of Neurology*, **43**, 558–564.

Stensman, R., Ursing, B. (1971) 'Epilepsy precipitated by hot water immersion.' *Neurology*, **21**, 559–562.

Stellman, G.R., Bannister, C.M., Hillier, V. (1986) 'The incidence of seizure disorder in children with acquired and congenital hydrocephalus.' *Zeitschrift für Kinderchirurgie*, **41** (Suppl. 1), 38–41.

Stephenson, J.B.P. (1978*a*) 'Reflex anoxic seizures ('white breath-holding'): nonepileptic vagal attacks.' *Archives of Disease in Childhood*, **53**, 193–200.

—— (1978*b*) 'Ocular compression in reflex anoxic seizures.' *Archives of Disease in Childhood*, **53**, 693.

—— (1978*c*) 'Non-epileptic television syncope.' *British Medical Journal*, **1**, 1622.

—— (1978*d*) 'Two types of febrile seizure: anoxic (syncopal) and epileptic mechanisms differentiated by oculocardiac reflex.' *British Medical Journal*, **2**, 726–728.

—— (1979*a*) 'Atropine methonitrate in management of near-fatal reflex anoxic seizures.' *Lancet*, **2**, 955.

—— (1979*b*) 'Concept of non-epileptic "anoxic" seizure threshold and its relation to age.' *Archives of Disease in Childhood*, **54**, 802. (*Abstract.*)

—— (1980) 'Reflex anoxic seizures and ocular compression.' *Developmental Medicine and Child Neurology*, **22**, 380–386.

—— (1983*a*) 'Febrile convulsions and reflex anoxic seizures.' *In:* Rose, F.C. (Ed.) *Research Progress in Epilepsy.* London: Pitman.

—— (1983*b*) 'Reactions to pertussis vaccine.' *Lancet*, **1**, 1218.

—— (1985*a*) 'Reflex anoxic seizures.' *Archives of Disease in Childhood*, **60**, 288.

—— (1985*b*) 'Prolonged expiratory apnoea in children.' *Lancet*, **2**, 953.

—— (1988) 'A neurologist looks at neurological disease temporally related to DTP immunization.' *Tokai Journal of Experimental and Clinical Medicine*, **13** (Suppl.), 157-164.

—— Byrne, K.E. (1983) 'Pyridoxine responsive epilepsy: expanded pyridoxine dependency?' *Archives of Disease in Childhood*, **58**, 1034.

—— Hainsworth, I.R., (1966) 'Ketotic hypoglycaemia.' *Proceedings of the Association of Clinical Biochemists*, **5**, 80–81.

—— King, M.D. (1989) *Handbook of Neurological Investigations in Children.* London: Butterworths.

—— Ounsted, C. (1982) 'Febrile convulsions.' *In:* Milton, A.S. (Ed.) *Handbook of Experimental Pharmacology, Vol. 60.* Berlin: Springer–Verlag.

Steptoe, A., Wardle, J. (1988) 'Emotional fainting and the psychophysiologic response to blood and injury: autonomic mechanisms and coping strategies.' *Psychosomatic Medicine,* **50**, 402–417.

Stern, S., Tzivoni, D. (1976) 'Atrial and ventricular asystole for 19 seconds without syncope.' *Israel Journal of Medicine,* **12**, 28–33.

Stevens, H. (1987) 'Syncope, seizures and stress.' *Stress Medicine,* **3**, 41–50.

—— Fazekas, J.F. (1955) 'Experimentally induced hypotension.' *Archives of Neurology and Psychiatry,* **73**, 416–424.

Stokes, W. (1846) 'Observations in some cases of permanently slow pulse.' *Dublin Quarterly Journal of Medical Science,* **2**, 73–85.

Storstein, O. (1949) 'Adams–Stokes attacks caused by ventricular fibrillation in a man with an otherwise normal heart.' *Acta Medica Scandinavica,* **133**, 437–441.

Strandjord, R.E. (1987) 'Differential diagnosis of epilepsy.' *In:* Dam, M., Johanessen, S.I., Nilsson, B., Sillanpää, M. (Eds.) *Epilepsy: Progress in Treatment.* New York: Wiley.

Strasburg, B., Lam., W., Swiryn, S., Bauernfeind, R., Scagliotti, D., Palileo, E., Rosen, K. (1982) 'Symptomatic spontaneous paroxysmal AV nodal block due to localized hyperresponsiveness of the AV node to vagotonic reflexes.' *American Heart Journal,* **103**, 795–801.

Suhren, O., Bruyn, G.W., Tuynman, J.A. (1966) 'Hyperexplexia: a hereditary startle syndrome.' *Journal of the Neurological Sciences,* **3**, 577–605.

Symonds, C. (1950) *In:* 'Discussion on faints and fits.' *Proceedings of the Royal Society of Medicine,* **43**, 507–510.

Szatmary, L.J. (1984) 'Autonomic blockade and sick sinus syndrome. New concept in the interpretations of electrophysiological and Holter data.' *European Heart Journal,* **5**, 637–648.

—— Czakoc, E., Solti, F., Szaboc, Z. (1984) 'Autonomic sinus node dysfunction and its treatment.' *Acta Cardiologica,* **39**, 209–220.

—— Jouve, A., Pinot, J.J., Torresani, J. (1983) 'Comparative study of electrophysiological and Holter monitoring data in estimating sinoatrial function.' *Cardiology,* **70**, 184–193.

Tardieu, M., Khoury, W., Navelet, Y., Questiaux, E., Landrieu, P. (1986) 'Un syndrome spectaculaire et bénin de "convulsions néonatales": les myoclonies du sommeil profond.' *Archives Françaises de Pédiatrie,* **43**, 259-260.

Tassinari, C.A., Bureau-Paillas, M., Dalla Bernardina, B. (1976) 'Syndrome avec apnées centrales périodiques (syncopés par arret respiratoire).' *Revue d'Electroencephalographie et de Neurophysiologie Clinique,* **6**, 79–87.

Temkin, O. (1971) *The Falling Sickness, 2nd Edn.* Baltimore, MD: Johns Hopkins Press.

Tizes, R. (1976) 'Cardiac arrest following routine venepuncture.' *Journal of the American Medical Association,* **236**, 1846–1847.

Trimble, M.R. (1986) 'Pseudoseizures.' *Neurological Clinics,* **4**, 531-548.

Tucker, J.S., Yoe, R.H. (1956) 'Simultaneous EEG-EKG recording: a study of a case with complete heart-block and paroxysmal ventricular tachycardia.' *Electroencephalography and Clinical Neurophysiology,* **8**, 129–132.

Twomey, J.A., Espir, M.L. (1980) 'Paroxysmal symptoms as the first manifestations of multiple sclerosis.' *Journal of Neurology, Neurosurgery and Psychiatry,* **43**, 296–304.

Vanasse, M., Bedard, P., Andermann, F. (1976) 'Shuddering attacks in children: an early clinical manifestation of essential tremor.' *Neurology,* **26**, 1027–1030.

Varadi, A., Gara, A., Solti, F. (1983) 'Evaluation of syncope.' *British Medical Journal,* **286**, 1900.

Verret, S., Steele, J.C. (1971) 'Alternating hemiplegia in childhood: a report of eight patients with complicated migraine beginning in infancy.' *Pediatrics,* **47**, 675–680.

Verrill, P.J., Aellig, W.H. (1970) 'Vasovagal faint in the supine position.' *British Medical Journal,* **4**, 348.

Vingerhoets, A.J.J.M., Schomaker, L.R.B. (1988) 'Emotional fainting: its physiological and psychological aspects.' *In:* Speilberger, C.D., Sarason, I.T. (Eds.) *Stress and Anxiety, Vol. 12.* Washington: Hemisphere.

Vigevano, F., Di Capua, M., Dalla Bernardina, B. (1989) 'Startle disease: an avoidable cause of sudden infant death.' *Lancet,* **1**, 216.

Volpe, J.J. (1989) 'Neonatal seizures: current concepts and revised classifications.' *Pediatrics,* **84**, 422–428.

Wahlström, G. (1978) 'The effects of atropine on the tolerance and the convulsions seen after withdrawal from forced barbital drinking in the rat.' *Psychopharmacology,* **59**, 123–128.

Walker, A.M., Jick, H., Perera, D.R., Knauss, T.A., Thompson, R.S. (1988) 'Neurologic events following diphtheria–tetanus–pertussis immunization.' *Pediatrics*, **81**, 345–349.

Wallace, S.J. (1988) *The Child with Febrile Seizures.* London: John Wright.

Wallin, B.G., Sundlöf, G. (1982) 'Sympathetic outflow to muscle during vasovagal syncope.' *Journal of the Autonomic Nervous System*, **6**, 287–291.

—— Westerberg, C.E., Sundlöf, G. (1984) 'Syncope induced by glossopharyngeal neuralgia: sympathetic outflow to muscle.' *Neurology*, **34**, 522–524.

Walsh, J.K., Farrell, M.K., Keenan, W.J., Lucas, M., Kramer, M. (1981) 'Gastroesophageal reflux in infants: relation to apnoea.' *Journal of Pediatrics*, **99**, 197–201.

Ward, D.E., Camm, A.J. (1988) 'QT interval syndromes' *Lancet*, **2**, 47–48.

Ward, O.C. (1964) 'A new familial cardiac syndrome in children.' *Journal of the Irish Medical Association*, **54**, 103–106.

Watanabe, K., Hara, K., Hakamada, S., Negoro, T., Sugiura, M., Matsumoto, A., Maehara, M. (1982) 'Seizures with apnea in children.' *Pediatrics*, **70**, 87–90.

—— Yamamoto, N., Negoro, T., Takaesu, E., Kozabura, A., Furune, S., Takahashi, I. (1987) 'Benign complex partial epilepsies in infancy.' *Pediatric Neurology*, **3**, 208–211.

Weiner, von C., Stünkel, S. (1982) 'Ventrikuläre Tachyarrythmien im Kindersalter.' *Fortschritte der Medizin*, **100**, 1541–1544.

Weinstein, I.R. (1982) 'Atropine . . . bradycardia . . . asystole . . . ? arrest: case report.' *Anesthesia Progress*, **29**, 112–114.

Weiss, S., Ferris, E.B., Jr. (1934) 'Adams–Stokes syndrome with transient complete heart block of vasovagal reflex origin.' *Archives of Internal Medicine*, **54**, 931–951.

Wennevold, A., Melchior, J.C., Sandoe, E. (1965) 'Adams–Stokes syndrome in children without organic heart disease.' *Acta Medica Scandinavica*, **177**, 557–563.

Werlin, S.L., D'Souza, B.J., Hogan, W.J., Dodds, W.J., Arndorfer, R.C. (1980) 'Sandifer syndrome: an unappreciated clinical entity.' *Developmental Medicine and Child Neurology*, **22**, 374–378.

Wilkinson, M.J., Fagan, D.G. (1990) 'Postmortem demonstration of intrapulmonary shunting.' *Archives of Disease in Childhood*, **65**, 435–437.

Willemse, J. (1986) 'Benign idiopathic dystonia with onset in the first year of life.' *Developmental Medicine and Child Neurology*, **28**, 355–366.

Williams, B. (1976) 'Cerebrospinal fluid pressure changes in response to coughing.' *Brain*, **99**, 331–346.

Williams, C., Bevan, V.T. (1988) 'The secret observation of children in hospital.' *Lancet*, **1**, 780–781.

Williams, D. (1950) *In:* 'Discussion on fits and faints.' *Proceedings of the Royal Society of Medicine*, **43**, 510–514.

Williamson, P.D. (1986) 'Intensive monitoring of complex partial seizures: diagnosis and subclassification.' *Advances in Neurology*, **46**, 69-84.

Wilson, J.B. (1989) 'Epileptic seizures and smother-proof pillows.' *Lancet*, **1**, 389.

Wolf, P. (1985) 'The classification of seizures and the epilepsies.' *In:* Porter, R.J., Morselli, P.L. (Eds.) *The Epilepsies.* London: Butterworth.

Woody, R.C., Kiel, E.A. (1986) 'Swallowing syncope in a child.' *Pediatrics*, **78**, 507–509.

Yohai, D., Barnett, S.H. (1989) 'Absences and atonic seizures induced by piperazine.' *Pediatric Neurology*, **5**, 393-394.

Yule, W., Fernando, P. (1980) 'Blood phobia—beware.' *Behaviour Research and Therapy*, **18**, 587–590.

Ziegler, D.K., Lin, J., Bayer, W.L. (1978) 'Convulsive syncope: its relationship to cerebral ischemia.' *Transactions of the American Neurological Association*, **103**, 150–154.

INDEX